Cancer in Women

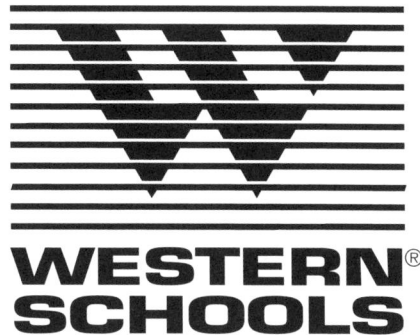

WESTERN SCHOOLS®

By
Ellen Carr, RN, MSN, AOCN

W P.O. Box 1930
Brockton, MA 02303
WESTERN SCHOOLS 1-800-438-8888

ABOUT THE AUTHOR

Ellen Carr, RN, MSN, AOCN, has been a healthcare and medical writer for more than 20 years. She specializes in assignments about clinical nursing, therapeutic and diagnostic technologies and patient advocacy. Ms. Carr is currently a medical and surgical oncology case manager at the Rebecca and John Moores University of California, San Diego (UCSD) Cancer Center. Ms. Carr continues to participate in local and national Oncology Nursing Society projects.

Ellen Carr has disclosed that she has no significant financial or other conflicts of interest pertaining to this course book.

ABOUT THE SUBJECT MATTER REVIEWER

Mary Louise Kanaskie, MS, RNC, AOCN, has been an oncology nurse for 25 years with experience in gynecologic oncology, medical oncology, and bone marrow transplant. As a nurse educator, she has designed, implemented, and continues to evaluate basic and advanced education programs and specialized courses related to oncology and medical/surgical nursing. Ms. Kanaskie presents courses on chemotherapy/biotherapy and oncology nursing core curriculum reviews annually. As an active member of the Oncology Nursing Society, she has served as Coordinator of the Staff Education Special Interest Group and has been a presenter at the National ONS Congress.

Mary Louise Kanaskie has disclosed that she has no significant financial or other conflicts of interest pertaining to this course book.

Copy Editor: Julie Munden

Indexer: Sylvia Coates

ISBN: 978-1-57801-103-2

IMPORTANT: Read these instructions *BEFORE* proceeding!

Enclosed with your course book, you will find the FasTrax® answer sheet. Use this form to answer all the final exam questions that appear in this course book. If you are completing more than one course, be sure to write your answers on the appropriate answer sheet. Full instructions and complete grading details are printed on the FasTrax instruction sheet, also enclosed with your order. Please review them before starting. *If you are mailing your answer sheet(s) to Western Schools, we recommend you make a copy as a backup.*

ABOUT THIS COURSE

A Pretest is provided with each course to test your current knowledge base regarding the subject matter contained within this course. Your Final Exam is a multiple choice examination. **You will find the exam questions at the end of each chapter.**

In the event the course has less than 100 questions, leave the remaining answer boxes on the FasTrax answer sheet blank. **Use a <u>black</u> pen to fill in your answer sheet.**

A PASSING SCORE

You must score 70% or better in order to pass this course and receive your Certificate of Completion. Should you fail to achieve the required score, we will send you an additional FasTrax answer sheet so that you may make a second attempt to pass the course. Western Schools will allow you three chances to pass the same course…*at no extra charge!* After three failed attempts to pass the same course, your file will be closed.

RECORDING YOUR HOURS

Please monitor the time it takes to complete this course using the handy log sheet on the other side of this page. See below for transferring study hours to the course evaluation.

COURSE EVALUATIONS

In this course book, you will find a short evaluation about the course you are soon to complete. This information is vital to providing Western Schools with feedback on this course. The course evaluation answer section is in the lower right hand corner of the FasTrax answer sheet marked "Evaluation," with answers marked 1–18. Your answers are important to us; please take a few minutes to complete the evaluation.

On the back of the FasTrax instruction sheet, there is additional space to make any comments about the course, the school, and suggested new curriculum. Please mail the FasTrax instruction sheet, with your comments, back to Western Schools in the envelope provided with your course order.

TRANSFERRING STUDY TIME

Upon completion of the course, transfer the total study time from your log sheet to question 18 in the course evaluation. The answers will be in ranges; please choose the proper hour range that best represents your study time. You **MUST** log your study time under question 18 on the course evaluation.

EXTENSIONS

You have two (2) years from the date of enrollment to complete this course. A six (6) month extension may be purchased. If after 30 months from the original enrollment date you do not complete the course, *your file will be closed and no certificate can be issued.*

CHANGE OF ADDRESS?

In the event you have moved during the completion of this course, please call our student services department at 1-800-618-1670, and we will update your file.

A GUARANTEE TO WHICH YOU'LL GIVE HIGH HONORS

If any continuing education course fails to meet your expectations or if you are not satisfied in any manner, for any reason, you may return it for an exchange or a refund (less shipping and handling) within 30 days. Software, video, and audio courses must be returned unopened.

Thank you for enrolling at Western Schools!

WESTERN SCHOOLS
P.O. Box 1930
Brockton, MA 02303
(800) 438-8888
www.westernschools.com

Cancer in Women

WESTERN SCHOOLS
P.O. Box 1930
Brockton, MA 02303

Please use this log to total the number of hours you spend reading the text and taking the final examination (use 50-min hours).

Date	Hours Spent
_____	_____
_____	_____
_____	_____
_____	_____
_____	_____
_____	_____
_____	_____
_____	_____
_____	_____
_____	_____
_____	_____
_____	_____
_____	_____

TOTAL [   ]

Please log your study hours with submission of your final exam. To log your study time, fill in the appropriate circle under question 18 of the FasTrax® answer sheet under the "Evaluation" section.

Cancer in Women

WESTERN SCHOOLS
CONTINUING EDUCATION EVALUATION

Instructions: Mark your answers to the following questions with a black pen on the "Evaluation" section of your FasTrax® answer sheet provided with this course. You should not return this sheet.

Please use the scale below to rate how well the course content met the educational objectives.

A Agree Strongly   **C Disagree Somewhat**
B Agree Somewhat   **D Disagree Strongly**

The course met the following educational objectives:

1. described the general trends associated with major cancers in women.

2. identified breast cancer's epidemiology, risk factors, prevention and detection strategies, and common staging schemas and treatments.

3. explained epidemiology, risk factors, prevention and detection strategies, and common staging schemas and treatments for endometrial cancer.

4. explained the epidemiology, risk factors, prevention and detection strategies, and common staging schemas and treatments for ovarian cancer.

5. explained epidemiology, risk factors, prevention and detection strategies, and common staging schemas and treatments for cervical cancer.

6. explained epidemiology, risk factors, prevention and detection strategies, and common staging schemas and treatments for lung cancer.

7. explained epidemiology, risk factors, prevention and detection strategies, and common staging schemas and treatments for colo-rectal cancer.

8. identified the psychosocial elements of the cancer patients experience, including the basis for the stress response, reactions to psychosocial interventions, anxiety, depression, and the benefits of social support.

9. indicated the psychologic, functioning, and fertility issues associated with sexuality of women with cancer.

10. listed some common complementary and alternative medicines (CAMs) and identified ways to evaluate the merit and usefulness of CAMs.

11. discussed ways for the nurse to evaluate and access content available on the Internet.

12. The content of this course was relevant to the objectives.

13. This offering met my professional education needs.

14. The objectives met the overall purpose and goal of the course.

15. The course was generally well-written and the subject matter explained thoroughly. (If no, please explain on the back of the FasTrax instruction sheet.)

16. The content of this course was appropriate for home study.

17. The final examination was well-written and at an appropriate level for the content of the course.

18. **PLEASE LOG YOUR STUDY HOURS WITH SUBMISSION OF YOUR FINAL EXAM.**
Please choose which best represents the total study hours it took to complete this 30-hour course.

A. Less than 25 hours

B. 25–28 hours

C. 29–32 hours

D. Greater than 32 hours

CONTENTS

Evaluation v

Figures and Tables xv

Pretest xix

Introduction xxiii

Chapter 1: Trends 1

    The Female Patient 1

    Trends: Women and Cancer 1

    Statistical Trends 3

    Summary 4

    Exam Questions 5

    References 7

Chapter 2: Breast Cancer 9

    Epidemiology 9

    Breast Anatomy 10

    Noninvasive Cancers 10

        Ductal Carcinoma In Situ (DCIS) 10

        Lobular Carcinoma In Situ (LCIS) 11

    Risk Factors 11

        Age 11

        Race 11

        Sex 11

        Personal History of Breast Cancer 12

        Family History 12

        Breast Changes 12

        Genetic Alterations 12

        Estrogen 12

        Late Childbearing 12

        Radiation Therapy 12

        Lifestyle 12

        Weight Gain and Lifestyle Factors 12

        Protective Effect 12

        Breastfeeding 12

        Prophylactic Mastectomy 12

        Unproven Risks 12

Hormone Therapy as Prevention 13

   Raloxifene 14

Screening 14

   Breast Self-Examination 14

   Clinical Breast Examination 15

   Mammography 15

      Mammography Screening 15

      False-Positives 16

      Screening Effect on Incidence and Mortality 16

Genetic Risk 17

   Assessing Risk 17

   Risk Assessment 18

   BRCA1 18

   BRCA2 18

   Counseling and Risk Models 18

Diagnosing Breast Cancer 19

Treatment 20

   Surgery 20

   Sentinel Lymph Node Biopsy (SLNB) 20

   Radiation Therapy 21

   Hormone Therapy 22

   Chemotherapy 22

   Biological Therapy 23

   Early-Stage Breast Cancer 23

   Stage III Breast Cancer 23

   Advanced Stage and Recurrent Breast Cancer 24

Rehabilitation 25

   Exercises 25

   Lymphedema 25

   Breast Reconstruction 25

   Breast Prosthesis 26

   Sexuality 26

Summary 26

Case Study: Breast Cancer 26

Exam Questions 29

References 31

Chapter 3: Endometrial Cancer **33**

   Introduction 33

Epidemiology 33

The Uterus 35

Tumor Development 35

Endometrial Cancer 35

Prevention 36

Risk Factors 36

Hormones 37

Endometrial Cancer and Colon Cancer 37

Tamoxifen 38

Detection 38

Diagnosis 39

Treatment 39

    Surgery 39

        Treatment-caused Menopause 39

    Radiation Therapy 41

        External Radiation 42

        Internal Radiation 42

    Hormone Therapy 42

    Chemotherapy 42

Summary 42

Case Study: Endometrial Cancer 43

Exam Questions 45

References 47

Chapter 4: Ovarian Cancer **49**

Introduction 49

Epidemiology 49

Overview: The Ovaries 51

Ovarian Cysts 51

Ovarian Cancer 51

Signs and Symptoms 52

Prevention 52

Risk Factors 52

    Risk Factors: Family Inheritance/Predisposition 53

Screening 54

    CA-125 Testing 55

    Other Markers 55

    Screening — Optimal Combination of Tests 55

Diagnosis, Treatment, and Prognosis 56

Surgery 57

Chemotherapy 58

Hormone Therapy 59

Radiation Therapy 59

Complications from Ovarian Cancer 59

Gene Therapy 59

Summary 59

Case Study: Ovarian Cancer 59

Exam Questions 63

References 65

Chapter 5: Cervical Cancer **67**

Introduction 67

Epidemiology 67

The Cervix, Cancer, and Risk Factors 68

Risk Factors 68

Human Papillomaviruses (HPVs) 69

Benign Tumor Treatments 69

Signs and Symptoms 70

Preinvasive Cervical Conditions 70

Assessment and Workup of CIN 71

Cervical Cancer 71

Screening 72

Nursing Role in Screening 72

Pap Test 73

Pap Test Technique 74

Interpretation 74

Diagnosis and Treatment 76

Surgery 77

Radiotherapy 77

Chemotherapy 79

Recurrent Cervical Cancer 79

Summary 80

Case Study: Cervical Cancer 80

Exam Questions 83

References 85

Chapter 6: Lung Cancer in Women **87**

Introduction 87

Epidemiology 87

Myths 87

Risk Factors: Smoking 89

   Teenagers and Smoking 90

   Women and Smoking 90

   Smoking and Other Health Issues 90

   Tobacco in the World 92

Other Risk Factors 92

Lung Cancer 92

   Genetic Carcinogenesis 95

Prevention and Detection Strategies 95

Signs and Symptoms 96

Diagnosis and Staging 96

Prognosis 98

Treatments 98

   Surgery 98

   Radiation Therapy 99

   NSCLC: Treatment of Stage III and Stage IV Disease 99

   SCLC and Chemotherapy 100

Complications 100

Summary 100

Case Study: Lung Cancer 100

Exam Questions 103

References 105

Chapter 7: Colorectal Cancer in Women **107**

Introduction 107

Epidemiology 107

   Colorectal Cancer and Women 109

Colorectal Cancer 109

   Genetic Origins 110

Risk Factors 110

   Polyps 111

   Personal and Family History 111

   Family History 112

   Other Lifestyle Risk Factors 112

      High-Fat Diet 112

      Cigarette Smoking 113

      Other Lifestyle Risks 113

Symptoms 113

Screening and Detection 113

Protective Strategies 115

Staging and Diagnosis 115

Treatments 116

   Surgery 116

   Chemotherapy 117

   Radiation Therapy 117

   Advanced Disease 117

   Metastatic Disease: Hepatic Involvement 118

Follow-up Care After Treatment 119

Summary 119

Case Study: Colorectal Cancer 119

Exam Questions 121

References 123

Chapter 8: Psychosocial Issues **125**

Introduction 125

Stress 126

Surviving Cancer and Psychosocial Issues 126

   Assessment and Screening 126

Psychosocial Distress and Adjustments 127

   Coping Theory — Stages for Cancer Patients 127

   Factors That Affect Coping 127

Selected Studies of Cancer Patients and Their Coping 129

Adjustment Disorders 131

   Prevalence 131

Anxiety 131

   Assessment and Screening 133

Depression 133

   Assessment and Screening 133

   Interventions 135

      Pharmacologic Intervention 136

Social Support and Interventions 137

   Other Support Interventions 141

Summary 141

Exam Questions 143

References 145

Chapter 9: Sexuality: Women With Cancer **149**

Introduction 149

Psychological Aspects 149

Issues of Functioning and Treatment 151

Treatments and Their Effects 152

    Fertility Issues 152

        Chemotherapy 152

        Radiation Therapy 152

        Pregnancy 153

        Preserving the Ability to Reproduce 153

Medication Factors 154

Assessment 154

Interventions 155

Summary 156

Exam Questions 157

References 159

Chapter 10: Complementary and Alternative Medicine 161

Introduction 161

CAMs as Options 163

Prevalence 163

Sound Foundation for Study 164

    Evaluation of Studies 165

Helpful CAMs in Cancer Patient Care 165

    CAMs in Practice, Two Abstracts 165

    Aromatherapy Program Curriculum 166

    CAMs in Community Practice 166

Patient Evaluation of CAMs 167

Summary 168

Exam Questions 169

References 171

Chapter 11: Health Care and the Internet 173

Internet — A Communication Tool 173

Finding Information 175

    Evaluating Internet-Based Information 175

Queries from Cancer Patients 177

E-mail to Communicate 179

Open Forums 179

Summary 180

Exam Questions 181

References 183

Appendix I: Cancer Resources for Patients and Their Families 185

Appendix II: Selected Internet Resources 189

Appendix III: Selected Nursing Diagnoses 191

Glossary 197

Index 207

Pretest Answer Key 213

FIGURES AND TABLES

Chapter 1: Trends

Figure 1-1 — Most Recent Age-adjusted Cancer Incidence Rates by Sex 2

Figure 1-2 — Leading Cancer Cases (Estimated) for Females, 2003 2

Figure 1-3 — Leading Cancer Deaths (Estimated) for Females, 2003 3

Chapter 2: Breast Cancer

Box 2-1 — Hormone Replacement Therapy (HRT) 13

Figure 2-1 — Breast Anatomy 11

Figure 2-2 — Breast Self Examination 14

Figure 2-3 — Surgical Procedures 21

Table 2-1 — Lifetime Probability of Being Diagnosed with Invasive Breast Cancer 10

Table 2-2 — Mortality Risk for Breast Cancer According to Age 10

Table 2-3 — Recommended Mammography Screening Guidelines 15

Table 2-4 — Risk Models 19

Table 2-5 — Staging Schemas 20

Table 2-6 — Hormone Therapies 22

Table 2-7 — Selected Chemotherapy Agents and Protocols 22

Table 2-8 — Early-Stage Treatment Options 23

Table 2-9 — Risk Categories For Women with Node-Negative Breast Cancer 23

Table 2-10 — Adjuvant Systemic Treatment Options for Women With Axillary Node-Negative

Breast Cancer 24

Table 2-11 — Treatment Options for Women with Axillary Node-Positive Breast Cancer 25

Chapter 3: Endometrial Cancer

Sidebar 3-1 — Hormone Replacement Therapy 41

Figure 3-1 — Estimated New Cancer Cases 34

Figure 3-2 — Estimated Cancer Deaths 34

Figure 3-3 — Uterus (and Endometrial Layer) 35

Table 3-1 — Endometrial Cancer Cell Types 36

Table 3-2 — Risk Factors for Endometrial Cancer 37

Table 3-3 — Endometrial Staging Summary 40

Chapter 4: Ovarian Cancer

Figure 4-1 — Estimated Cancer Deaths 50

Figure 4-2 — Estimated New Cancer Cases 50

Figure 4-3 — Anatomy 51

Table 4-1 — Risk Factors for Ovarian Cancer 53

Table 4-2 — BRCA1 and BRCA2 Mutations In Ovarian Cancers 53

Table 4-3 — Diagnostic Tests and Workup for Ovarian Cancer 56

Table 4-4 — Staging Criteria for Ovarian Cancer 57

Chapter 5: Cervical Cancer

Figure 5-1 — Anatomy 68

Table 5-1 — Risk Factors for Cervical Cancer 68

Table 5-2 — Signs and Symptoms of Cervical Cancer 70

Table 5-3 — Cervical Cancer Screening Guidelines 72

Table 5-4 — Pap Test Terms, Follow-up, and Testing Strategies 73

Table 5-5 — Pap Test Classifications of Abnormalities 75

Table 5-6 — Categories of Cell Abnormalities Based on the Bethesda System ...75

Table 5-7 — Causes of Inflamed Cervical Tissue 76

Table 5-8 — Cervical Cancer Staging 78

Table 5-9 — Staging — FIGO 79

Chapter 6: Lung Cancer in Women

Figure 6-1 — Growth in Lung Cancer 88

Figure 6-2 — Lung Cancer Incidence Compared to Other Cancers 88

Figure 6-3 — Lung Cancer Deaths Compared to Other Cancers 88

Figure 6-4 — Women — Lung Illnesses 89

Figure 6-5 — Cancer Deaths Internationally 92

Figure 6-6 — Anatomy of a Lung 94

Table 6-1 — Excerpts — Ways to Quit Smoking 91

Table 6-2 — Lung Cancer Risks 92

Table 6-3 — Lung Cancer Profile 93

Table 6-4 — Histopathologic Cell Types, Bronchogenic, and Lung Carcinomas ...94

Table 6-5 — Diagnostic Tests 96

Table 6-6 — Revised International System for Staging Lung Cancer 97

Table 6-7 — Performance Status 98

Table 6-8 — NSCLS/SCLC Chemotherapy Agents 99

Chapter 7: Colorectal Cancer in Women

Figure 7-1 — Most Recent Age-Adjusted Cancer Incidence and Death Rates by Sex ...108

Figure 7-2 — Leading Cancer Cases (Estimated) for Females, 2003 109

Figure 7-3 — Colon Anatomy 110

Table 7-1 — Race and Ethnicity — Incidence and Mortality 109

Table 7-2 — Criteria Identifying Hereditary Risk for Colorectal Cancer 111

Table 7-3 — Fecal Occult Blood Test (FOBT) Instructions 114

Table 7-4 — Colorectal Screening 115

Table 7-5 — Suggestions to Limit Risk of Colorectal Cancer 116

Table 7-6 — Colorectal Staging 116

Table 7-7 — Important Aspects of Ostomy Management 117

Table 7-8 — Common Chemotherapies for Colorectal Cancer and Common Adverse Effects 118

Chapter 8: Psychosocial Issues

Table 8-1 — Diagnostic Criteria for the Adjustment Disorders 128

Table 8-2 — Meaning in Ovarian Cancer Survivorship 130

Table 8-3 — Possible Causes of Anxiety 132

Table 8-4 — Symptoms of Anxiety 132

Table 8-5 — Commonly Prescribed Benzodiazepines 132

Table 8-6 — Questions to Assess Anxiety 133

Table 8-7 — Indicators of Depression 134

Table 8-8 — Examples of Assessment Questions for Depression and Suicide 134

Table 8-9 — Cancer-Related Risk Factors for Depression 135

Table 8-10 — Risk Factors: Suicide in Cancer Patients 135

Table 8-11 — Possible Medication-Based Causes of Depression 136

Table 8-12 — Common Antidepressants 136

Table 8-13 — Factors to Consider in Choosing an Antidepressant for Adult Cancer Patients 137

Table 8-14 — Common Physical Adverse Effects from Antidepressants 138

Table 8-15 — Selected On-Line Support Groups 139

Chapter 9: Sexuality: Women with Cancer

Table 9-1 — Coping with Changes That Affect Sexuality 151

Table 9-2 — Selected Causes or Sources of Sexual Dysfunction Related to Cancer Treatment 151

Table 9-3 — Selected Chemotherapy Agents That Affect Sexuality 153

Table 9-4 — Medications that Affect Sexual Response 154

Table 9-5 — Strategies for Helping Women with Sexual Function 155

Chapter 10: Complementary and Alternative Medicine

Table 10-1 — Selected Complementary and Alternative Medicines (CAMs) 162

Table 10-2 — Five Domains of CAMs 163

Table 10-3 — Selected CAM-related Studies 164

Table 10-4 — Criteria to Evaluate CAM Studies 164

Table 10-5 — Therapeutic Nature of Selected Essential Oils 166

Table 10-6 — Precautions When Using Essential Oils 166

Table 10-7 — Patient Satisfaction and Effectiveness Data 167

Table 10-8 — Questions to Ask When Considering CAMs 167

Table 10-9 — Selecting a CAM Practitioner 168

Table 10-10 — Evaluating Medical Resources on the Web 168

Chapter 11: Health Care and the Internet

Figure 11-1 — Search Engine Preferences 175

Table 11-1 — Trends — Integration of Tech Health Care Behaviors 174

Table 11-2 — Health on the Net Foundation (HON) 176

Table 11-3 — Health Organizations Developing Guidelines for Health Care Consumers to
Evaluate On-Line Sources of Health Information 177

Table 11-4 — Tips for Health Surfing On-Line 178

Table 11-5 — Types of Web Sites 178

Table 11-6 — Advantages and Disadvantages of Internet-Based Support Groups 180

PRETEST

1. Begin this course by taking the pretest. Circle the answers to the questions on this page, or write the answers on a separate sheet of paper. Do not log answers to the pretest questions on the FasTrax test sheet included with the course.

2. Compare your answers to the PRETEST KEY located in the back of the book. The pretest answer key indicates the course chapter where the content of that question is discussed. Make note of the questions you missed, so that you can focus on those areas as you complete the course.

3. Complete the course by reading each chapter and completing the exam questions at the end of the chapter. Answers to these exam questions should be logged on the FasTrax test sheet included with the course.

1. Strategies to reduce and manage lymphedema include

   a. massage only.

   b. wrapping of the extremity with an elastic sleeve or cuff only.

   c. exercises protecting the limb from injury and infection control.

   d. massage, wrapping, exercises, and prevention of infection.

2. For a premenopausal woman, the best time for breast self-examination is

   a. about a week before her period starts.

   b. about a week after her period ends.

   c. about 3 days after her period ends.

   d. about 2 weeks after her period ends.

3. In the United States, cancer of the endometrium accounts for this percentage of all gynecological cancers each year

   a. 25%.

   b. 40%.

   c. 50%.

   d. 75%.

4. A malignant condition of the endometrium is

   a. fibroid diseases.

   b. endometriosis.

   c. adenocarcinoma.

   d. the recurrence of cysts.

5. Ovarian cancer is the fourth leading killer of women and kills more women than these two gynecologic cancers combined

   a. breast and cervical.

   b. cervical and endometrial.

   c. breast and endometrial.

   d. lung and breast.

6. Stage II ovarian cancer is

   a. growth limited to both ovaries; no ascites.

   b. tumor of one or both ovaries with histologically confirmed implants of abdominal peritoneal surfaces, none exceeding 2 centimeters in diameter. Nodes negative.

   c. growth involving one or both ovaries with pelvic extension.

   d. growth involving one or both ovaries with distant metastasis.

7. When cervical cells become abnormal, they change in

    a. size, shape, and number of cells on the surface of the cervix.

    b. size, shape, and number of cells, only in the test tube.

    c. color only.

    d. number only.

8. A Papanicolaou (Pap) test appointment should be scheduled preferably in

    a. last half of the menstrual cycle.

    b. the first half of the menstrual cycle before ovulation but after completion of menses.

    c. 5 days after the first day of menses.

    d. 20 days after the last day of her period.

9. The leading cause of death in women due to malignancy is

    a. breast.

    b. colorectal.

    c. lung.

    d. skin.

10. If a woman stops smoking her risk of dying of lung cancer

    a. never changes.

    b. increases.

    c. decreases.

    d. is still not known.

11. Smokers who stop smoking can significantly reduce their risk of dying of lung cancer if they have stopped smoking for at least

    a. 5 years.

    b. 10 years.

    c. 15 years.

    d. 20 years.

12. For women in the United States, colorectal cancer is the

    a. main cause of death.

    b. 2nd leading cause of death.

    c. 3rd leading cause of death.

    d. equal to breast cancer statistics in the cause of death.

13. A supportive cognitive or behavior intervention to offer women diagnosed with cancer is

    a. antiemetics.

    b. narcotics.

    c. biofeedback.

    d. bone marrow transplant.

14. Studies about support indicate that the most important tool a nurse can offer the patient is the ability to

    a. ask a question.

    b. develop a plan of action.

    c. listen.

    d. document.

15. The P-LI-SS-IT model is an acronym for the levels of

    a. Planning, Limited Information, Specific Suggestion, and Idealism.

    b. Permission, Limited Information, Specific Suggestion, and Intensive Therapy.

    c. Prioritizing, Limited Ideas, Some Suggestions, and Ideal Timing.

    d. Permission, Levels of Intervention, Specific Suggestions, Ideas, and Treatment.

16. Those being treated for cancer may wish to preserve their reproductive options. Therefore, a first step to start a plan is to

    a. immediately start tissue banking.

    b. choose to cryopreserve embryos.

    c. seek counseling about options.

    d. seek counseling about losing their ability to be parents.

17. Strategies to cope with sexual dysfunction include

    a. avoiding physical recovery, including diet and physical activities.

    b. omit your partner in discussions.

    c. avoid romance.

    d. use a water-soluble lubricant (Astroglide, K-Y jelly, Lubrin), if needed.

18. Examples of complementary and alternative therapies categories are

    a. medical.

    b. vocational.

    c. mind-body interventions.

    d. topical.

19. Examples of manual healing methods are

    a. acupressure, reflexology, and Reiki.

    b. macrobiotic diets and transcutaneous electrical nerve stimulation.

    c. music and prayer.

    d. echinacea, ephedra, and evening primrose.

20. A disadvantage of an Internet support group is

    a. inability to access body language.

    b. always available for a person to seek support.

    c. time limited.

    d. limited geographical reach.

INTRODUCTION

The experience of a woman diagnosed with cancer is distinctive. Not only may the sites of her diagnosis be uniquely female — ovarian, cervical, endometrial — but her illness experience can be different from that of a man.

This fully-referenced course reviews many of the major concepts in nursing care when women are diagnosed with malignancies. The course provides a foundation for the generalist nurse about specific gynecologic cancers in women, which have significant incidence and/or death rates — breast, endometrial, ovarian, and cervical cancers.* It also reviews cancers that have high incidence or death rates for women — cancers of the lung and colorectum. Case studies for these cancers highlight the experience of the female patient with cancer.

In providing a context for the experience of women diagnosed with a major illness, the course reviews concepts important to the woman's healthcare experience. These concepts are psychosocial support, sexuality, the use of complementary and alternative therapies, and the use of the Internet as a major source of information and support.

The course also provides a quick reference about nursing diagnoses for the care of women with cancer. This section highlights interventions specific to surgery, radiation therapy, and chemotherapy treatments. The course also offers a listing of resources and credible Web sites for further information about cancers in women.

---

* Cancers of the vagina and vulva are not included in this course because of their overall low incidence rates.

CHAPTER 1

TRENDS

CHAPTER OBJECTIVE

After completing this chapter, the reader will be able to describe trends associated with major cancers in women.

LEARNING OBJECTIVES

After studying this chapter, the reader will be able to

1. cite general trends concerning cancer diagnosis, incidence, and death.

2. specify one epidemiological trend affecting women diagnosed with cancer, based on cancer statistics.

3. identify two issues women have identified as important to their nursing care.

THE FEMALE PATIENT

Researchers tell us that most women rely on a psychosocial framework to provide support and sustenance when they are fighting illness (Ekwall, Ternestedt, & Sorbe, 2003; Schaefer, Ladd, Gergits, & Gyauch, 2001). Because of this context of care, women may look at issues affected by their disease differently than men. Among those issues are their body image, femininity, sexuality, reproductive capability, symptom management, well-being, self-concept, emotional health and spir-

itual reliance, and overall satisfaction with care. (Ekwall et al., 2003; Velji & Fitch, 2001).

Woman, in general, have a distinct approach to decision-making, relationships, prognosis, and quality of life. It follows that health care providers can take cues from these assumptions about a woman's experience and support her with information, open communication, and help with coping when she is ill (Halstead & Hull, 2001; Ekwall et al., 2003; Schaefer et al., 2001). Toward providing that foundation for excellent care for women with cancer, nurses should be aware of general trends that affect women diagnosed with the disease.

TRENDS: WOMEN AND CANCER

Cancer is the second leading cause of death in the United States, following cardiovascular disease. It affects three of every four families. During 2000, an estimated 1,220,100 persons in the United States were diagnosed with cancer; 552,200 persons died from a cancer diagnosis. (Figure 1-1 shows the most recent age-adjusted cancer incidence and death rates by sex.) One-half of new cases of cancer occur in people age 65 and older (ACS, 2003).

About 491,400 individuals who get cancer in a given year are expected to be alive 5 years after diagnosis, based on age-adjusted statistics for all cancers.

FIGURE 1-1: MOST RECENT AGE-ADJUSTED CANCER INCIDENCE RATES BY SEX

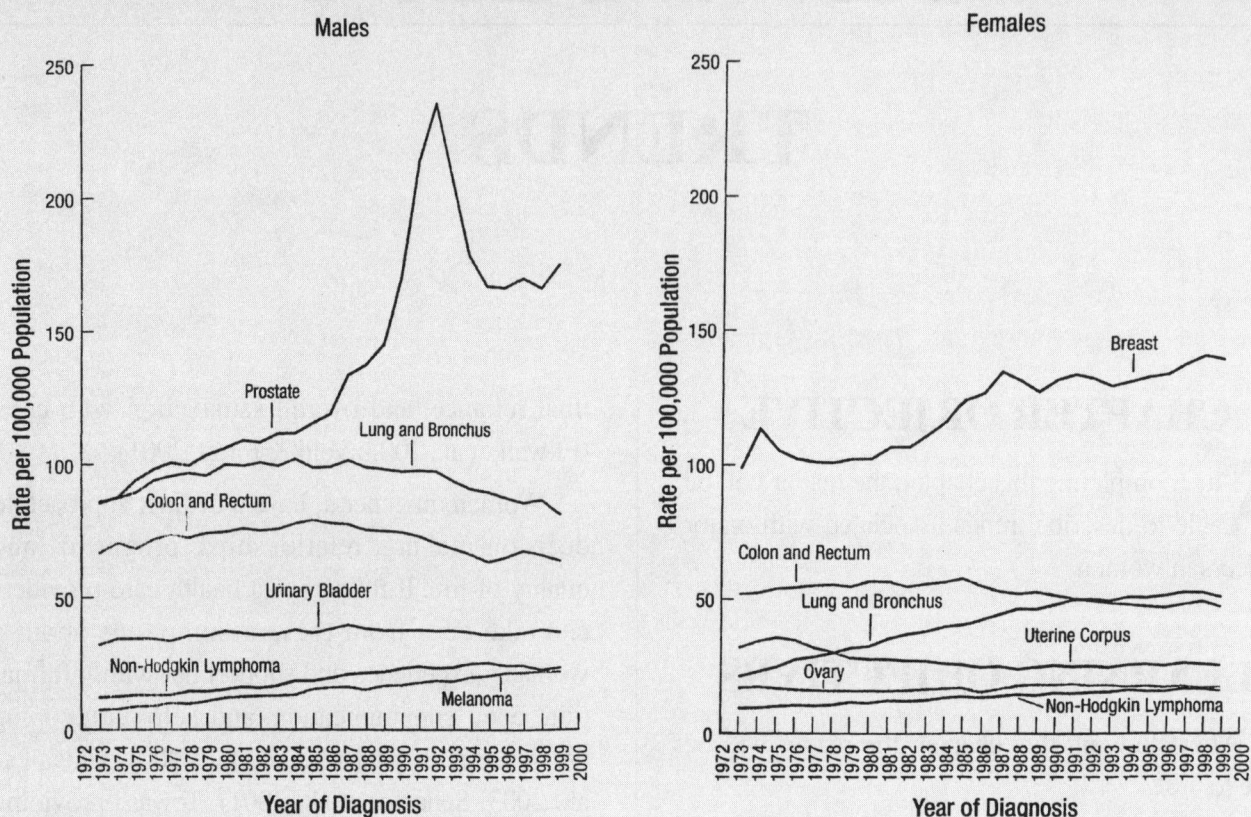

Note. From "Cancer Statistics, 2003," by A. Jemal, T. Murray, A. Samuels, A. Ghafoor, E. Ward, & M.J. Thun, 2003, *CA Cancer Journal for Clinicians, 53*, pp. 5-26. Reprinted with permission.

This rate means that the chance of a person recently diagnosed with cancer being alive in 5 years is 60% compared to the general public (ACS, 2003).

In America, one half of all men and one third of all women will develop cancer during their lifetimes. Figure 1-2 shows the leading cancer cases in females. The lifetime probability of developing cancer is higher in men (43.5%) compared to women (38.5%), but breast cancer incidence rates indicate that women are more likely to develop cancer before age 60 (ACS, 2003). Today, millions of people are living with cancer or have been cured of the disease.

Breast cancer — although sometimes diagnosed in men — is predominantly a woman's disease. Breast cancer is the most common new cancer diagnosed in women (ACS, 2003). What we know about breast cancer and a woman's response helps us to understand other cancers in women.

Because breast cancer is the second most frequently cited cancer in women — second to lung cancer — women are concerned with ways to prevent, diagnose, and treat that particular cancer diag-

FIGURE 1-2: LEADING CANCER CASES (ESTIMATED) FOR FEMALES, 2003

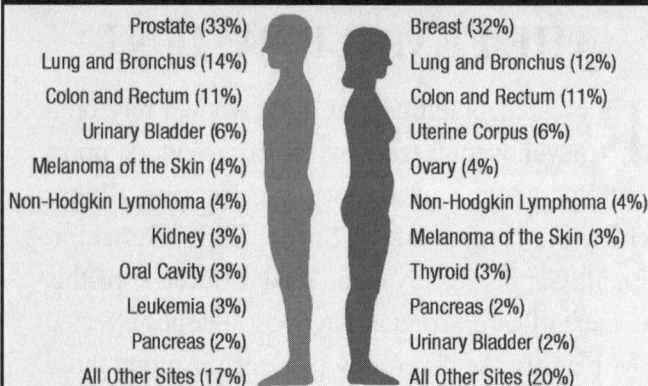

Prostate (33%)	Breast (32%)
Lung and Bronchus (14%)	Lung and Bronchus (12%)
Colon and Rectum (11%)	Colon and Rectum (11%)
Urinary Bladder (6%)	Uterine Corpus (6%)
Melanoma of the Skin (4%)	Ovary (4%)
Non-Hodgkin Lymohoma (4%)	Non-Hodgkin Lymphoma (4%)
Kidney (3%)	Melanoma of the Skin (3%)
Oral Cavity (3%)	Thyroid (3%)
Leukemia (3%)	Pancreas (2%)
Pancreas (2%)	Urinary Bladder (2%)
All Other Sites (17%)	All Other Sites (20%)

Excludes basal and squamous cell skin cancers and in situ carcinomas except urinary bladder.

Note: Percentages may not total 100 percent due to rounding.

Note. From "Cancer Statistics, 2003," by A. Jemal, T. Murray, A. Samuels, A. Ghafoor, E. Ward, & M.J. Thun, 2003, *CA Cancer Journal for Clinicians, 53*, pp. 5-26. Reprinted with permission.

nosis. (Figure 1-3 shows the leading causes of cancer death in women.) For African American women, the interest is heightened. Breast cancer is the leading killer of African American women with cancer (ACS, 2003).

Extensive cancer research in recent years has increased what we know about cancer prevention. The risk of developing some types of cancer can be clearly reduced by changes in a person's lifestyle. It cannot be emphasized enough: The best reduction behaviors are quitting smoking, eating healthier, and staying active and fit. And, we know that the sooner a cancer is found and the sooner treatment begins, the better a patient's chances are of control or cure of the disease.

STATISTICAL TRENDS

When reviewing statistics on cancers in women, several trends emerge.

- For breast cancer, screening, earlier detection, and more effective treatments have led to a decline in the death rate for breast cancer. Breast cancer incidence rates continue to climb, due in part to a wider use of mammography. White women, 50-64 years, have a higher rate of new breast cancer cases (ACS, 2003).

- Smoking and lifestyle are major issues for women with cancer. For 40 years breast cancer was the major cause of cancer death in women. Now lung cancer is the most common cause of cancer death for women (as well as men). Figure 1-3 shows the death rates for cancers that affect women. In 1987 (for the first time since cancer statistics were recorded), more women died of lung cancer than breast cancer. Since 1992, the rates of lung cancer death have leveled off for women. Still, it is the leading cause of cancer death in women (ACS, 2003).

  Because of a lag in smoking cessation trends, lung cancer death rates for women

FIGURE 1-3: LEADING CANCER DEATHS (ESTIMATED) FOR FEMALES, 2003

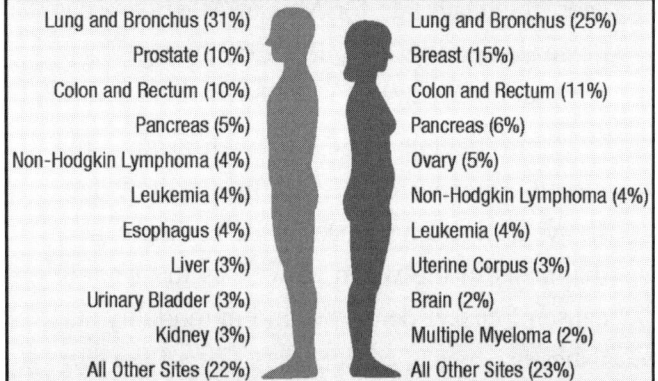

Lung and Bronchus (31%)	Lung and Bronchus (25%)
Prostate (10%)	Breast (15%)
Colon and Rectum (10%)	Colon and Rectum (11%)
Pancreas (5%)	Pancreas (6%)
Non-Hodgkin Lymphoma (4%)	Ovary (5%)
Leukemia (4%)	Non-Hodgkin Lymphoma (4%)
Esophagus (4%)	Leukemia (4%)
Liver (3%)	Uterine Corpus (3%)
Urinary Bladder (3%)	Brain (2%)
Kidney (3%)	Multiple Myeloma (2%)
All Other Sites (22%)	All Other Sites (23%)

Excludes basal and squamous cell skin cancers and in situ carcinomas except urinary bladder.
Note: Percentages may not total 100 percent due to rounding.
Note. From "Cancer Statistics, 2003," by A. Jemal, T. Murray, A. Samuels, A. Ghafoor, E. Ward, & M.J. Thun, 2003, *CA Cancer Journal for Clinicians, 53,* pp. 5-26. Reprinted with permission.

increased 0.8% per year between 1992 and 1998. There has been a gradual slowing of death rates from this cancer in women over the past 3 decades. Death rates for men decreased 1.9% per year between 1992 and 1998. Still the type of cancers that women contract are strongly affected by the number of women who smoke or have smoked in their past (ACS, 2003).

- Cancer affects all populations in the United States, but especially African American women. In the United States, the death rate for all cancers is about one third higher in African Americans than in Whites (Jemal, Murray, Samuels, Ghafoor, Ward, & Thun, 2003). The most common cancers among African American women are breast cancer (31%), lung cancer (12%), and colon and rectum cancers (12%). (ACS, 2003) About 63,500 African Americans died from cancer in 2003.

- Lung cancer accounts for the largest number of cancer deaths among both men (30%) and women (21%), followed by prostate cancer in men (19%) and breast cancer in women (19%). For both men and women, cancer of the colon and rectum and cancer of the pancreas are expected to rank third and fourth as leading causes of cancer death. But for all cancers or sites, the death rate for African Americans has decreased during 1991-1997, on average 1.1% per year (ACS, 2001).

Lung cancer affects women around the world. International epidemiological data shows us that lung cancer is the leading cancer diagnosis in the world as well as the leading cause of cancer death. Second in mortality statistics is stomach cancer, with 37% of the cancer deaths reported occurring in China. Breast cancer is the third most common cancer in women and ranks fifth as the leading cause of cancer death. Worldwide estimates have breast cancer representing 14.1% of cancer deaths in females (ACS, 2003; Jemal, 2003).

SUMMARY

Nurses caring for women with cancer should be aware of the special context of care and focus for the female patient. Emotional support, information, open communication, and help with coping are key to the woman's experience. Trends continue to develop related to cancer in women. Breast and lung cancer are the major cancers in women with the highest incidence rates. Lung, colorectal, and ovarian cancer are the major killers of women diagnosed with cancer. Lifestyle issues contribute to cancers in women, as they do with men — the most predominant external factor is smoking. Hereditary factors, which continue to be studied and clarified, may also play a role in the development of some cancers in women.

EXAM QUESTIONS

CHAPTER 1
Questions 1-6

1. The leading cause of death from cancer in women is

    a. breast cancer.

    b. ovarian cancer.

    c. lung cancer.

    d. colon cancer.

2. The two most common cancers in women are

    a. endometrial and breast cancer.

    b. breast and colon cancer.

    c. lung and breast cancer.

    d. lung and colon cancer.

3. Studies tell us that most women want their care to include a recognition of

    a. well-being.

    b. aggressive treatment options.

    c. the overall importance of diet.

    d. legal rights.

4. A cancer diagnosis affects

    a. 3 of 10 families.

    b. 1 of 2 families.

    c. 1 of 5 families.

    d. 3 of 4 families.

5. More than 50% of new cancer cases affect people over age

    a. 65.

    b. 75.

    c. 50.

    d. 80.

6. Using 5 years after diagnosis as a benchmark, for all cancers

    a. 3 in 10 patients are expected to survive to their 5th anniversary past diagnosis.

    b. 4 in 10 patients are expected to survive to their 5th anniversary past diagnosis.

    c. 5 in 10 patients are expected to survive to their 5th anniversary past diagnosis.

    d. 6 in 10 patients are expected to survive to their 5th anniversary past diagnosis.

REFERENCES

American Cancer Society (ACS). (2003). Cancer Facts & Figures 2003. Atlanta: Author.

Ekwall, E., Ternestedt, B-M, & Sorbe, B. (2003). Important aspects of health care for women with gynecologic cancer. *Oncology Nursing Forum, 30*(2):313-319.

Halstead, M.T., & Hull, M. (2001). Struggling with paradoxes: The process of spiritual development in women with cancer. *Oncology Nursing Forum, 28*(10):1534-1544.

Jemal, A., Murray, T., Samuels, A., Ghafoor, A., Ward, E., & Thun, M.J. (2003). Cancer Statistics, 2003. *CA Cancer Journal for Clinicians, 53*(1):5-26.

Schaefer, K.M., Ladd, E., Gergits, M.A., & Gyauch, L. (2001). Backing and forthing: The process of decision making by women considering participation in a breast cancer prevention trial. *Oncology Nursing Forum, 28*:703-709.

Velji, R., & Fitch, M. (2001). The experience of women receiving brachytherapy for gynecologic cancer. *Oncology Nursing Forum, 28*(4): 743-751.

CHAPTER 2

BREAST CANCER

CHAPTER OBJECTIVE

After completing this chapter on breast cancer, the reader will be able to discuss the disease's epidemiology, risk factors, prevention and detection strategies, and common staging schemas and treatments.

LEARNING OBJECTIVES

After studying this chapter, the reader will be able to

1. recognize the main risk factors for breast cancer.

2. cite histologic terms for breast cancers.

3. identify advantages of mammography screening.

4. list tests included in the diagnostic workup of breast cancer.

5. describe the role that chemotherapy plays as a treatment for breast cancer.

6. describe the role that tamoxifen plays as a treatment for breast cancer.

7. recognize treatment options for early stage, node-negative breast cancer.

8. recognize treatment options for advanced stage breast cancer.

EPIDEMIOLOGY

Breast cancer is the most commonly diagnosed cancer in women, second to skin cancer. And in 2003 in the United States, breast cancer was the second leading cause of cancer deaths after lung cancer. In 2003, an estimated 211,300 new cases of invasive disease were diagnosed and 40,000 died of breast cancer. In 2003, 68,800 women died of lung cancer (ACS, 2003a). Breast cancer also occurs in men. An estimated 1,300 cases were diagnosed in men in 2003.

For the past few years, early detection and new treatment options have improved the outlook for breast cancer as a major health issue — long-term survival rates have risen and mortality is somewhat less. Most women diagnosed with early stage breast cancer become long-term survivors. Death rates from breast cancer declined significantly during 1992 to 1996, with the largest decreases in younger women — specifically in African American and Caucasian women.

For an average 40-year-old woman, the risk of developing breast cancer in the next 10 years is less than 1 in 60. For an average 70-year-old woman her 10-year-risk of developing breast cancer is 1 in 25. Table 2-1 lists the statistical probability of developing invasive breast cancer and Table 2-2 lists the mortality rates according to age.

Although age-adjusted breast cancer incidence rates are higher in Caucasian women than in

TABLE 2-1: LIFETIME PROBABILITY OF BEING DIAGNOSED WITH INVASIVE BREAST CANCER

from age 30 to age 40	1 out of 252
from age 40 to age 50	1 out of 68
from age 50 to age 60	1 out of 35
from age 60 to age 70	1 out of 27
Ever	1 out of 8

Note. From National Cancer Institute (NCI). (2003a). *Breast Cancer: Prevention.* CancerNet (PDQ®) Web sites for health professionals. Retrieved March 1, 2003, from http://www.nci.nih.gov/cancerinfo/pdq/prevention/breast/healthprofessional

African American women, mortality rates are higher in African American women. Among breast cancer cases diagnosed during 1992-1998, 64% of Caucasian women but only 53% of African American women had localized disease. Both breast cancer incidence and mortality are lower among Hispanic and Asian/Pacific Islander women than among Caucasian and African American women (NCI, 2003a). This might be due to limitations in gathering statistics.

Medicaid recipients and uninsured patients of all races have been shown to have later-stage breast cancer at diagnosis, and that survival from the time of diagnosis is shorter (NCI, 2003b).

BREAST ANATOMY

Figure 2-1 shows the basic breast anatomy.

Histological classifications of breast tumor cells are

• Noninvasive cancer (examples include ductal carcinoma in situ [DCIS], lobular carcinoma in situ [LCIS])

• Invasive cancers (examples include invasive ductal carcinoma, invasive lobular carcinoma, mucinous carcinoma, medullary carcinoma)

• Miscellaneous breast cancers (Examples include inflammatory breast cancer, Paget's disease).

The most common type of breast cancer is ductal carcinoma. It begins in the lining of the ducts.

NONINVASIVE CANCERS

Ductal Carcinoma In Situ (DCIS)

DCIS is a noninvasive neoplasm that originates from the breast ducts. It can progress to invasive cancer. Sometimes this condition is a precursor to

TABLE 2-2: MORTALITY RISK FOR BREAST CANCER ACCORDING TO AGE

For women age:	Chance of dying of breast cancer in the next 10 years	Chance of dying from any cause in the next 10 years
40-44	0.3% (1 in 333)	2.1% (1 in 48)
45-49	0.4% (1 in 250)	3.3% (1 in 30)
50-54	0.6% (1 in 167)	5.1% (1 in 20)
55-59	0.7% (1 in 143)	8.1% (1 in 12)
60-64	0.8% (1 in 125)	12.0% (1 in 8)
65-69	1.0% (1 in 100)	18.0% (1 in 6)
70-74	1.1% (1 in 91)	27.0% (1 in 4)
75-79	1.2% (1 in 83)	41.0% (1 in 2)
80-84	1.2% (1 in 83)	67.0% (2 in 3)
85+	1.1% (1 in 91)	79.0% (4 in 5)

(adapted from Woloshin & Schwartz, 1999).

Note. From National Cancer Institute (NCI). (2003b). *Breast Cancer: Screening.* CancerNet (PDQ®) Web sites for health professionals. Retrieved March 1, 2003, from http://www.nci.nih.gov/cancerinfo/pdq/screening/breast/healthprofessional/#Section_1

FIGURE 2-1: BREAST ANATOMY

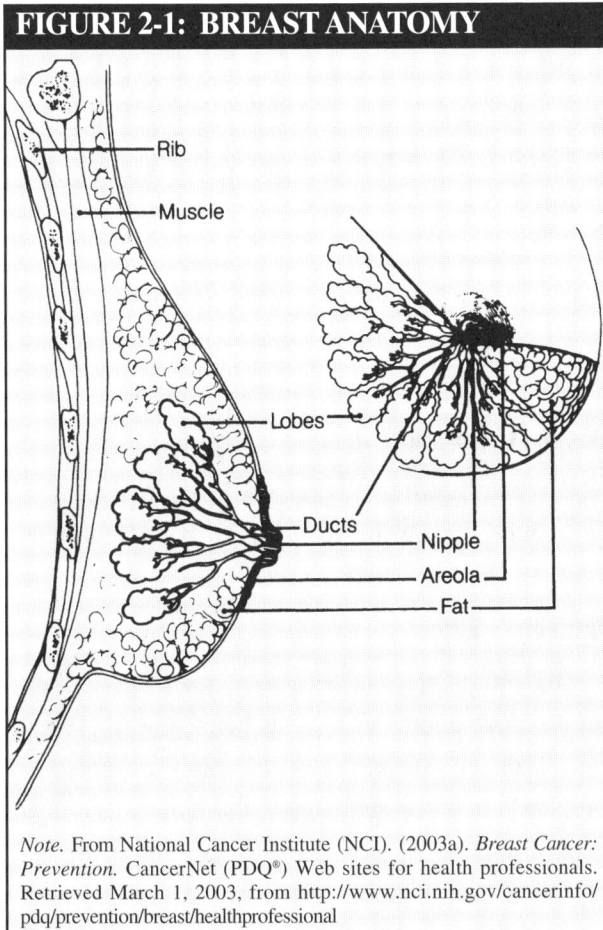

Note. From National Cancer Institute (NCI). (2003a). *Breast Cancer: Prevention.* CancerNet (PDQ®) Web sites for health professionals. Retrieved March 1, 2003, from http://www.nci.nih.gov/cancerinfo/pdq/prevention/breast/healthprofessional

invasive cancer. Screening mammography identified DCIS in about 30% of breast malignancies (NCI, 2003b).

Subtypes of DCIS include micropapillary, papillary, solid, cribriform, and comedo. Comedo-type DCIS appears to be more aggressive, with a higher probability of associated invasive ductal carcinoma (NCI, 2003b).

To date, DCIS treatment options (when localized) include mastectomy or breast-conserving surgery (lumpectomy) plus radiation. Studies continue to look at whether lumpectomy or radiation alone can be a safe alternative treatment for various early stages of DCIS.

Lobular Carcinoma In Situ (LCIS)

Women who are diagnosed with LCIS are at an increased risk for developing invasive breast cancer.

This risk remains for a long time — studies have reported the risk remains for at least 20 years.

But most of the subsequent cancers that develop from LCIS as an early tumor marker are ductal rather than lobular.

Most women with LCIS can be managed without additional local therapy after biopsy.

RISK FACTORS

Clarity on the causes of breast cancer is elusive. We know that breast cancer cannot be caused or exacerbated by trauma to the breast (NCI, 2003a, Gasalberti, 2002).

Defining risk factors for breast cancer continues to be problematic. Women who get breast cancer do not necessarily have the risk factors mentioned here, but studies have suggested they put women at greater risk (NCI, 2003a) Therefore a combination of these factors appear to increase a woman's risk of breast cancer.

Age

We know that breast cancer risks increase with age. (Breast cancer is uncommon < 35 years; risk increases > 60 years.) (NCI, 2003a; Barnes, Grizzle, Grubbs, & Partridge, 2002). Approximately 77% of women with breast cancer are over age 50 (ACS, 2003b).

Race

Incidence rates are higher for Caucasian women than other ethnic groups, although these statistics may be skewed by study methodologies, which looked at Caucasian women more often than any other group. Even taking into account economic factors (better access to care), Caucasian women were not always diagnosed early (Bibb, 2001; ACS, 2003b).

Sex

Men can develop breast cancer, but this disease is about 100 times more common among women than men.

Personal History of Breast Cancer

Risk increases for women who have been diagnosed with breast cancer in the same or opposite breast before. Previous history of breast cancer increases a woman's risk three- to four-fold (ACS, 2003b).

Family History

Risk increases if a woman's mother, sister, or daughter had breast cancer, especially when premenopausal (first-degree relative doubles the risk) (ACS, 2003b). See Genetic Risk section in this chapter.

Breast Changes

Certain breast changes such as atypical hyperplasia LCIS (see above) increase risk. On mammogram, breasts have a high proportion of dense lobular and ductal tissue.

Genetic Alterations

For some women, changes in certain genes (BRCA1, BRCA2, and others) increase the risk. Estimates of increased risk for these women are 50% to 85% of developing breast cancer during their lifetime (ACS, 2003b). (See Chapter 4, Ovarian Cancer, Family Inheritance/Predisposition; and Genetic Risk section in this chapter.)

Estrogen

Long-term exposure to estrogen increases the risk. This includes women who began menstruation before age 12, experienced menopause after age 55, never had a full-term pregnancy, or took hormone replacement therapy for long periods. See Chapter 3, Endometrial Cancer (HRT Box) and adjacent Box 1-HRT.

Late Childbearing

Risk increases if a woman is age 30 or older at the time of the first child birth (NCI, 2003a).

Radiation Therapy

Radiation therapy exposure before age 30 increases the risk (for example, for Hodgkin's disease) (NCI, 2003a).

Lifestyle

Relative risk of breast cancer increases by about 7% for each 10 gram (1 drink) per day compared to the risk for women who drink no alcohol (NCI, 2003a).

Weight Gain and Lifestyle Factors

Especially after menopause, risk increases for those who follow high-fat diets, have sedentary lifestyles, and smoke (NCI, 2003a).

Protective Effect

To mitigate risk factors, researchers are looking at protective agents as well as behaviors to prevent breast cancer. Among areas of focus are exercise, diet, and chemoprotective agents. No one strategy, or combination of strategies, to date, has emerged to prevent breast cancer (Barnes et al., 2002).

These factors suggest a protective effect against breast cancer, but little hard data is available.

Breastfeeding

For every 12 months of breastfeeding a woman lowers her risk of breast cancer by 4.3% (ACS, 2003b).

Prophylactic Mastectomy

Women at inherited risk to develop invasive breast cancer may choose to have prophylactic mastectomies. The advantage of this strategy is not clear. Few prospective data exist regarding the benefit of prophylactic mastectomy among these women (ACS, 2003b; NCI, 2003a).

Unproven Risks

No evidence, to date, supports these factors as risks for breast cancer (ACS, 2003b; NCI, 2003a; NCI, 2003b; NCI, 2003d)

• Antiperspirants

• Underwire bras

BOX 2-1: HORMONE REPLACEMENT THERAPY (HRT)

Conflicting data exist regarding the association between postmenopausal hormone replacement therapy (HRT) and breast cancer. Looking at many studies, conclusions emerged for women who had used HRT for 5 years or more after menopause. Risk decreased when women stopped their HRT. Five years after stopping HRT, previous HRT use for these women was not a risk factor (NCI, 2003e).

Studies of family history of breast cancer and the use of HRT has mixed outcomes, either suggesting an increased risk or no risk (NCI, 2003e). No data exist about HRT use on breast cancer among carriers of BRCA1 or BRCA2 mutations.

Clarity about breast cancer and the use of oral contraceptives is also mixed. Some studies show a slight increase in breast cancer risk with their use. Yet studies show no increased risk 10 years after the woman stops taking oral contraceptives (NCI, 2003e).

Some studies recommend that HRT should never be given to breast cancer survivors. Others believe that some women may not be put at risk for breast cancer and that the benefits of HRT toward menopausal symptoms or a protective agent for osteoporosis outweigh the risk (ACS, 2003b). Studies to clarify the impact of HRT on breast cancer in women continue.

- Induced abortion
- Breast implants
- Night work

HORMONE THERAPY AS PREVENTION

Tamoxifen (Nolvodex®) is a frequently used hormone to help prevent breast cancer. It blocks the action of estrogen in breast tissue, thereby preventing estrogen to stimulate the proliferation of breast cells (ACS, 2003b).

Tamoxifen has been shown to decrease the risk of developing breast cancer in women with LCIS. Women treated with tamoxifen had a reduced rate of several benign breast diseases, including atypical hyperplasia, a condition in which noncancerous cells multiply to an abnormal extent. These results also suggest that tamoxifen can reduce the incidence of atypical hyperplasia, which can develop into invasive breast cancer (Dienger, 2004; NCI, 2003f).

Studies have confirmed the benefit of adjuvant tamoxifen in estrogen receptor positive (ER+) premenopausal women. (See Box 2-1: Hormone Replacement Therapy [HRT] above.) A study pub-

lished in 2003 reported that women at high risk for breast cancer who took tamoxifen were 28% less likely to be diagnosed with benign breast conditions (Tan-Chiu et al., 2003). In another study from the Breast Cancer Prevention Trial (BCPT), women who took tamoxifen for 5 years had a 49% reduction in new cases of breast cancer (Dienger, 2004; NCI, 2003f).

Results from the National Surgical Adjuvant Breast and Bowel Project (NSABP) B-14 study, which compared 5 years of adjuvant tamoxifen to 10 years of adjuvant tamoxifen for women with early-stage breast cancer, indicate no advantage for continuation of tamoxifen beyond 5 years in women with node-negative, ER+ breast cancer (Dienger, 2004; Fisher et al., 2001). The optimal duration of tamoxifen treatment for node-positive women is still controversial and is being studied in ongoing clinical trials (NCI, 2003f).

Tamoxifen may cause weight gain, hot flashes, vaginal discharge or irritation, nausea, and irregular periods. Women who are still menstruating and having irregular periods may become pregnant more easily when taking tamoxifen (NCI, 2003f). Blood clots and development of cataracts are also rare but significant adverse effects.

Some studies show that tamoxifen can slightly increase the risk of developing endometrial cancer. (Risk increases 2-7 times that of a woman not taking tamoxifen.) (See Chapter 3, Endometrial Cancer.)

Tamoxifen is also used to treat metastatic breast cancer. (See Treatment: Hormone Therapy section in this chapter.)

Raloxifene

In addition to tamoxifen, another antiestrogen type agent, raloxifene, is being studied as a preventive hormonal agent. Its intended advantage is to reduce the incidence of both breast and uterine cancers. The study evaluating the efficacy of tamoxifen and raloxifene in postmenopausal women is the STAR trial (Study of Tamoxifen and Raloxifene). The goal of the trial is to follow more than 20,000

women on these preventive hormonal agents for 5-10 years.

So far study results show that raloxifene does not reduce the frequency of hot flashes associated with menopause and, like estrogen, it increases the risk of blood clots (ACS, 2003b).

SCREENING

Screening methods for breast cancer include the following:

Breast Self-Examination

Breast self-examination (BSE) has long been a means for patients to have control and an early awareness of breast changes. (Figure 2-2 shows the American Cancer Society's [ACS] recommended method of BSE.) We do not know if women who practice BSE universally practice with good tech-

FIGURE 2-2: BREAST SELF-EXAMINATION

If you regularly examine your own breasts, you will probably notice changes. The best time for breast self-examination (BSE) is about a week after your period ends, when your breasts are not tender or swollen. If you are not having regular periods, do BSE on the same day every month.

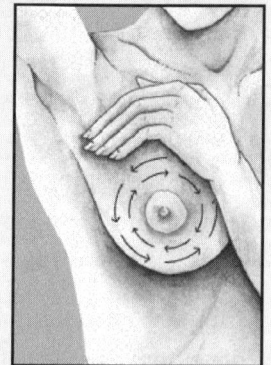

- Lie down with a pillow under your right shoulder and place your right arm behind your head.

- Use the finger pads of the three middle fingers on your left hand to feel for lumps in the right breast. Press firmly enough to know how your breast feels. A firm ridge in the lower curve of each breast is normal. If you're not sure how hard to press, talk with your doctor or nurse.

- Move around the breast in an up-and-down line, a circular, or a wedge pattern. Be sure to do it the same way every time, check the entire breast area, and remember how your breasts feel from month to month.

- Repeat the exam on your left breast, using the finger pads of the right hand. (Move the pillow to under your left shoulder.)

- Repeat the examination of both breasts while standing, with one arm behind your head. The upright position makes it easier to check the upper and outer part of the breasts (toward your armpit). This is where about half of breast cancers are found. You might want to do this part of the BSE while you are standing in the shower. Some breast changes can be felt more easily when your skin is wet and soapy.

- For added safety, you can check your breasts for any dimpling of the skin, changes in the nipple, redness, or swelling while standing in front of a mirror right after your BSE each month.

- If you find any changes, see your doctor right away.

Note. From American Cancer Society, Cancer Reference Information, Detailed Guide, Breast Cancer (2003b). Retrieved from http://www.cancer.org/docroot/CRI/CRI_2_3x.asp?dt=5

nique. Women in some studies have indicated that they practice BSE less frequently and less thoroughly because of a fear of "looking for trouble" (Gasalberti, 2002). We also don't know if BSE is truly effective in reducing breast cancer incidence and mortality rates (Machia, 2004; NCI, 2003b; Barnes et al., 2002).

Despite BSE being an accepted and effective strategy for early breast cancer prevention, studies report that BSE is not as widely practiced as desired (Machia, 2004; NCI, 2003b). The evidence is limited about whether BSE is actually practiced by many women at risk for breast cancer. Thus, BSE as a widely-accepted method of prevention is in question.

Clinical Breast Examination

Clinical breast examination (CBE) is a manual breast examination performed by a trained clinician. Although recommended at regular intervals for women at risk for breast cancer, studies are limited that prove that CBE is effective in reducing incidence and mortality (NCI, 2003b). CBE is recommended especially for women who carry the BRCA1 or BRCA2 high-risk mutation. (See Genetic Risk section in this chapter.)

Mammography

A mammogram is a low-dose x-ray of the breast. Screening mammography is widely used to look for breast disease in women who are asymptomatic. Mammograms can show masses, cysts, or small deposits of calcium in the breast. Although most calcium deposits are benign, microcalcifications may be an early sign of cancer.

Although breast x-rays have been performed for more than 70 years, modern mammography has only existed since 1969 — the first year x-ray units, specifically for breast imaging, were available. Modern mammography equipment designed for breast x-rays uses low levels of radiation, usually a dose of about 1 mGy to 2 mGy (100-200 mrad) per view or 2 mGy to 4 mGy (200-400 mrad) per two-view examination. Mammography has never been shown to be harmful to women or increase their risk of contracting breast cancer.

To put the x-ray dose for mammography in perspective, if a woman had yearly mammograms beginning at age 40 — continuing until she was age 90 — she would receive 20 to 40 rads of radiation. If treated with radiation therapy for breast cancer, she would receive several thousands rads. Another way to clarify the risk: One mammogram exposes a woman to about the same amount of radiation as flying from New York to California on a commercial jet (ACS, 2003b).

Mammography Screening

In the general population, strong evidence suggests that regular mammography screening of women age 50-59 leads to a 25-30% reduction in breast cancer mortality (NCI, 2003b). Table 2-3 lists the latest mammogram recommendations,

---

TABLE 2-3: RECOMMENDED SCREENING GUIDELINES

- Women between the ages of 20 and 39 should have a clinical breast examination (CBE) by a health professional every 3 years. (Monthly breast self-examination is encouraged for all women age 20 and older.)

- Women in their 40s should be screened every 1-2 years with mammography and have a CBE every year.

- Women age 50 and older should be screened every 1-2 years.

- Women who are at higher than average risk of breast cancer should seek expert medical advice about whether they should begin screening before age 40 and the frequency of screening.

(ACS, 2003a; NCI, 2003b)

accompanied by CBE recommendations, from the National Cancer Institute (NCI) and ACS.

For women who begin mammographic screening at age 40 through 49, a 17% reduction in breast cancer mortality is seen, based on 15 years of data after the start of screening. The reduction rate is lower for women 30-49 with a first-degree relative with breast cancer (due to the lower sensitivity rate of mammography for the younger woman) (NCI, 2003b).

Studies have concurred that the positive predictive value of mammography increases with age and is highest among older women and among women with a family history of breast cancer. Other studies show that CBE or CBE with mammogram have been more effective than mammogram alone in detecting breast cancers over time (Machia, 2004; NCI, 2003b).

No data exist regarding relative benefits or risks of screening mammography among female carriers of a BRCA1 or BRCA2 mutation, male carriers of a BRCA2 mutation, and women at inherited risk for breast cancer. The Cancer Genetics Studies Consortium Task Force of the NIH has recommended that for female carriers of a BRCA1 or BRCA2 high-risk mutation, annual mammography begin between age 25-35 years (NCI, 2003b).

The best use of mammograms is to have women have their films taken at a consistent location so that comparisons can be made. The experience of the radiologist reviewing films is also important.

False-Positives

Approximately 10% of women will require additional mammograms due to false-positives. Yet only 8-10% of those women will need a biopsy, and 80% of those biopsies will be benign (ACS, 2003b).

Mammography sensitivity ranges between 70-90%, depending on the woman's age and the densi-

ty of her breasts, which is affected by her genetic predisposition, hormone status, and diet. In studies based on an average sensitivity of 80%, mammograms will miss approximately 20% of breast tumors during screening (false-negatives) (Machia, 2004; NCI, 2003b).

A retrospective analysis of 61,273 screening mammograms showed that 3.3% of studies had false-positives due to superimposition of normal breast structures. About one half of these false-positives could be eliminated with two-view studies and 29% by additional diagnostic imaging (NCI, 2003b).

Under the Mammography Quality Standards Act (MQSA) enacted by Congress in 1992, all facilities that perform mammography must be certified by the U.S. Food and Drug Administration (FDA). This mandate has resulted in improved mammography technique, lower radiation dose, and better training of personnel.

Screening Effect on Incidence and Mortality

Widespread screening for breast cancer does not affect overall mortality. Its absolute benefit for breast cancer mortality appears to be small.

A 1995 study (Harris & Leininger, 1995) attempted to put the advantage of screening in perspective. The study estimated the outcomes of 10,000 women age 50-70 who underwent a single-screen mammogram. Mammograms were normal (true-negatives and false-negatives) in 9,500 women. Of the 500 abnormal screens, between 466 and 479 were false-positives, and 100 to 200 of these women underwent invasive procedures. The remaining 21 to 34 abnormal screens were true-positives, indicating breast cancer.

Some of the women in the study died of breast cancer, in spite of mammographic detection and optimal therapy, and some lived long enough to die of other causes, even if the cancer was not screen-detected. Based on this study's data, the number of extended lives attributable to mammographic detection was between 2 and 6 (NCI, 2003b).

Based on this researcher's analysis, one life may be extended per 1,700–5,000 women screened and followed for 15 years. Using the same analysis for 10,000 women age 40-49, assuming the same 500 abnormal examinations, an estimated 488 of these will be false-positives, and 12 will indicate breast cancer. Of these 12, there will probably be only 1-2 lives extended. Thus, for women aged 40-49, only 1-2 lives may be extended per 5,000 to 10,000 mammograms.

Two large population-based trials offer insight as to why the merits of widespread screening programs are inconclusive. One study concluded that screening can offer a statistically significant breast cancer mortality reduction of 18-32% (Duffy et al., 2002). The other reported a "statistically nonsignificant reduction" of 16-20% in favor of screening (Jonsonn et al., 2001). It is worth noting that conclusions from both studies were skewed by advances in adjuvant breast cancer therapy.

GENETIC RISK

Although risk factors for breast cancer are not yet clear or definitive, family history has emerged as an important risk factor for breast and ovarian cancer. After gender and age, for some women, a positive family history is the strongest known predictive risk factor for breast cancer.

For some women with a family history of breast cancer, the woman carries a genetic heritage that is compatible with autosomal dominant inheritance of cancer susceptibility. Several genes that create this susceptibility have been identified. These mutations are rare, however, and are estimated to account for no more than 5-10% of breast cancer cases overall.

Approximately 50% of susceptible individuals inherit the predisposing genetic alteration that is associated with breast cancer. The susceptibility may be inherited through either the mother's side or the father's side of the family.

This knowledge suggests that there are other background genetic factors that contribute to breast cancer occurrence.

Assessing Risk

Genetic testing and counseling can help women look at their own family history, which may increase their susceptibility to breast cancer. The focus of counseling is usually on women with mothers or sisters with breast cancer. Additional focus is on a second-degree relative with breast cancer.

It is important to know the age of the family member when diagnosed. Generally, the younger the age of the affected relative (for example, under 50), the greater the risk posed to relatives (also under 50). Risk also increases with the number of affected first- and second-degree relatives (Clark, 2004; NCI, 2003d).

Studies show that families with a history of ovarian cancer can be at risk for breast cancer. The presence of both breast and ovarian cancer in a family increases the likelihood that family members carry a cancer-predisposing mutation (Clark, 2004). (See Chapter 4, Ovarian Cancer.)

Establishing genetic risk is difficult because a woman's family history may be spotty or a reported family history can be incorrect. For instance, some women may be unaware of relatives affected with cancer or family members may have died of illnesses not known to the family. Studies also indicate that it may be especially difficult to gather family history about breast cancer from the father's side of the family; those family members may be distant and the father may have lost contact with that history (Clark, 2004; NCI, 2003d).

Risk Assessment

Pedigree analysis of the family history establishes if there is a dominant inheritance pattern. Sometimes a specific cancer susceptibility syndrome can be isolated.

So far, the syndromes most associated with an autosomal dominant inheritance of breast cancer risk are hereditary breast and ovarian cancer due to BRCA1 or BRCA2 mutations, Li-Fraumeni syndrome due to p53 mutations, and Cowden syndrome due to PTEN mutations (Clark, 2004; NCI, 2003d).

BRCA1

In 1990, a susceptibility gene for breast cancer was mapped by genetic linkage. BRCA1 appears to be responsible for disease in 45% of families with multiple cases of breast cancer only, and up to 90% of families with both breast and ovarian cancer. Approximately 1 in 800 individuals in the general population may carry a pathogenic mutation in BRCA1 (Clark, 2004; NCI, 2003d).

BRCA2

A second breast cancer susceptibility gene, BRCA2, was localized in families with multiple cases of breast cancer that were not linked to BRCA1. Mutations in BRCA2 are thought to account for approximately 35% of multiple case breast cancer families, and are also associated with male breast cancer, ovarian cancer, prostate cancer, and pancreatic cancer (Clark, 2004; NCI, 2003d).

Studies have shown that the likelihood of finding a BRCA1 or BRCA2 mutation was more than 50% if the patient had bilateral breast cancer, both breast and ovarian cancer, a diagnosis of breast cancer before age 40, and relatives with both breast and ovarian cancer (NCI, 2003d; Clark 2004).

BRCA1 and BRCA2 gene mutations produce different clinical phenotypes of characteristic malignancies and, in some instances, associated nonmalignant abnormalities. Several other genetic syndromes that may include breast cancer are being studied.

Counseling and Risk Models

Genetic counseling can help a woman decide whether testing would be appropriate for her. Also, genetic counseling before and after genetic testing is extremely important in helping women understand and deal with the possible test results.

Two models for predicting breast cancer risk — the Claus model and the Gail model — are listed in Table 2-4. Neither the Gail model nor the Claus model were designed to be used to predict the likelihood of a woman having a BRCA1 or BRCA2 mutation. Table 2-4 also reviews factors considered when determining BRCA1 or BRCA2 mutations.

The field of genetic testing is growing, but the limits of what can be verified by testing cannot be overemphasized. Many issues surface with testing and prompt numerous questions that either have no answers or ambiguous or speculative answers. Among questions that are prompted are what type of extra screening is needed, the recommended timetable of screening, appropriate immediate treatment options, appropriate long-term treatment options, what information is needed to pass on to family members, which family members need the information, how best to deal with psychosocial stress and distress by women and family members (who know limited genetic information), and what are appropriate decision-making strategies (Clark 2004; NCI, 2003d).

Additional challenges emerge with genetic counseling and the testing of women for breast cancer. Some studies have shown that even counseling does not dissuade women at low to moderate risk from the belief that BRCA1 testing is crucial to their future health and health decisions (Clark 2004; NCI, 2003d).

TABLE 2-4: RISK MODELS

The risk models described here calculate the probability of developing breast cancer for women with a family history of breast cancer.

Claus Model

Risk based on assumption that a rare autosomal dominant mutation can be inherited, using

- a woman's current age
- the number of first-degree and second-degree relatives with breast cancer
- age of cancer onset in first-degree and second-degree relatives.

(NOTE: The model does not take into account exposures, behavioral factors, or reproductive histories that increase risk. Not suitable for use in women who belong to high-risk families, containing three or more women with breast cancer.)

Gail Model

Risk based on known nongenetic risk factors and some family history, such as

- current age
- age at menarche
- age at first live birth
- number of previous breast biopsies
- presence of atypical hyperplasia
- number of first-degree relatives (mother or sister) with breast cancer.

(NOTE: This model does not consider data about second-degree relatives, paternal relatives, or age of onset of breast cancer in the affected relative.)

Models to determine *BRCA1* or *BRCA2* Mutation

Risk based on

- breast cancer diagnosed at an early age
- bilateral breast cancer
- a history of both breast and ovarian cancer
- the presence of breast cancer in one or more male family members.
- Family history characteristics associated with an increased likelihood of carrying a BRCA1 or BRCA2 mutation include:
  - multiple cases of breast cancer in the family
  - both breast and ovarian cancer in the family
  - one or more family members with two primary cancers
  - Ashkenazi Jewish background.

Note. From National Cancer Institute (NCI). (2003d). *Genetics of Breast and Ovarian Cancer.* CancerNet (PDQ®) Web sites for health professionals. Retrieved on March 1, 2003, from http://www.cancer.gov/cancerinfo/pdq/genetics/breast-and-ovarian

DIAGNOSING BREAST CANCER

When suspicious masses are found on BSE, CBE, or mammography, diagnostic strategies are considered. The diagnostic workup often includes ultrasound and biopsy. Biopsies can be fine-needle, needle, or surgical.

Additional imaging technologies used to determine a diagnosis include digital mammography, magnetic resonance imaging (MRI), and positron emission tomography (PET). Further tests to detect the spread of cancer include x-rays, bone scans, liver scans, and lung scans.

A more specific use of ultrasound is stereotactic needle biopsy. This technique allows computers to map the exact location of the mass using mammograms taken from two angles. A computer then guides the needle to the right spot.

Estrogen and progesterone receptor tests (see Treatments: Hormone Therapy in this chapter) indicate whether the woman's hormones affect the cancer's growth. With a positive test result, the cancer is likely to respond to hormone therapy.

20   *Chapter 2–*
Cancer in Women

Other diagnostic strategies in use or study include testing for the human epidermal growth factor receptor-2 or HER-2 gene. This mutation is associated with a higher risk of breast cancer and some specific treatments can follow. Also being studied are tumor markers in the blood and further technology to offer more specificity such as ductal lavage.

(NOTE: Ductal lavage is for women at high risk for breast cancer. Cells from the inside of the milk ductal system are evaluated for atypical cells. Results from ductal lavage can indicate whether a woman requires closer surveillance or more aggressive preventive strategies.)

TREATMENT

Staging emerges from the diagnostic workup. Staging is based on the existence and size of a malignant tumor (T), whether malignant cells have spread to lymph nodes (L), and whether malignant cells have spread distant to the primary tumor (M = metastasis). Numbers are added to staging schemas to provide more specific information about the tumor and its behavior. For example, a Stage IIB tumor can be a tumor 2-5 cm (T2) or > 5 cm (T3) with involvement in the axillary lymph node (N1) or no involvement (N0) and no metastasis (M0). Table 2-5 highlights staging criteria for breast cancer. Standard local treatments are surgery and radiation therapy. Systemic treatments are hormone therapy, chemotherapy, and biological therapy.

Surgery

Surgery is the classic local treatment. Figure 2-3 shows various surgical procedures in the workup and treatment of breast cancer. Breast-sparing surgeries include lumpectomy and segmental (partial) mastectomy. During surgery, axillary lymph nodes are removed to determine cancer spread.

TABLE 2-5: STAGING SCHEMAS

Breast cancer stage grouping

	T (Tumor)	N (Nodes)	M (Metastasis)
Stage 0	Tis N0	M0	
Stage 1	T1	N0	M0
Stage IIA	T0	N1	M0
	T1	N1	M0
	T2	N0	M0
Stage IIB	T2	N1	M0
	T3	N0	M0
Stage IIIA	T0	N2	M0
	T1	N2	M0
	T2	N2	M0
	T3	N2	M0
	T3	N2	M0
Stage IIIB	T4	N0, N1, N2	M0
Stage IIIC	Any T	N3	M0
Stage IV	Any T	Any N	M1

Breast cancer survival by stage

Stage	5-year relative survival rate
0	100%
I	98%
IIA	88%
IIB	76%
IIIA	56%
IIIB	59%
IV	16%

Note. From National Cancer Institute (NCI). (2003c). *Breast Cancer: Treatment.* CancerNet (PDQ®) Web sites for health professionals. Retrieved March 1, 2003, from http://www.nci.nih.gov/cancerinfo/pdq/treatment/breast/healthprofessional

Reprinted with permission from the American Joint Committee on Cancer (AJCC) staging system.

Sentinel Lymph Node Biopsy (SLNB)

Approximately 70% of women with early-stage breast cancer at the time of surgery will have no evidence of regional lymph node involvement. Therefore, determining who is likely to have negative nodes before extensive lymph node harvesting will spare women these potential complications of lymphedema. (See Lymphedema in this chapter.)

Toward reducing these complications, clinical practice is evolving toward more frequent use of

FIGURE 2-3: SURGICAL PROCEDURES

Lymph Node Dissection

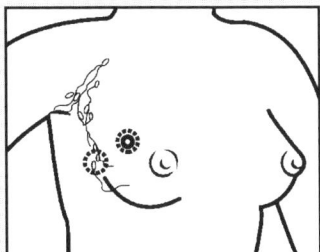

In *lumpectomy*, the surgeon removes the breast cancer and some normal tissue around it. (Sometimes an excisional biopsy serves as a lumpectomy.) Often, some of the lymph nodes under the arm are removed.

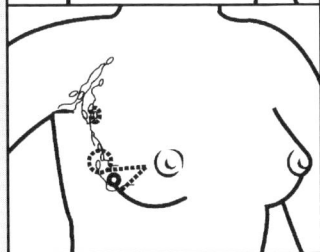

In *segmental mastectomy*, the surgeon removes the cancer and a larger area of normal breast tissue around it. Occasionally, some of the lining over the chest muscles below the tumor is removed as well. Some lymph nodes under the arm may also be removed.

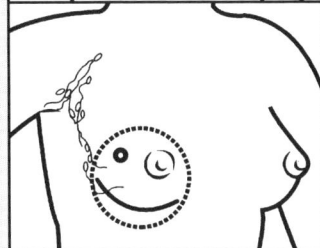

In *total (simple) mastectomy*, the surgeon removes the whole breast. Some lymph nodes under the arm may also be removed.

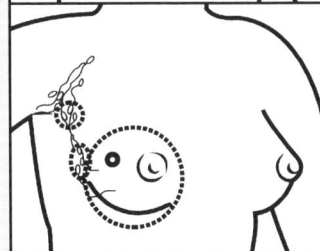

In *modified radical mastectomy*, the surgeon removes the whole breast, most of the lymph nodes under the arm, and, often, the lining over the chest muscles. The smaller of the two chest muscles also may be taken out to help in removing the lymph nodes.

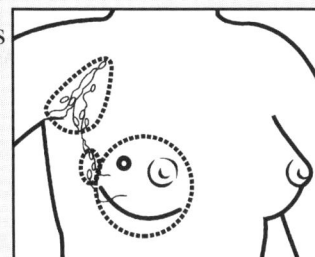

Note. From National Cancer Institute (NCI). (2003c). *Breast Cancer: Treatment.* CancerNet (PDQ®) Web sites for health professionals. Retrieved March 1, 2003, from http://www.nci.nih.gov/cancerinfo/pdq/treatment/breast/healthprofessional

sentinel lymph node biopsy (SLNB). The technique reduces the number of lymph nodes that must be removed during breast cancer surgery.

To have SLNB, before surgery the doctor injects a radioactive substance near the tumor. The injected contrast substance flows through the lymphatic system to the first lymph node or nodes where cancer cells are likely to have spread (the "sentinel" node or nodes). The doctor uses a scanner to locate the radioactive substance in the sentinel nodes. The surgeon can make a small incision and remove only the nodes with radioactive material (NCI, 2003c).

SLNB has been shown to significantly minimize the morbidity associated with axillary lymph node dissection while providing accurate diagnostic and prognostic information (Fraker, 2004; Baron et al., 2002).

Radiation Therapy

Radiation therapy can be used alone, before or after surgery, or with chemotherapy or hormone therapy. Therapy is generated from external radiation beams, delivered daily over a few weeks, or from radiation implants, that stay in for a few days.

For the treatment of some invasive breast cancer, studies over the past 10 years have shown that radiation therapy with lumpectomy is considered as effective a treatment as mastectomy (Perun, 2004; NCI, 2003c). Radiation therapy with lumpectomy has been shown to improve survival when provided as an adjunct to breast-conserving surgery. For patients with > 4 positive lymph nodes, studies have shown that with radiation therapy after surgery, local and regional recurrence can be reduced as much as 40% compared to surgery alone (Perun, 2004).

Hormone Therapy

Hormone therapy generally should be considered as initial treatment for a postmenopausal patient with newly diagnosed metastatic disease if the patient's tumor is estrogen receptor positive (ER+), progesterone receptor positive (PR+), or ER/PR-unknown.

A blood test can indicate if a woman can bind estrogen or progesterone to the ER or PR sites on the nuclear cell membrane of breast tumor tissue. If binding can occur, then breast tumor cells are stimulated. Hormonal therapy attempts to compete with estrogen or reduce the amount of circulating estrogen that stimulates breast tumor development.

Approximately 80% of breast tumors in postmenopausal women are ER+, but only 50-70% in premenopausal women indicate ER expression (Dienger, 2004). About 30% of ER+ tumors are progesterone receptor negative (PR–). Fewer than 5% of estrogen receptor negative (ER–) tumors are PR+. Women with both ER+ and PR+ status are the best candidates for hormone therapy (Dienger, 2004).

Hormone therapy is especially indicated if the woman's disease involves only bone and soft tissue and if she has not received adjuvant antiestrogen therapy (for example, tamoxifen) or has been off of antiestrogen therapy for more than 1 year (Dienger, 2004; NCI, 2003f).

As treatment in addition to tamoxifen, several agents are used to block the effect of estrogen or

TABLE 2-6: HORMONE THERAPIES

Tamoxifen (Nolvadex®)

Toremifene (Fareston®)

Fulvestrant (Faslodex®)

Aromatase Inhibitors: Three drugs that stop estrogen production have been approved for use in treating breast cancer called letrozole (Femara®), anastrozole (Arimidex®), and exemestane (Aromasin®).

Megestrol acetate (Megace®)

TABLE 2-7: SELECTED CHEMOTHERAPY AGENTS AND PROTOCOLS

Neoadjuvant and adjuvant protocols for breast cancer, include

- cyclophosphamide (Cytoxan®), methotrexate (Amethopterin, Mexate, Folex®), and fluorouracil (Fluorouracil, 5-Fu, Adrucil® [abbreviated CMF])

- cyclophosphamide, doxorubicin (Adriamycin®), and fluorouracil (abbreviated CAF)

- doxorubicin (Adriamycin®) and cyclophosphamide (abbreviated AC)

- doxorubicin (Adriamycin®) and cyclophosphamide with paclitaxel (Taxol®)

- doxorubicin (Adriamycin®), followed by CMF

- cyclophosphamide, epirubicin (Ellence™), and fluorouracil.

Other chemotherapy drugs used for treating women with breast cancer include docetaxel (Taxotere®), vinorelbine (Navelbine®), gemcitabine (Gemzar®), capecitabine (Xeloda®), topotecan, and irinotecan.

lowering estrogen levels. Table 2-6 lists some of these hormone therapies.

Chemotherapy

Neoadjuvant (before surgery) and adjuvant (after surgery) chemotherapy protocols are offered as systemic therapies to boost the effectiveness of surgery and radiation and to treat tumors that have metastasized. Table 2-7 lists common chemotherapy agents and protocols for breast cancer.

Biological therapy

Biological therapies are designed to capitalize on the body's natural defenses against cancer.

For example, trastuzumab (Herceptin®) is a monoclonal antibody that targets breast cancer cells that have too much of the protein human epidermal growth factor receptor-2 (HER-2). By blocking HER-2, trastuzumab slows or stops the growth of these cells. The drug may be given by itself or along with chemotherapy. Approximately 25% of patients with breast cancer have tumors that overexpress HER-2/neu (NCI, 2003c).

Patients with metastatic breast cancer with substantial overexpression of HER-2/neu are candidates for treatment with the combination of trastuzumab and paclitaxel or for clinical studies of trastuzumab combined with taxanes and other chemotherapeutic agents.

Determining the appropriate course of treatment for women with breast cancer is a challenge due to the nature of the (various) types of diseases and the woman's goals of treatment and quality of life.

Early-Stage Breast Cancer

Table 2-8 lists treatment options for women with early-stage breast cancer. Treatments include local-regional surgeries and/or adjuvant radiation therapy for node negative breast cancers. Factors taken into account to determine treatment are

---

TABLE 2-8: EARLY-STAGE TREATMENT OPTIONS

Stage I, II, or early III breast cancer

Local-regional treatment

- breast-conserving therapy (lumpectomy, breast irradiation, and surgical staging of the axilla)
- modified radical mastectomy (removal of the entire breast with level I-II axillary dissection) with or without breast reconstruction
- sentinel lymph node biopsy, under clinical evaluation.

Adjuvant radiation therapy postmastectomy in axillary node-positive tumors

- one to three nodes: unclear role for regional radiation (infra- and supraclavicular nodes, internal mammary nodes, axillary nodes, and chest wall)
- more than 4 nodes or extranodal involvement: regional radiation is advised.

Note. From National Cancer Institute (NCI). (2003c). *Breast Cancer: Treatment.* CancerNet (PDQ®) Web sites for health professionals. Retrieved March 1, 2003, from http://www.nci.nih.gov/cancerinfo/pdq/treatment/breast/healthprofessional

---

tumor size, ER/PR status, and tumor grade. Table 2-9 shows risk categories for negative axillary lymph node breast cancer. Table 2-10 reviews adjuvant systemic treatment options for women with axillary node-negative breast cancer.

Stage III Breast Cancer

Typically smaller stage IIIA breast cancers may be removed by lumpectomy or modified radical mastectomy. Adjuvant systemic therapy and radia-

---

TABLE 2-9: RISK CATEGORIES FOR WOMEN WITH NODE-NEGATIVE BREAST CANCER

	Low-risk (has all listed factors)	Intermediate-risk (risk classified between the other 2 categories)	High-risk (has at least 1 listed factor)
Tumor size	</= 1 cm	1-2 cm	> 2 cm
ER or PR status	positive	positive	negative
Tumor grade	grade 1	grade 1-2	grade 2-3

Note. From National Cancer Institute (NCI). (2003c). *Breast Cancer: Treatment.* CancerNet (PDQ®) Web sites for health professionals. Retrieved March 1, 2003, from http://www.nci.nih.gov/cancerinfo/pdq/treatment/breast/healthprofessional

TABLE 2-10: ADJUVANT SYSTEMIC TREATMENT OPTIONS FOR WOMEN WITH AXILLARY NODE-NEGATIVE BREAST CANCER

Patient group	Low-risk	Intermediate-risk	High-risk
Premenopausal, ER+ or PR+	None or tamoxifen	Tamoxifen plus chemotherapy, tamoxifen alone, ovarian ablation, GnRH analogue*	Chemotherapy plus tamoxifen, chemotherapy plus ablation or GnRH analogue*, chemotherapy plus tamoxifen plus ovarian ablation or GnRH*, or ovarian ablation alone or with tamoxifen or GnRH alone or with tamoxifen
Premenopausal, ER– or PR–	N/A	N/A	Chemotherapy
Postmenopausal, ER+ or PR+	None or tamoxifen	Tamoxifen plus chemotherapy, tamoxifen alone	Tamoxifen plus chemotherapy, tamoxifen alone
Postmenopausal, ER– or PR–	N/A	N/A	Chemotherapy
>70 years of age	None or tamoxifen	Tamoxifen alone, tamoxifen plus chemotherapy	Tamoxifen; consider chemotherapy if ER– or PR–

*Note: This treatment option is under clinical evaluation.

Note. From National Cancer Institute (NCI). (2003c). *Breast Cancer: Treatment.* CancerNet (PDQ®) Web sites for health professionals. Retrieved March 1, 2003, from http://www.nci.nih.gov/cancerinfo/pdq/treatment/breast/healthprofessional

tion therapy usually follow surgery. Tamoxifen is given for hormone receptor-positive tumors.

Larger stage IIIA as well as stage IIIB and IIIC cancers may be treated with neoadjuvant chemotherapy. Then a modified radical mastectomy or lumpectomy follows, with or without reconstruction. Additional adjuvant chemotherapy and radiation therapy can follow surgery. Tamoxifen is given for hormone receptor-positive tumors.

Table 2-11 reviews treatment options for women with axillary node-positive breast cancer.

Advanced Stage and Recurrent Breast Cancer

Treatment options include surgery, radiation therapy, and neoadjuvant chemotherapy. Anthracycline-based chemotherapy and/or taxane-based therapy is standard. Treatment for metastatic breast cancer will usually involve hormone therapy and/or chemotherapy with or without trastuzumab (Herceptin).

Radiation therapy and/or surgery may be indicated for patients with limited symptomatic metastasis. All patients with metastatic or recurrent breast cancer should be considered candidates for ongoing clinical trials.

TABLE 2-11: TREATMENT OPTIONS FOR WOMEN WITH AXILLARY NODE-POSITIVE BREAST CANCER	
Patient group	**Treatments**
Premenopausal, ER+ or PR+	Chemotherapy plus tamoxifen, chemotherapy plus ovarian ablation/GnRH analogue, chemotherapy plus tamoxifen plus ovarian ablation/GnRH analogue*, ovarian ablation alone or with tamoxifen or GnRH alone or with tamoxifen
Premenopausal, ER– or PR–	Chemotherapy
Postmenopausal, ER+ or PR+	Tamoxifen plus chemotherapy, tamoxifen alone
Postmenopausal, ER– or PR–	Chemotherapy
>70 years of age	Tamoxifen alone; consider chemotherapy if receptor-negative

*Note: This treatment option is under clinical evaluation.

Note. From National Cancer Institute (NCI). (2003c). *Breast Cancer: Treatment.* CancerNet (PDQ®) Web sites for health professionals. Retrieved March 1, 2003, from http://www.nci.nih.gov/cancerinfo/pdq/treatment/breast/healthprofessional

Recurrent breast cancer is often responsive to therapy, although treatment is rarely curative at this stage of disease. Patients with local-regional breast recurrence may become long-term survivors with appropriate therapy.

Treatment to relieve symptoms depends on where the cancer has metastasized. For example, pain due to bone metastases may be treated with external beam radiation therapy and/or bisphosphonates such as pamidronate (Aredia®). See Appendix III for further review of Nursing Diagnoses.

REHABILITATION

A woman recovering from treatment for breast cancer faces some unique challenges because of her disease. Among them are the need for post-surgery exercises (for patients undergoing mastectomy or lumpectomy), management of lymphedema, and facing the possibility of further surgery for reconstruction.

Exercises

For mastectomy or lumpectomy patients, exercising the arm and shoulder after surgery can help a woman regain motion, balance, and strength.

Properly targeted and paced exercises can reduce pain and stiffness in her neck and back. These exercises typically start slowly within a 1-2 days after surgery. In time, exercising can be more active and part of a woman's normal routine (NCI, 2003c).

Lymphedema

For women who have had extensive axillary lymph node dissections as part of their mastectomies, lymphedema may be a troubling chronic adverse effect.

Strategies to reduce and manage lymphedema include special techniques in massage, wrapping of the extremity with an elastic sleeve or cuff, exercises protecting the limb from injury, and infection control. Special physical therapists coordinate care of lymphedema patients.

Breast Reconstruction

Patients with total mastectomies may choose to pursue reconstructive surgery at the time of the original mastectomy or later after healing. Breast implants with a rectus muscle or other flap are applied to the reconstructed area. Implants are typically saline filled. Some techniques begin with tissue expanders that are injected with saline, which allow the tissue to stretch over time. A permanent implant is then placed.

Silicone implants are available only through restricted clinical trials approved by the FDA (NCI, 2003c).

Following breast reconstruction, the chest wall and node regions may be treated with radiation therapy.

Breast Prosthesis

Women can choose to wear specially made bras or prosthesis after surgery. Many options are available, so women usually need to go through a period of customizing and special fittings of available garments to accommodate their needs.

Sexuality

Breast cancer surgery and treatment affects the woman's sexuality. Chapter 9 reviews some of the issues of sexuality.

Researchers have studied postmastectomy patients, especially related to their sexuality. Body image, not surprisingly, is a major concern of these women. Support and education for these women is key to their rehabilitation and ability to go on with their lives.

SUMMARY

Screening, early detection, and more effective treatments have led to a decline in the death rate for breast cancer. Breast cancer incidence rates continue to climb, due in part to a wider use of mammography. Noninvasive or preinvasive forms of breast cancer — DCIS and LCIS are the focus of BSE, CBE, and mammography. Definitive risk factors for breast cancer are elusive, but we do know that breast cancer is a disease of aging. Genetic predispositions to breast cancer have also been identified. Early stage breast cancer is treated with surgery and radiation therapy. More advanced cancers follow multimodality protocols that also

include chemotherapy, hormone therapies, and biological therapies.

The period after treatment can be especially complicated with women facing issues of reconstruction. Lymphedema and other complications from treatment (pain, body image changes, depression) have been identified as issues that require nursing management and support.

CASE STUDY: BREAST CANCER

BB is a 65-year-old Hispanic woman, who presents to her primary care physician with symptoms of the flu (fever and chills). The physician takes a throat swab and sends it to cytology for evaluation. Before BB leaves, he asks if he can do a Clinical Breast Exam (CBE). (BB said she had not had a mammogram "for a while.") The physician also ordered a mammogram.

On CBE, the physician noted a fixed, irregular nodule on her outer right breast. Mammogram results came back suspicious for an opaque, irregular mass on the outer right breast.

BB was scheduled for an ultrasound guided fine needle aspirate (FNA). Results indicated invasive ductal carcinoma. Further workup included a bone scan, chest x-ray, and magnetic resonance imaging (MRI).

After weighing her options with her primary physician, a breast surgeon, and radiation oncologist, BB opted to have a lumpectomy, followed by adjunctive radiation therapy. The lumpectomy procedure was unremarkable. (The excised nodule was 4 cm x 2 cm.) Based on sentinel node mapping, BB was found to have no positive nodes. BB's breast cancer was staged at Stage IIB (T2 N1M0). She went home about 4 hours after the procedure.

Postoperatively, BB experienced some pain that resolved within a few days. She also had some nausea because of anesthesia, which resolved with-

in 2 days of the procedure. She was instructed to reduce physical activity involving her right side for 7-10 days.

Radiation therapy began 4 weeks after surgery. A total of 5000 cGy was given (25 fractions) over a 6 weeks (5 times/week). BB complained of skin irritation from the radiation therapy, which started 2 weeks after her therapy began. She was counseled to manage her mild erythema by washing with gentle soap and water, avoiding heat and using unscented creams on her breast. The erythema resolved about 2 weeks after her treatments ended.

At 3 months postradiation therapy, BB had another mammogram. The results were negative for any new masses. As part of her new vigilance about breast health, BB began to be more conscientious with BSE and had a nurse practitioner provide a CBE every 6 months.

Continued follow-up every 6 months showed no new breast masses. Under a federal-sponsored program, BB had a yearly mammogram.

Additional information:

BB started menopause at 50. (She believes she started menstruation at 13.) Her other health problems are obesity (50 pounds overweight), hypertension, and gout.

BB loves to cook for her family. She makes traditional Mexican dishes that use oils, fat, and spices for flavor. She also uses medication, which a local "herb" doctor in her neighborhood has recommended.

BB is a widow and the grandmother of seven. She splits her time between living with two of her daughters, who have families but work outside of the home. BB helps with housework and errands for her daughters, but she finds that her energy fades during the day and she does not have the stamina she had before her lumpectomy and radiation therapy.

One of BB's granddaughters has urged BB to ask about ovarian cancer, because the granddaughter says that she had heard that women with breast cancer "can get" ovarian cancer.

She is pleased with her recovery, but states she has second thoughts about whether she should have had her breast removed as treatment. She says some days she believes she should just have both breasts removed. Her physician has prescribed tamoxifen for her (because she was shown to be ER+) but she admits that she forgets some days to take her pills. Since Medicare does not cover her prescription and BB is on a fixed income, she is reluctant to spend money for medication.

Family and religion are extremely important to BB. Since her diagnosis of breast cancer was made, she has attended religious services more frequently. She cries easily around her family. She says she has trouble sleeping and cannot concentrate. She says she feels low more days than not.

EXAM QUESTIONS

CHAPTER 2
Questions 7-14

7. The main risk factors for breast cancer are

    a. sex, age, and obesity.

    b. sex, age, and personal history of breast cancer.

    c. sex, age, and breast implants.

    d. sex, age, and use of antiperspirants.

8. A type of noninvasive breast cancer is

    a. Paget's disease.

    b. medullary carcinoma.

    c. DCIS.

    d. mucinous carcinoma.

9. Breast cancer screening using mammography is most advantageous for women age

    a. 20-30.

    b. 30-40.

    c. 40-50.

    d. over 50.

10. An initial diagnostic workup for breast cancer should include

    a. CBE, mammography, ultrasound, and biopsy.

    b. PET scan only.

    c. a CA-125 blood test.

    d. stereotactic needle biopsy.

11. Neoadjuvant chemotherapy as a treatment for breast cancer is scheduled

    a. before surgery.

    b. during surgery.

    c. after surgery.

    d. as a sole modality.

12. Tamoxifen

    a. can only be used as a preventive treatment for cancer.

    b. is a new treatment with no track record.

    c. only prescribed with patients who are ER–.

    d. has been shown to be effective for women who are ER+.

13. When staging early stage breast cancer, factors that lead to appropriate treatment are

    a. the age of the woman.

    b. family members with breast cancer.

    c. if the patient had smoked.

    d. the number of positive lymph nodes.

14. Standard treatment for advanced stage breast cancer includes

    a. anthracycline-based and/or taxane-based chemotherapy.

    b. progressive hormonal therapy.

    c. investigational drugs alone.

    d. watch and wait monitoring.

REFERENCES

American Cancer Society (ACS). (2003a). *Cancer Facts & Figures 2003.* Atlanta: Author.

American Cancer Society (ACS). (2003b). Cancer Reference Information, Detailed Guide, Breast Cancer. Retrieved May 1, 2003, from http://www.cancer.org/docroot/CRI/CRI_2_3x.asp?dt=5

American Joint Commission on Cancer (AJCC). (2002). Breast Cancers. *AJCC Cancer Staging Handbook* (6th ed.) (pp. 221-240). New York: Springer-Verlag.

Baron, R.H., Fey, R.H., Raboy, R., Thaler, H.T., Borgen, P.I., Templber, L.K.F, et al. (2002). Eighteen sensations after breast cancer surgery: A comparison of sentinel lymph node biopsy and axillary lymph node dissection. *Oncology Nursing Forum, 29*(4):651-659.

Barnes, M.B., Grizzle, W.E., Grubbs, C.J., & Partridge, E.E. (2002). Paradigms for primary prevention of breast carcinoma. *CA Cancer Journal for Clinicians, 52:*216-225.

Bibb, G. (2001). The relationship between access and stage at diagnosis of breast cancer in African American and Caucasian women. *Oncology Nursing Forum, 28*(4):711-719.

Clark, P. (2004). Nongenetic and heritable risk factors. In K. Dow (Ed.), *Contemporary issues in Breast Cancer* (pp. 10-24). Sudbury, MA: Jones & Bartlett Publishers.

Dienger, M.J. (2004). Hormonal therapy in advanced and metastatic disease. In K. Dow (Ed.), *Contemporary Issues in Breast Cancer* (pp. 175-186). Sudbury, MA: Jones & Bartlett Publishers.

Duffy, S.W., Tabár, L., Chen, H.H., Holmquist, M., Yen, M.F., Abdsalah, S., et al. (2002). The impact of organized mammography service screening on breast carcinoma mortality in seven Swedish counties. *Cancer, 95*(3):458-469.

Fisher, B., Dignam, J., Bryant, J., & Wolmark, N. (2001). Five versus more than five years of tamoxifen for lymph node-negative breast cancer: updated findings from the National Surgical Adjuvant Breast and Bowel Project B-14 randomized trial. *Journal of the National Cancer Institute, 93*(9):684-690.

Fraker, T. (2004). Diagnosis and staging. In K. Dow (Ed.), *Contemporary Issues in Breast Cancer* (pp. 58-77). Sudbury, MA: Jones & Bartlett Publishers.

Gasalberti, D. (2002). Early detection of breast cancer by self-examination: The influence of perceived barriers and health conception. *Oncology Nursing Forum, 29*(9):1341-1347.

Harris, R., & Leininger L. (1995). Clinical strategies for breast cancer screening: Weighing and using the evidence. *Annals of Internal Medicine, 122*(7):539-47.

Jonsson, H., Nyström, L., Törnberg, S., et al. (2001). Service screening with mammography of women aged 50-69 years in Sweden: Effects on mortality from breast cancer. *Journal of Medical Screening, 8*(3):152-60.

Machia, J. (2004). Screening and early detection. In K. Dow (Ed.), *Contemporary Issues in Breast Cancer* (pp. 45-47). Sudbury, MA: Jones & Bartlett Publishers.

National Cancer Institute (NCI). (2003a). *Breast Cancer: Prevention.* CancerNet (PDQ®) Web sites for health professionals. Retrieved March 1, 2003, from http://www.nci.nih.gov/cancer info/pdq/prevention/breast/healthprofessional

National Cancer Institute (NCI). (2003b). *Breast Cancer: Screening.* CancerNet (PDQ®) Web sites for health professionals. Retrieved March 1, 2003, from http://www.nci.nih.gov/cancer info/pdq/screening/breast/healthprofessional/ #Section_1

National Cancer Institute (NCI). (2003c). *Breast Cancer: Treatment.* CancerNet (PDQ®) Web sites for health professionals. Retrieved March 1, 2003, from http://www.nci.nih.gov/cancerin-fo/pdq/treatment/breast/healthprofessional

National Cancer Institute (NCI). (2003d). *Genetics of Breast and Ovarian Cancer.* CancerNet (PDQ®) Web sites for health professionals. Retrieved March 1, 2003, from http://www. cancer.gov/cancerinfo/pdq/genetics/breast-and-ovarian

National Cancer Institute (NCI). (2003e). *Menopause Hormone Use: Questions and Answers.* Retrieved July 2, 2003, from http:// www.cancer.gov/newscenter/estrogenplus

National Cancer Institute (NCI). (2003f). *Tamoxifen Lowers Risk of Benign Breast Disease in Some Women.* Retrieved March 1, 2003, from http://www.cancer.gov/ clinicaltrials/results/tamoxifen-and-benign-breast-disease0102

Perun, J. (2004). Radiation therapy. In K. Dow (Ed.), *Contemporary Issues in Breast Cancer* (pp. 110-133). Sudbury, MA: Jones & Bartlett Publishers.

Tan-Chiu, E., Wang, J., Costantino, J.P., Paik, S., Butch, C., Wickerham, D.L., Fisher, B., & Wolmark, N. (2003). Effects of tamoxifen on benign breast disease in women at high risk for breast cancer. *Journal of National Cancer Institute, 95*(4):302-307.

Woloshin, S., Schwartz, L.M. (1999). How can we help people make sense of medical data? *Eff Clin Prac,* 2(4):176-83.

CHAPTER 3

ENDOMETRIAL CANCER

CHAPTER OBJECTIVE

After completing this chapter on endometrial cancer, the reader will be able to discuss the disease's epidemiology, risk factors, prevention and detection strategies, and common staging schemas and treatments.

LEARNING OBJECTIVES

After studying this chapter, the reader will be able to

1. recognize the main risk factors for endometrial cancer.

2. cite terms that describe abnormal endometrial cells or their spread so that the cancer can be staged.

3. describe the role that hormone replacement therapy (HRT) plays as a treatment for endometrial cancer.

4. list tests included in the diagnostic workup of endometrial cancer.

5. recognize radiation therapy strategies to treat endometrial cancer.

6. identify adverse effects that women may experience after a hysterectomy.

INTRODUCTION

Endometrial cancer is the most common gynecologic cancer and is highly curable if detected early. The chapter will review those factors that increase a woman's risk for endometrial cancer and update the issues related to HRT and endometrial cancer. The standard treatment for endometrial cancer is surgery, sometimes accompanied by radiation therapy or chemotherapy.

EPIDEMIOLOGY

Cancer of the endometrium is the most common gynecologic malignancy and accounts for 6% of all cancers in women and 3% of all cancer deaths. (See Figure 3-1 and Figure 3-2.) Based on 2003 statistics, 40,100 new cases were estimated (ACS, 2003; NCI, 2003a). It is the fourth most common cancer in women and accounts for almost one-half of the new cases of gynecological cancer diagnosed each year (Reuters, 2001). Endometrial cancer is highly curable and the mortality rate has declined about 25% from 1974 to the present.

Endometrial cancer increases with advancing age in most but not all racial and ethnic groups, with the exceptions being Chinese and Filipino women. Relative overall survival at 1 year from diagnosis is 98% with 5-year survival rate at 84%. If detected when the disease is localized, women with endometrial cancer have a 96% survival rate

FIGURE 3-1: ESTIMATED NEW CANCER CASES

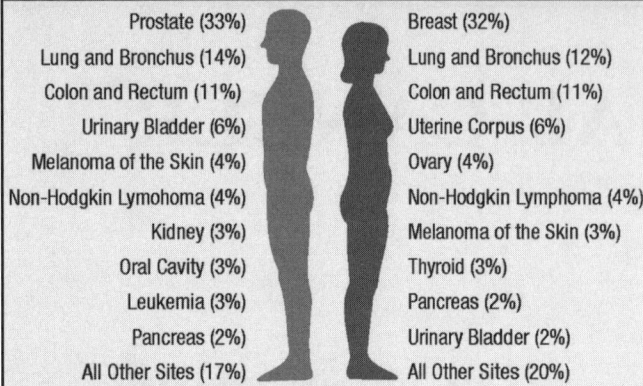

Prostate (33%)	Breast (32%)
Lung and Bronchus (14%)	Lung and Bronchus (12%)
Colon and Rectum (11%)	Colon and Rectum (11%)
Urinary Bladder (6%)	Uterine Corpus (6%)
Melanoma of the Skin (4%)	Ovary (4%)
Non-Hodgkin Lymohoma (4%)	Non-Hodgkin Lymphoma (4%)
Kidney (3%)	Melanoma of the Skin (3%)
Oral Cavity (3%)	Thyroid (3%)
Leukemia (3%)	Pancreas (2%)
Pancreas (2%)	Urinary Bladder (2%)
All Other Sites (17%)	All Other Sites (20%)

Excludes basal and squamous cell skin cancers and in situ carcinomas except urinary bladder.
Note: Percentages may not total 100 percent due to rounding.
Note. From "Cancer Statistics, 2003," by A. Jemal, T. Murray, A. Samuels, A. Ghafoor, E. Ward, & M.J. Thun, 2003, *CA Cancer Journal for Clinicians, 53,* pp. 5-26. Reprinted with permission.

FIGURE 3-2: ESTIMATED CANCER DEATHS

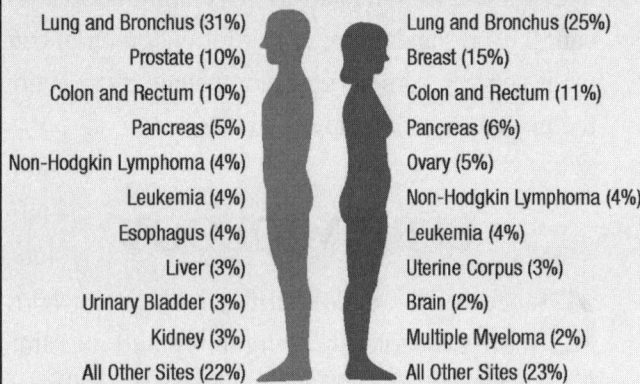

Lung and Bronchus (31%)	Lung and Bronchus (25%)
Prostate (10%)	Breast (15%)
Colon and Rectum (10%)	Colon and Rectum (11%)
Pancreas (5%)	Pancreas (6%)
Non-Hodgkin Lymphoma (4%)	Ovary (5%)
Leukemia (4%)	Non-Hodgkin Lymphoma (4%)
Esophagus (4%)	Leukemia (4%)
Liver (3%)	Uterine Corpus (3%)
Urinary Bladder (3%)	Brain (2%)
Kidney (3%)	Multiple Myeloma (2%)
All Other Sites (22%)	All Other Sites (23%)

Excludes basal and squamous cell skin cancers and in situ carcinomas except urinary bladder.
Note: Percentages may not total 100 percent due to rounding.
Note. From "Cancer Statistics, 2003," by A. Jemal, T. Murray, A. Samuels, A. Ghafoor, E. Ward, & M.J. Thun, 2003, *CA Cancer Journal for Clinicians, 53,* pp. 5-26. Reprinted with permission.

at 5 years. When detected as a regional disease at 5 years, women have a survival rate of 64%; when detected as a distant disease, 26% (ACS, 2003; NCI, 2003a).

Endometrial cancer generally matches breast cancer for its ethnic incidence and mortality trends. The age-adjusted incidence rate is highest in Hawaiians, Whites, Japanese, and Blacks. The lowest incidence rates are in Koreans, Vietnamese, and American Indian women (ACS, 2003; NCI, 2003c).

Although incidence is higher in White women, death rates are twice as high for Black women compared to White women (7.0 vs. 3.9 per 100,000). At all stages, White women have a greater rate of survival than Black women, with survival by White women surpassing that of Black women by 15% (NCI, 2003c). Age-adjusted mortality rates in the United States are highest among Hawaiian women, followed by Black women (ACS, 2003). Mortality among White, Hispanic, Chinese, Japanese, and Filipino women is less than one-half the rate for Hawaiian women. Some experts speculate that higher mortality rate for Blacks and Hawaiian women may be related to their lack of access to care (NCI, 2003c; Dolinsky, 2002).

Despite reductions reported in epidemiological statistics, some evidence suggests that endometrial cancer incidence rates are rising. Since 1987, there has been a 128% increase in the number of new cases of endometrial cancer. But the number of new cases diagnosed per year climbed only 10% during the same time period (NCI, 2003a; Reuters, 2002).

One theory about the cause of the statistical rise is the report in the decline of more treatable endometrial cancers versus those that are more resistant to treatment (Rueters, 2001). (See Risk Factors section in this chapter.) Endometrial cancer, related to estrogen levels, is highly treatable. Other types of endometrial cancer with a different biological basis have been shown to respond less to treatments (NCI, 2003b; Reuters, 2001).

In addition, delays in treating endometrial cancer — due to access and insufficient treatment — may be the cause of increased incidence and mortality rates (Reuters, 2001; NCI, 2003b). Also, statistics about the incidence of endometrial cancer can be skewed if women who have undergone a hysterectomy are counted or not counted in the incidence rates.

THE UTERUS

The uterus has two separate parts, which have structural and functional differences. The cervix is the entry channel into the main part of the uterus — also called the uterine corpus. The uterus is the hollow, pear-shaped sac, which carries a developing embryo until birth. A slight narrowing between the cervix and corpus uterus separates these two structures called the isthmus. Figure 3-3 shows the endometrial anatomy (Paniscotti, 2000c; Walczak, 2000a).

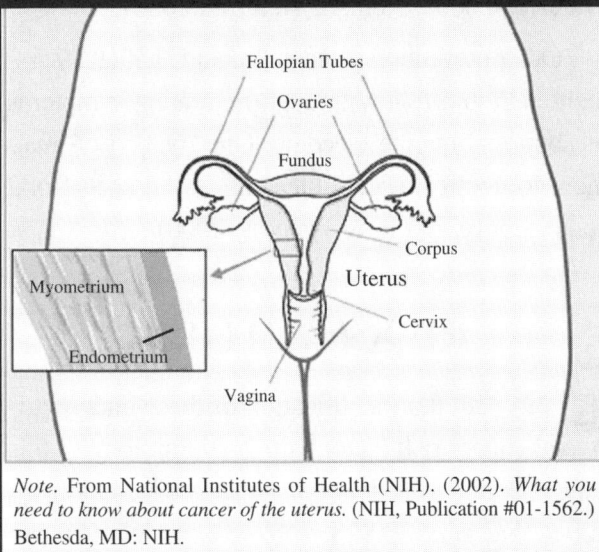

FIGURE 3-3: UTERUS (AND ENDOMETRIAL LAYER)

Note. From National Institutes of Health (NIH). (2002). *What you need to know about cancer of the uterus.* (NIH, Publication #01-1562.) Bethesda, MD: NIH.

The endometrium is the inner epithelial lining of a woman's uterine corpus. The endometrium tissue thickens each month during the menstrual cycle in women of childbearing age, then sloughs off when the woman's hormone levels change.

TUMOR DEVELOPMENT

The most common type of cancer of the uterus begins in the endometrium. (Frequently uterine cancer and endometrial cancer are interchangeable terms.)

Benign tumors that form in the uterus are called fibroids. They grow in the muscle layer (outer layer of the uterus). If a woman is to develop fibroids, that woman is typically in her 40s. As the woman reaches menopause, fibroids are likely to decrease or disappear (NCI, 2003b).

Fibroids typically do not cause symptoms. Yet those that press on adjacent organs may cause bleeding, vaginal discharge, or spur on frequent urination. Sometimes the best treatment for fibroids is to have them removed surgically (NCI, 2003b; Paniscotti, 2000c).

Another benign condition of the uterus is endometriosis. This is when the endometrial tissue grows outside of the uterus. The condition can cause painful menstrual periods, abnormal vaginal bleeding, and infertility. Endometriosis is most common in women in their 30s or 40s, who have never been pregnant. Treatment strategies for endometriosis include surgery or HRT (NCI, 2003b; Paniscotti, 2000e; Walczak, 2000a).

Endometrial hyperplasia is an increase in cells lining the uterus. It is most common in women over age 40. Sometimes hyperplasia develops into malignant cells. Symptoms of hyperplasia include heavy menstrual periods, bleeding between periods, and bleeding after menopause (Dolinsky, 2002; NCI, 2003b; Paniscotti, 2000b).

ENDOMETRIAL CANCER

Symptoms of endometrial cancer are

- Unusual vaginal bleeding or discharge
- Difficult or painful urination
- Pain during intercourse
- Pain in the pelvic area.

The most common endometrial cancer cell type is endometrioid adenocarcinoma, originating from malignant glandular epithelial tissue. Table 3-1 summarizes other endometrial cancer cell types. Endometrial cancers are rarely squamous or undifferentiated cell types.

TABLE 3-1: ENDOMETRIAL CANCER CELL TYPES

I.   Endometrioid (75%-80%)

    A. Ciliated adenocarcinoma

    B. Secretory adenocarcinoma

    C. Papillary or villoglandular

    D. Adenocarcinoma with squamous differentiation

      1. Adenoacanthoma

      2. Adenosquamous

II.   Uterine papillary serous (<10%)

III. Mucinous (1%)

IV.   Clear cell (4%)

V.   Squamous cell (< 1%)

VI.   Mixed (10%)

VII. Undifferentiated

(NCI, 2003b; Paniscotti, 2000b)

For conditions that may become cancer, clinicians may recommend that the woman undergo a hysterectomy (removal of the uterus) or take exogenous hormones that include progesterone (NIH, 2002; Dolinsky, 2002).

Once uterine cancer develops, it can metastasize to nearby lymph nodes, nerves or blood vessels, or to the vagina, lungs, liver, brain, and bones. Patients with deep muscle invasion and high-grade tumors and/or intraperitoneal disease have a significant risk of nodal spread to pelvic nodes (20-60%) and para-aortic nodes (10-30%) (NCI, 2003b; Dolinsky, 2002; Paniscotti, 2000e).

Once a woman is diagnosed and treated for early stage endometrial cancer, hormone receptor status is an important prognostic indicator. A pivotal study has reported that patients with progesterone receptor levels greater than 100 had a 3-year disease-free survival rate of 93% compared with 36% for levels less than 100 (NCI, 2003b; Liu & Jacobs, 2001).

PREVENTION

For years, surgery — specifically hysterectomy — has been the key strategy to prevent endometrial cancer. However, reducing the risk of endometrial cancer is preferable. So prevention efforts have targeted ways to reduce risk factors for endometrial cancer.

Risk factor prevention strategies include weight loss and other risk reductions. (See Risk Factors section in this chapter.) The focus has also been on prescribing HRT (progestins added to estrogens) and helping women to stop smoking. Smoking appears to play a role in many cancers, including endometrial cancer (NCI, 2003a; Paniscotti, 2000b; Walczak, 2000c, Nolte & Walczak, 2000).

Other prevention strategies include a high assessment alert and follow-through in treating symptoms of abnormal uterine bleeding. One method of treatment to control uterine bleeding is the use of oral contraceptives (Nolte & Walczak, 2000).

RISK FACTORS

Even with the identification of these endometrial cancer risk factors, the epidemiology of this cancer is not well defined (NCI, 2003a; Dolinsky, 2002; Walczak, 2000b). Table 3-2 reviews known risk factors associated with endometrial cancer. These should be considered as a group of risk factors — usually no one factor carries a supreme risk. But multiple risk factors combining as cofactors appear to increase risks for women (NCI, 2003b; Dolinsky, 2002; Walczak, 2000b).

Suggested endometrial cancer risk factors include obesity (> 20 pounds overweight), nulliparity, late menopause (after age 52), diabetes, hypertension, infertility, irregular menses, failure of ovulation, a history of breast or ovarian cancer, adenomatous hyperplasia, prolonged use of exogenous estrogen therapy, and tamoxifen use (Walczak, 2000b).

TABLE 3-2: RISK FACTORS FOR ENDOMETRIAL CANCER

- Obesity (> 20 pounds overweight)

- Nulliparity

- Late menopause (after age 52)

- Diabetes

- Hypertension

- Infertility

- Irregular menses

- Failure of ovulation

- A history of breast or ovarian cancer

- Adenomatous hyperplasia

- Prolonged use of exogenous estrogen therapy

- Tamoxifen use

(NCI, 2003a; Paniscotti, 2000a; Walczak, 2000b)

In one study a woman was shown to have an 87% risk of developing endometrial cancer if she is age 70 or older, childless, has diabetes and presents with abnormal vaginal bleeding (Paniscotti, 2000a; Walczak, 2000b). If the woman presents only with abnormal bleeding but not the rest of these risk factors, her risk of developing endometrial cancer plummets to 3% (Panisocotti, 2000a; Walczak, 2000b). In another study a woman who is obese, nulliparous and experiencing a late menopause, has a five-fold increase of developing endometrial cancer (NCI, 2003a).

Obesity, brought on by polycystic ovarian syndrome, physical inactivity, and a diet high in saturated fat, increases the risk of endometrial cancer (NCI, 2003a; Paniscotti, 2000b; Walczak, 2000b). One study estimated that the risk of overweight women developing endometrial cancer was 26-47% (NCI, 2003a).

(NOTE: Diet modification to reduce total body weight may reduce the risk of developing endometrial cancer. Also, physical activity — as a means to reduce weight — can reduce the risk of endometri-

al cancer. The duration and intensity of exercise quantified to risk reduction is not yet known (NCI, 2003a; Paniscotti, 2000c; Walczak, 2000b).

HORMONES

Increased hormone metabolism is a risk factor, but thought to be related to obesity because body size plays a role in the conversion of androgen to estrogen (Bradley, 2001; Walczak, 2000a). Because fat cells provide an excellent harbor to store estrogen, the more obese the woman, the higher the estrogen level and thus the higher the risk of developing endometrial cancer. Fat cells provide a slow, constant means to deliver estrogen to the woman's body. In some obese women, their levels of estradiol or progesterone are high or inappropriate. Presenting symptoms for women with abnormal hormone levels are irregular menses (Bradley, 2001; Paniscotti, 2000d; Walczak, 2000a).

Tamoxifen, a drug that is widely used to treat breast cancer, appears to have estrogen-like effects on the uterus, and may also be associated with increased risk of endometrial cancer. But when menopausal women take estrogen replacement therapy along with progesterone, the risk related to endometrial cancer decreases (NCI, 2003d; Bradley, 2001; Paniscotti, 2000e; Walczak, 2000a).

Also during menopause, the ovaries can continue to secrete testosterone and androstenedione (androgen). Androstenedione is converted to estrone, which is carcinogenic when in large amounts. Women who develop endometrial cancer have been shown to have a greater conversion of androstenedione to estrone.

ENDOMETRIAL CANCER AND COLON CANCER

Women with a family history of endometrial cancer and colorectal cancer (nonpolyposis varieties) have an increased risk of developing endometrial cancer. Women with hereditary non-polyposis colorectal cancer (HNPCC) syndrome have a markedly increased risk of endometrial cancer compared to women in the general population.

Among women who are HNPCC mutation carriers, the estimated cumulative incidence of endometrial cancer ranges from 20-60% (NCI, 2003a; Liu & Jacobs, 2001).

The risk for these women is estimated at 4-11% of women for the time period, which is about 2 decades earlier than would usually be expected. Overall, a family history of endometrial cancer is present in about 5% of all cases and a family history of colorectal cancer in about 2% (NCI, 2003a; Paniscotti, 2000e; Walczak, 2000a). (See Chapter 7, Colorectal Cancer.)

TAMOXIFEN

Tamoxifen is a member of a group of drugs known as a selective estrogen receptor modulator (SERM). Tamoxifen, a treatment for breast cancer (see Chapter 2, Breast Cancer), acts as an anti-estrogen on breast tissue and serves as a weak estrogenic agent on endometrial tissue. Thus, with endometrial tissue, it contributes to the thickening of the endometrium, leading to tissue changes from polyps to hyperplasia and then to cancer cells (Walczak, 2000a).

Recent data from the breast cancer prevention trial (see Chapter 2, Breast Cancer) indicate that women who take tamoxifen have a 2.5% increased risk of developing endometrial cancer. (If a woman has had a hysterectomy and is taking tamoxifen, she is not at increased risk because her endometrium has been removed.) (Reuters, 2002; Walczak, 2000a). Women over age 50 who take tamoxifen are at greatest risk. However, in this trial, it is worth noting that endometrial cancer was detected at Stage I disease (NCI, 2003d; Bradley, 2001).

Despite the evidence linking tamoxifen to an increased endometrial cancer risk, the advantage of tamoxifen in preventing recurrence of breast cancer is significant. Therefore, cancer specialists have concluded that the benefits to breast cancer patients, in suppression of breast cancer recurrence, substantially outweigh the risks (NCI, 2003d; Paniscotti, 2000e; Walczak, 2000a).

Clinical trials are ongoing to determine the appropriate and most effective strategies of surveillance of women on tamoxifen so that they will not get endometrial cancer. Because of this increased risk, clinicians should weigh the advantages and disadvantages, specific to each patient's situation. All patients on tamoxifen should have regular follow-up pelvic examinations and should be examined if there is any abnormal uterine bleeding (NCI, 2003d; Walczak, 2000a).

DETECTION

To detect endometrial cancer, a tissue biopsy is necessary. The Papincoloaou smear is not reliable as a screening procedure for endometrial cancer.

Hyperplasia or the overgrowth of the endometrial lining of the uterus may present as abnormal bleeding. Endometrial hyperplasia can precede endometrial carcinoma. Hyperplasia is categorized as simple (cystic without atypia), complex (adenomatous without atypia), and atypical (simple cystic with atypia or complex adenomatous with atypia).

Histopathologic analysis of the biopsied cells is important to staging and treatment decisions. The degree of tumor differentiation is also important. The pattern of spread is partially dependent on the degree of cellular differentiation. Well-differentiated tumors tend to limit their spread to the surface of the endometrium; myometrial extension is less common (NCI, 2003b; Dolinsky, 2002; Walczak, 2000a).

In patients with poorly differentiated tumors, myometrial invasion is more frequent and is linked to lymph node involvement. Metastatic spread typically is due to the pelvic and para-aortic nodes. Distant metastases is most common to the lungs, inguinal and supraclavicular nodes, liver, bones, brain, and vagina (NCI, 2003b; Walczak, 2000a).

Progesterone receptor levels are important to diagnosis and when deciding treatment options. One report found progesterone receptor levels to be the single most important prognostic indicator of 3-year survival in clinical stage I and II disease. Patients with progesterone receptor levels greater than 100 had a 3-year disease-free survival of 93% compared with 36% for a level less than 100 (NCI, 2003b; Couto, 2001).

Oncogene expression, deoxyribonulceic acid (DNA) ploidy, and the fraction of cells in S-phase have also been found to be prognostic indicators of clinical outcome (NCI, 2003b; Liu & Jacobs, 2001; Walczak, 2000a). These characteristics indicate a more highly malignant cell type.

DIAGNOSIS

Workup of a woman who presents with symptoms of endometrial cancer can include

- blood and urine tests

- pelvic examination (to check the vagina, uterus, bladder, and rectum)

- transvaginal ultrasound (to show if the endometrium looks thicker)

- biopsy (to check for cancer and hyperplasia, a physician removes a tissue sample from the uterine lining. In some cases, the biopsy procedure is a dilation and curettage [D&C]. Endometrial biopsy is 90% effective in detecting cancer cells [NCI, 2003b]). (Postmenopausal women at high risk for endometrial cancer should have regular biopsies.)

The choice of treatment for endometrial cancer depends on the size of the tumor, the stage of the disease, whether female hormones affect tumor growth, and the tumor grade. The grade determines differences between normal and abnormal cells. Grading the tumor can also indicate how quickly the cells are growing. Low-grade cancers typically grow slower than high-grade tumors.

Staging is key to directing treatment decisions. Table 3-3 lists staging schema for endometrial cancer from two accepted sources — the American Joint Committee on Cancer (AJCC) and the International Federation of Gynecology and Obstetrics (FIGO).

TREATMENT

Surgery

Most women with uterine cancer are treated with surgery. Removal of only the uterus is called a hysterectomy. When the uterus, both fallopian tubes, and both ovaries are removed, the procedure is called a bilateral salpingo-oophorectomy (Walczak, 2000a). During surgery, the surgeon removes selected lymph nodes to check for tumor spread.

After a hysterectomy, women usually have some pain and feel extremely tired, but most return to their normal activities within 4-8 weeks after surgery. Postoperative adverse effects can include GI disturbance, and bladder and bowel problems. These symptoms will pass in time (Paniscotti, 2000e; Walczak, 2000a).

Appendix III reviews nursing diagnoses for gynecological surgery and suggests interventions in care.

Treatment-caused Menopause

A woman who has had a hysterectomy does not have menstrual cycles and, obviously, cannot conceive. Removal of the ovaries causes menopause to start immediately.

Symptoms of menopause include hot flashes; surgically-initiated menopause can cause more severe hot flashes. Hormone replacement therapy (HRT) may be prescribed to alleviate the severity of the symptoms (See Sidebar 3-1). However, HRT is a risk factor for endometrial cancer. Therefore, the prescribing of HRT is controversial and not for all women (NCI, 2003b; Bradley, 2001; Paniscotti, 2000e).

For some women, a hysterectomy can affect sexual intimacy because of the perceived loss of their female identity. Clinicians, family members, and friends should offer support for women facing these psychological adjustments (Chapter 8,

---

TABLE 3-3: ENDOMETRIAL STAGING SUMMARY

American Joint Committee on Cancer (AJCC) (2002):

Stage I – The cancer is only in the body of the uterus. It is not in the cervix.
*   Stage IA: tumor limited to endometrium
*   Stage IB: invasion to less than one half of the myometrium
*   Stage IC: invasion to greater than one half of the myometrium

Stage II – The cancer has spread from the body of the uterus to the cervix.
*   Stage IIA: endocervical glandular involvement only
*   Stage IIB: cervical stromal invasion

Stage III – The cancer has spread outside the uterus, but not outside the pelvis (and not to the bladder or rectum). Lymph nodes in the pelvis may contain cancer cells.
*   Stage IIIA: tumor invades serosa and/or adnexa and/or positive peritoneal cytology
*   Stage IIIB: vaginal metastases
*   Stage IIIC: metastases to pelvic and/or para-aortic lymph nodes

Stage IV – The cancer has spread into the bladder or rectum. Or it has spread beyond the pelvis to other body parts.
*   Stage IVA: tumor invasion of bladder and/or bowel mucosa
*   Stage IVB: distant metastases, including intra-abdominal and/or inguinal lymph nodes

Endometrial cancer can be grouped with regard to the degree of differentiation of the adenocarcinoma, as follows:
*   G1: 5% or less of a nonsquamous or nonmorular solid growth pattern
*   G2: 6% to 50% of a nonsquamous or nonmorular solid growth pattern
*   G3: more than 50% of a nonsquamous or nonmorular solid growth pattern

Federation of Gynecology and Obstetrics (FIGO) (2002)
*   Stage IA G123: tumor limited to endometrium
*   Stage IB G123: invasion to less than one half of the myometrium
*   Stage IC G123: invasion to more than one half of the myometrium
*   Stage IIA G123: endocervical glandular involvement only
*   Stage IIB G123: cervical stromal invasion
*   Stage IIIA G123: tumor invades serosa and/or adnexa, and/or positive peritoneal cytology
*   Stage IIIB G123: vaginal metastases
*   Stage IIIC G123: metastases of pelvic and/or para-aortic lymph nodes
*   Stage IVA G123: tumor invasion of bladder and/or bowel mucosa
*   Stage IVB: distant metastases including intra-abdominal and/or inguinal lymph nodes

(AJCC, 2002; Shepherd, 1989)

Psychosocial Issues, and Chapter 9, Sexuality: Women With Cancer, further identifies issues related to treatment and sexuality.)

Radiation Therapy

Radiation therapy treatment alone is an option when the cancer is localized to cells in a specific area. In earlier stage endometrial cancers, when the cells are considered high-grade, radiation treatment is coupled with surgery. These cancers can be staged at I, II, or III (NIH, 2000; Brown, Lewis & Axiak, 2000). Radiation therapy to the cancerous area can shrink the tumor before or after surgery.

SIDEBAR 3-1: HORMONE REPLACEMENT THERAPY

In postmenopausal women, estrogen levels are reduced — about one tenth of the level in pre-menopausal women (NCI, 2003e). Progesterone is nearly eliminated. The low levels of estrogen after menopause are produced by the adrenal glands and fat cells. Estrogen use, with or without progestin, approximately doubles the estrogen level of a postmenopausal woman. Therefore, even with hormone treatment, estrogen and progesterone levels of a postmenopausal woman are not at the natural levels of a pre-menopausal woman (NCI, 2003e; Liu & Jacobs, 2001).

Symptoms of menopause may include hot flashes, night sweats, sleeplessness, and vaginal dryness. Therefore, women have enthusiastically embraced hormone replacement therapy (HRT) as a means to offset those symptoms.

Postmenopausal HRT either includes estrogen alone or in combination with progestin (to offset the decrease in natural hormones after menopause). Estrogen is a natural hormone manufactured primarily by the ovaries. It affects the development and maintenance of secondary sex characteristics such as breasts in females and affects many aspects of a woman's physical and emotional health (Paniscotti, 2000e; Walczak, 2000a).

Progestins are preparations that have effects similar to those of the natural hormone progesterone, which is primarily responsible for regulating the reproductive cycle. Among women who use postmenopausal hormones, women who have had their uterus removed use estrogen alone, whereas women with a uterus take a combination of estrogen plus progestin (Paniscotti, 2000e; Walczak, 2000a).

About 8 million women in the United States take estrogen alone and about 6 million women take the combined hormone regimen (NCI, 2003d). One estimate reports that 45% of U.S. women born between 1897 and 1950 used postmenopausal hormones for at least 1 month and 20% used 5 or more years (NCI, 2003d).

Generally, standard postmenopausal hormones for women who have undergone a hysterectomy (surgical removal of uterus) have been given estrogen alone, whereas women who have not undergone this procedure have been given the estrogen-progestin combination (NCI, 2003d; Bradley, 2001).

Since the mid-1970s, estrogen therapy (alone) has been shown to increase the incidence of endometrial cancer. To reduce that risk, women are prescribed a combination estrogen and progesterone, known as HRT. Thus, HRT has been thought to have a protective effect against endometrial cancer, as well as the use of oral contraceptives. One study has estimated that the risk of endometrial cancer decreases by approximately 40% with the use of oral contraceptives. Other studies have reported an equally significant statistical range of risk reduction (NCI, 2003d).

Progesterone should be used a minimum of 12 days per month. Still, hormone replacement therapy should not be used longer than 5 years as a means to reduce the symptoms of menopause. (Bradley, 2001; Paniscotti, 2000e; Walczak, 2000a).

Either exogenous or endogenous estrogen may lead to endometrial hyperplasia (adenomatous hyperplasia). Studies have not been able to clarify if the hyperplasia is triggered by atypical cells or the if it advances on its own (Walczak, 2000a).

This is done in cases when the woman is a poor surgical candidate due to preexisting health problems.

Some patients need both external and internal radiation therapies. Both therapies can be used when the tumor is large and fixed to the pelvic wall and other critical structures. Clinicians use two types of radiation therapy to treat endometrial cancer.

External Radiation

External radiation therapy is delivered in fractionated doses each day over several weeks. The radiation beams emit from machines. No internal radiation sources are put into the woman's body.

Internal Radiation

In internal radiation therapy, tiny tubes containing a radioactive substance are inserted through the vagina and implanted in the endometrium of the woman, where it stays for a few days. The radiation sources can be placed intracavity or interstitial. To protect others from radiation exposure, the patient may be isolated from visitors. Nurses caring for the patient should limit their time with the patient. Once the implant is removed, the woman has no radioactivity in her body (NIH, 2002).

Adverse effects may occur, depending on the treatment target and dose. Those adverse effects can include dry, reddened skin and hair loss in the treated area, loss of appetite, and extreme tiredness. In addition, the woman may feel dryness, itching, tightening, and burning in the vagina. And radiation may cause diarrhea or frequent and uncomfortable urination (NCI, 2003b; NIH, 2002).

Nurses can support patients through these adverse effects with appropriate interventions. (See Appendix III, Nursing Diagnoses: Radiation Therapy.)

Hormone Therapy

Hormones can attach to receptors, causing changes in uterine tissue. To properly prescribe hormone therapy, the woman's estrogen and progesterone receptors are tested via a blood test. If the tissue has receptors, the woman is more likely to respond to hormone therapy (See Sidebar 3-1) (NCI, 2003b; Bradley, 2001; Paniscotti, 2000a).

Hormone therapy is a treatment option when a woman is not a candidate for surgery or radiation therapy. It is also a treatment for metastatic disease.

Women undergoing progesterone treatment may retain fluid, have an increased appetite, and gain weight. In addition, women still menstruating may have changes in their cycle.

Chemotherapy

Effective chemotherapy treatment options for endometrial cancer are limited. No standard protocol for metastatic uterine cancer has emerged, although doxorubicin has been shown to be active alone or in combination with other chemotherapies. Paclitaxel is another chemotherapy that has been included in chemotherapy protocols for endometrial cancer (NCI, 2003b; Couto, 2001).

SUMMARY

Endometrial cancer is a highly curable cancer when detected early. It is the most common of the gynecologic cancers. Atypical pain or uterine bleeding are early symptoms of this cancer. Women especially at increased risk for this cancer usually present with a combination of factors — obesity, nulliparity, and smoking. Because estrogen plays a role in endometrial cancer development, HRT can be a preventive strategy and treatment. Controversies associated with HRT (estrogen alone) focus on its advantages to offset treatment-triggered menopause, while increasing the risks of endometrial cancer. Standard treatment for endometrial cancer remains surgery, although radiation therapy plays a therapeutic role alone or in combination with surgery. Chemotherapy regimens are used as treatment for advanced stage endometrial cancers.

CASE STUDY: ENDOMETRIAL CANCER

CC is a 63-year-old Asian woman who presents to her primary care physician with intermittent vaginal bleeding for 3 months. Occasionally, she said the discharge was yellow and watery. She also reports pain on urination, and has had problems with swelling in her abdomen, so that her skirts and pants are tight.

On pelvic examination, her clinician evaluated the size, shape, and consistency of her uterus. She was scheduled for a D&C to obtain a sufficient endometrial biopsy. CC also underwent a vaginal probe ultrasonography, color flow Doppler, chest x-ray, and blood work (complete blood count [CBC]; metabolic, renal, and liver panel; CA-125 levels.) The pathology report indicated that CC has endometrial adenocarcinoma.

CC's surgeon performed a total abdominal hysterectomy, bilateral salpingo-oophorectomy, and lymph node biopsy, where further staging of her tumor followed. Pathologic and staging results indicated T1c disease (AJCC staging) or Stage 1C (FIGO staging). She discussed further treatment with her surgeon and oncologist and opted to have her care team manage her with close observation rather than add radiation therapy or chemotherapy as treatment now.

After surgery, CC had periods of diarrhea and fatigue. She also experienced estrogen deficiency, manifested by vaginal dryness (dyspareunia). Her postoperative pain was controlled with Vicodin® and a stool softener. Her appetite and energy gradually returned and she was back at work part-time as a 6th grade teacher's aid 4 weeks after surgery.

Following surgery, CC dutifully went to follow-up checks every 2-3 months for the next 2 years. During the 3rd year, follow-up was every 6 months. (Checks included a pelvic examination, chest x-ray, CBC, and metabolic panel. Every 6 months for the first year posttreatment, she had a transvaginal ultrasound.)

Additional Information

CC's medical history is remarkable for the use of unopposed estrogens for 10 years, no pregnancies (nulliparity), and menopause, which began after age 55. The challenge of HRT now, is weighing the risks and benefits of treatment for her hot flashes, irritability, and developing osteoporosis compared with the risk of breast cancer with HRT use. She intends to discuss this issue with her physician so that she can decide what is best for her.

CC's social network is limited. She lives alone with her cats. She has a niece, who lives nearby and looks in on her every 2 weeks. Her social support group is limited to a few neighbors and some teachers at her school. She plans to retire within the next 4 months and live on her fixed income that is supplemented with Social Security checks. She fears that her medical bills will overwhelm her ability to stay healthy in her post-retirement years.

She says she uses Japanese herbs for her well-being and practices Reiki. In addition, CC has decided to boost her immune system with supplements that she has heard about on late-night television info-mercials.

EXAM QUESTIONS

CHAPTER 3

Questions 15-23

15. The risk factors for endometrial cancer include

    a. hypotension, early menopause, infertility.

    b. obesity (> 20 pounds overweight), no children, history of breast or ovarian cancer.

    c. many children, early menopause.

    d. weight loss, early menopause, productive cough.

16. Endometrial cancer affected by estrogen levels

    a. is highly treatable with surgery and hormonal therapies.

    b. is rare.

    c. is determined by computed tomography scan.

    d. first presents with symptoms of nausea and headache.

17. Tamoxifen is a treatment for breast cancer but has also been linked to an increased risk of endometrial cancer. Cancer specialists have concluded that the

    a. benefits of tamoxifen in preventing recurrence of breast cancer outweigh the risks.

    b. risk of taking tamoxifen outweighs the benefit, therefore tamoxifen should be taken off the market.

    c. risk increases in patients who have had a hysterectomy.

    d. risk is the same for all patients with breast cancer.

18. The most frequent endometrial cancer cell type is

    a. endometrioid adenocarcinoma.

    b. uterine papillary serous.

    c. squamous cell.

    d. clear cell.

19. In Stage III endometrial cancer, the tumor has

    a. spread outside the uterus but not to the bladder.

    b. remains confined to the uterus.

    c. invaded the bladder.

    d. spread only to the cervix.

20. Women who take HRT for menopausal symptoms can reduce their risk of endometrial cancer by taking

    a. estrogen alone.

    b. a combination of estrogen and progesterone for period of time (less than 5 years).

    c. progesterone 1 day per month.

    d. a combination of estrogen and progesterone intermittently over a period of a year.

21. A typical test included in the diagnostic workup for endometrial cancer is the

    a. transvaginal ultrasound.

    b. colonoscopy.

    c. bone scan.

    d. CA-125 blood test.

22. Radiation therapy for endometrial cancer

    a. can shrink the tumor only if it is administered before surgery.

    b. is the lone modality of therapy.

    c. can only be delivered with external beam radiation.

    d. is preferred over chemotherapy because radiation is more effective.

23. A women recovering from a hysterectomy may typically experience

    a. GI disturbance, pain, fatigue.

    b. neutropenia, alopecia, and fatigue.

    c. tachycardia, anemia, and insomnia.

    d. hot flashes, pain, and rashes.

REFERENCES

American Cancer Society. (2003). *Cancer Facts and Figures 2003*. Atlanta: Author.

American Joint Commission on Cancer (AJCC). (2002). Gynecological sites: Corpus uteri. *AJCC Cancer Staging Handbook* (6th ed.), (pp. 299-306). New York: Springer-Verlag.

Bradley, C.S. (2001). *Estrogen replacement therapy after treatment for endometrial cancer*. University of Pennsylvania Cancer Center. Retrieved March 1, 2003, from Oncolink http://www.oncolink.com/types/article.cfm?c=6&s=18&ss=140&id=6031

Brown, D., Lewis, L.C., & Axiak, A. (2000). Use of radiation in gynecologic and breast malignancies. In G.J. Moore-Higgs (Ed.), *Women and Cancer* (2nd ed.), (pp. 436-438). Sudbury, MA: Jones & Bartlett Publishers.

Couto, S. (2001). *Uterine Cancer: Traditional methods and new directions for treating endometrial cancer*. CancerSource. Retrieved March 1, 2003, from http://wwwcancersourcemd.com

Dolinsky, C. (2002). *Endometrial Cancer: The Basics*. Retrieved March 1, 2003, from http://www.oncolink.com/types/article.cfm?c=6&s=18&ss=137&id=8227

Eriksson, J.H., & Frazier, S., (2000). Epithelial cancers of the ovary and fallopian tube. In G.J. Moore-Higgs (Ed.), *Women and Cancer* (2nd ed.), (pp. 186-232). Sudbury, MA: Jones & Bartlett Publishers.

Jemal, A., Murray, T., Samuels, A., Ghafoor, A., Ward, E., & Thun, M.J. (2003). Cancer Statistics, 2003. *CA Cancer Journal for Clinicians, 53*(1):5-26.

Liu, P., & Jacobs, A.J. (2001). *Endometrial Cancer and Inheritance*. Retrieved March 1, 2003, from http://www.oncolink.com/types/article.cfm?c=6&s=18&ss=138&id=6032

National Cancer Institute (NCI). (2003a). *Endometrial Cancer: Prevention*. CancerNet (PDQ®) Web sites for health professionals. Retrieved March 1, 2003, from http://www.nci.nih.gov/cancerinfo/pdq/prevention/endometrial/health/professional

National Cancer Institute (NCI). (2003b). *Endometrial Cancer: Treatment*. CancerNet (PDQ®) Web sites for health professionals. Retrieved March 1, 2003, from http://www.nci.nih.gov/cancerinfo/pdq/treatment/endometrial/health/professional

National Cancer Institute (NCI). (2003c). *Endometrium: U.S. Racial/Ethnic Cancer Patterns*. Retrieved March 1, 2003, from http://www.nci.nih.gov/statistics/cancertype/endometrium-racial-ethnic

National Cancer Institute (NCI). (2003d). *Questions and Answers: Use of Hormones After Menopause*. Retrieved March 1, 2003, from http://www.nci.nih.gov/newscenter/estrogenplus

National Cancer Institute (NCI). (2003e). *Questions and Answers: The Study of Tamoxifen and Raloxifene (STAR)*. Retrieved March 1, 2003, from http://cis.nci.nih.gov/fact/4_19.htm

National Institutes of Health (NIH). (2002). *What You Need to Know about Cancer of the Uterus*. (NIH, Publication #01-1562.) Bethesda, MD: NIH.

NANDA. (2001). *Nursing Diagnoses: Definitions and Classification, 2001-2003.* Philadelphia: North American Nursing Diagnosis Association.

Nolte, S., & Walczak, J. (2000). Screening and prevention of gynecologic malignancies. In G.J. Moore-Higgs (Ed.), *Women and Cancer* (2nd ed.) (p. 36). Sudbury, MA: Jones & Bartlett Publishers.

Paniscotti, B. (2000a). Cancer of the endometrium. In G.J. Moore-Higgs (Ed.), *Women and Cancer* (2nd ed.) (pp. 162-184). Sudbury, MA: Jones & Bartlett Publishers.

Paniscotti, B. (2000b). Nursing management for cancer of the endometrium. In *Women and Cancer: A Gynecologic Oncology Nursing Perspective.* Retrieved March 1, 2003, from CancerSource, http://www.cancersourcemd.com

Paniscotti, B. (2000c). Uterine cancer: Cancer of the endometrium pathophysiology. In *Women and Cancer: A Gynecologic Oncology Nursing Perspective.* Retrieved March 1, 2003, from CancerSource, http://www.cancersourcemd.com

Paniscotti, B. (2000d). Uterine cancer: Diagnosis of cancer of the endometrium. In Women and *Cancer: A Gynecologic Oncology Nursing Perspective.* Retrieved March 1, 2003, from CancerSource, http://www.cancersourcemd.com

Paniscotti, B. (2000e). Uterine cancer: Treatment of cancer of the endometrium. In Women and *Cancer: A Gynecologic Oncology Nursing Perspective.* Retrieved March 1, 2003, from CancerSource, http://www.cancersourcemd.com

Reuters Health Information. (2001) *Rate of endometrial cancer deaths climbs sharply* (published 09/21/2001). Retrieved March 1, 2003, from http:/www.reuters.com

Shepherd, J. (1989). Revised FIGO staging for gynaecological cancer. *Br J Obstet Gynaecol 96*(8):889-92.

Walczak, J.R. (2000a). Endometrial cancer. In C.H. Yarbro, M.H. Frogge, M. Goodman, & S.L. Groenwald (Eds.), *Cancer Nursing: Principles and Practice* (5th ed.), (pp. 1168-1178). Boston: Jones & Bartlett Publishers.

Walczak, J. (2000b). Endometrial cancer risk factors. In *Women and Cancer: A Gynecologic Oncology Nursing Perspective.* Retrieved March 1, 2003, from CancerSource, http://www.cancersourcemd.com

Walczak, J. (2000c). Endometrial cancer screening methods. In *Women and Cancer: A Gynecologic Oncology Nursing Perspective.* Retrieved March 1, 2003, from CancerSource, http://www.cancersourcemd.com

CHAPTER 4

OVARIAN CANCER

CHAPTER OBJECTIVE

After completing this chapter, the reader will be able to discuss the epidemiology, risk factors, prevention and detection strategies, common staging schemas, and treatments for ovarian cancer.

LEARNING OBJECTIVES

After studying this chapter, the reader will be able to

1. identify trends in cure rates for ovarian cancer.

2. describe the purpose of the ovaries.

3. recognize ovarian cancer risk factors.

4. identify signs and symptoms for ovarian cancer.

5. list detection strategies used in the workup for ovarian cancer.

6. describe tests that are ordered when diagnosing ovarian cancer.

7. identify concepts related to autosomal dominant predisposition, when related to ovarian cancer inheritance.

8. cite treatment options for advanced stage ovarian cancer.

9. recognize chemotherapy agents used to treat ovarian cancer.

INTRODUCTION

Ovarian cancer is one of the deadliest gynecological cancers. Unfortunately, when women present with ovarian cancer it has progressed to a more advanced stage of malignancy. The focus of this chapter is on the known risks for ovarian cancer and standard treatments. Because of the high morbidity of an ovarian cancer diagnosis, the initial workup and continuing follow-up after treatment stages are key elements to providing care.

EPIDEMIOLOGY

Ovarian cancer is the 4th leading cause of cancer death in women (ACS, 2003). It is the most deadly of the gynecological cancers, killing more women than cervical and endometrial cancers combined (NCI, 2003c). In the United States in 2003, at least 14,300 deaths were due to ovarian cancer (ACS, 2003). (See Figure 4-1.) Morbidity is high because approximately 70% of the women who are diagnosed with ovarian carcinoma will present as Stage III or IV disease (ACS, 2003).

In 2003, new ovarian cancer cases were estimated at 25,400. (See Figure 4-2.) The incidence rate for ovarian cancer is about 4% of all diagnosed women's cancers (ACS, 2003). Ovarian cancer is the 5th leading incidence of cancer in women (NCI, 2003c). Yet the rate of incidence has slightly

FIGURE 4-1: ESTIMATED CANCER DEATHS

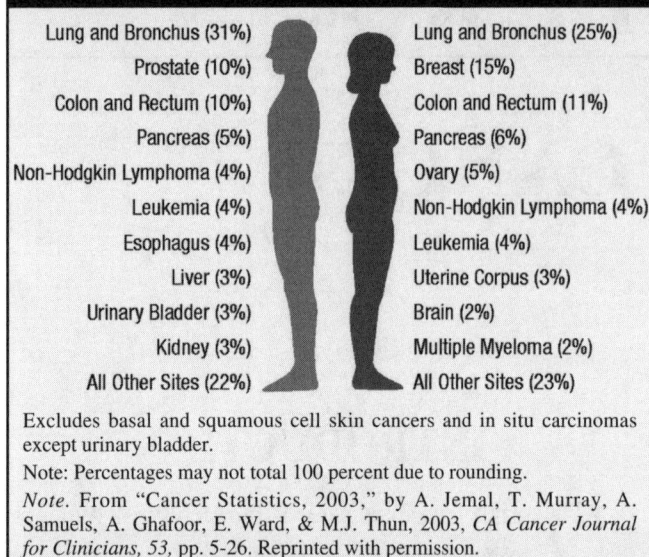

Lung and Bronchus (31%)	Lung and Bronchus (25%)
Prostate (10%)	Breast (15%)
Colon and Rectum (10%)	Colon and Rectum (11%)
Pancreas (5%)	Pancreas (6%)
Non-Hodgkin Lymphoma (4%)	Ovary (5%)
Leukemia (4%)	Non-Hodgkin Lymphoma (4%)
Esophagus (4%)	Leukemia (4%)
Liver (3%)	Uterine Corpus (3%)
Urinary Bladder (3%)	Brain (2%)
Kidney (3%)	Multiple Myeloma (2%)
All Other Sites (22%)	All Other Sites (23%)

Excludes basal and squamous cell skin cancers and in situ carcinomas except urinary bladder.

Note: Percentages may not total 100 percent due to rounding.

Note. From "Cancer Statistics, 2003," by A. Jemal, T. Murray, A. Samuels, A. Ghafoor, E. Ward, & M.J. Thun, 2003, *CA Cancer Journal for Clinicians, 53,* pp. 5-26. Reprinted with permission.

FIGURE 4-2: ESTIMATED NEW CANCER CASES

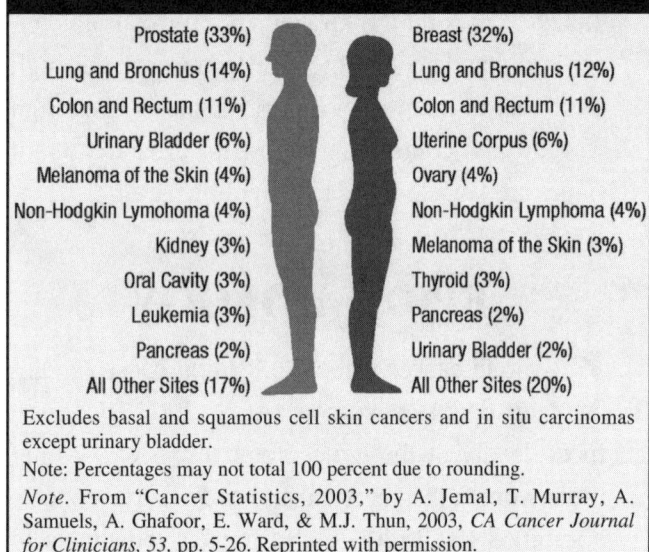

Prostate (33%)	Breast (32%)
Lung and Bronchus (14%)	Lung and Bronchus (12%)
Colon and Rectum (11%)	Colon and Rectum (11%)
Urinary Bladder (6%)	Uterine Corpus (6%)
Melanoma of the Skin (4%)	Ovary (4%)
Non-Hodgkin Lymohoma (4%)	Non-Hodgkin Lymphoma (4%)
Kidney (3%)	Melanoma of the Skin (3%)
Oral Cavity (3%)	Thyroid (3%)
Leukemia (3%)	Pancreas (2%)
Pancreas (2%)	Urinary Bladder (2%)
All Other Sites (17%)	All Other Sites (20%)

Excludes basal and squamous cell skin cancers and in situ carcinomas except urinary bladder.

Note: Percentages may not total 100 percent due to rounding.

Note. From "Cancer Statistics, 2003," by A. Jemal, T. Murray, A. Samuels, A. Ghafoor, E. Ward, & M.J. Thun, 2003, *CA Cancer Journal for Clinicians, 53,* pp. 5-26. Reprinted with permission.

declined over the period from 1989-1999 by 0.7% (ACS, 2003).

The latest epidemiological incidence rates for ovarian cancer are highest in developed, industrialized countries, with the exception of Japan. For example in 2002, women born and living in Sweden had an incidence rate of 14.9 cases per 100,000 compared to a low of 2.7 cases per 100,000 women born and living in Japan (ACS, 2003).

In the United States, the highest ovarian cancer incidence rates are among American Indian women, followed by White, Vietnamese, Hispanic,

and Hawaiian women. Rates are lowest among Korean and Chinese women. Over all age groups, White woman have a higher incidence rate of ovarian cancer compared to Blacks, Asians, and Hispanics (NCI, 2003b).

In 2002, incidence rates for ovarian cancer in the United States were 13.3 cases per 100,000 women. Women who migrated to an industrialized country increased their ovarian cancer risk. Offspring of Japanese immigrants to the United States have an increased risk of developing ovarian cancer compared to their mothers living in Japan. This phenomena suggests that dietary and environmental factors play a role in ovarian cancer incidence rates (NCI, 2003b).

For all ethnic classifications, ovarian cancer is a cancer of aging. The highest incidence age-group for ovarian cancer is women in their 70s, with a rate of 57 cases per 100,000 women in the 75-79 age-group, compared to 16 cases per 100,000 women in the 40-44 age-group (NCI, 2003c).

If there are any bright stories in the tale of ovarian cancer, it is in the short-term gains of aggressive therapy once a woman is diagnosed. When women present with ovarian cancer, survival at the 1-year anniversary is now 80%, due to aggressive surgery or chemotherapy administration. Nevertheless, the majority of ovarian cancer patients relapse. Over the past 30 years, advances in treatment for advanced-stage ovarian cancer have not improved long-term survival rates (ACS, 2002; NCI, 2003d; NCI, 2003e).

Relative overall survival of all stages of ovarian cancer at 5 years is 53%. If detected when the disease is localized, women have a 95% survival rate at 5 years or are 3 times more likely to survive than women with distant disease (NCI, 2003d; NCI, 2003e). When ovarian cancer is detected as regional disease, the survival rate at 5 years is 81%; with distant disease at diagnosis being 31% (ACS, 2003). For women under age 65, their survival rate at 5 years is 65.8%. Women over age 65 have a survival rate at 5 years of 33.2% (ACS, 2003). Age-adjusted mortality rate is highest among White women in all age groups, followed by Hawaiian women, and Black women.

OVERVIEW: THE OVARIES

A woman's ovaries have two roles: to produce eggs and to produce the female hormones — estrogen and progesterone — which are integral to reproduction. In addition to being part of the reproduction process, estrogen and progesterone contribute to the female characteristic changes seen in puberty: development of breasts, body shape, and body hair. These hormones also regulate the menstrual cycle.

Each of the two ovaries lies on adjacent sides of the uterus. The uterus is the hollow sac that holds a growing embryo as it becomes a fetus. (See Figure 4-3.) Each ovary is the size of an almond. Every month when a woman menstruates, one of the ovaries releases an egg in a process called ovulation. The egg travels from the ovary to the uterus through the fallopian tube.

FIGURE 4-3: ANATOMY

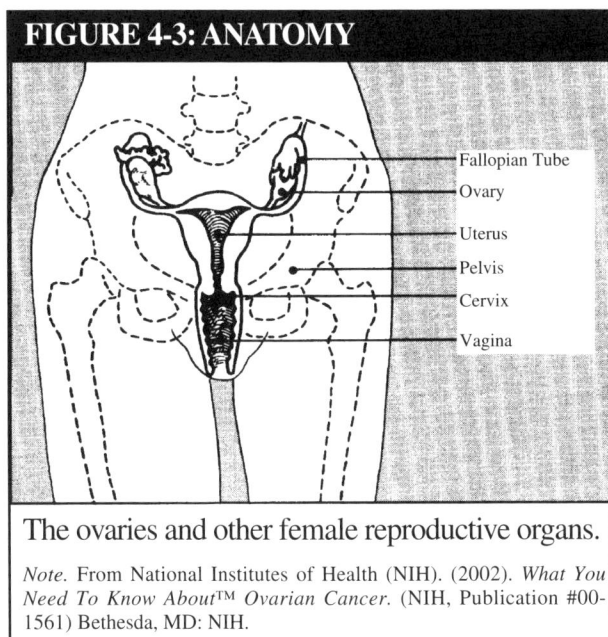

The ovaries and other female reproductive organs.

Note. From National Institutes of Health (NIH). (2002). *What You Need To Know About™ Ovarian Cancer.* (NIH, Publication #00-1561) Bethesda, MD: NIH.

OVARIAN CYSTS

As with other cancer cell processes, ovarian cancer cells can grow, divide, and produce more cells, creating tumors that can be benign or malignant. Benign tumors do not spread to other parts of the body and do not threaten the woman's life (NCI, 2003e).

A variation of benign ovarian growth is the ovarian cyst — a fluid filled sac that can form on the surface of the ovary. Cysts usually occur in younger women. Often ovarian cysts go away on their own. If they do not, a surgeon may remove them.

OVARIAN CANCER

When a tumor becomes malignant, cells in these tumors are abnormal and divide unchecked. Most malignant ovarian cancers begin on the surface cells of the ovaries in the epithelial layer. Epithelial ovarian cancer makes up about 90% of all ovarian cancers that occur in older women (Dolinsky, 2002).

Nonepithelial ovarian cancer can also emerge from the eggs. These are germ cell tumors from the embryonic layers of ectoderm, mesoderm, and endoderm. These tumors also can arise from the supportive tissue around the ovary called stromal tumors, which are activated by the hormones estrogen, androgen, progestin, and corticosteroids. These forms of ovarian cancer typically occur in younger women (< age 30) and even during adolescence. Nonepithelial ovarian tumors are rare — germ cell tumors equal 5% and stromal tumors equal 5% (Dolinsky, 2002).

Ovarian cancer cells can invade and damage nearby tissues or can metastasize to other organs through shedding or traveling through the lymphatic system. When ovarian cancer cells shed, they can form new tumors on the peritoneum (the large membrane that lines the abdomen) and on the diaphragm (the thin muscle that separates the chest from the abdomen). When this occurs, fluid accumulates creating ascites. In this case, the woman's abdomen becomes bloated and distended (NIH, 2002).

SIGNS AND SYMPTOMS

Signs and symptoms of ovarian cancer can be vague. In general, women report symptoms as the ovarian cancer tumor cells grow. These symptoms include

- abdominal swelling or abdominal pain
- vaginal bleeding between periods or after menopause
- bloating, gas, indigestion, or cramps
- pelvic pain
- loss of appetite
- feeling full after a small meal, or feeling full quickly
- changes in bowel or bladder habits
- weight loss or weight gain

(NCI, 2003d).

PREVENTION

Unfortunately, no definitive strategies exist for women to avoid ovarian cancer. General strategies to prevent ovarian cancer match those for other gynecologic malignancies. They include having an annual pelvic examination, reducing dietary fat, increasing dietary intake of vitamin A, and using oral contraceptives for birth control in younger women (Nolte & Walczak, 2000).

What is known — with increasing evidence — is a list of risk factors, which increase a woman's tendency to develop ovarian cancer. These risk factors, listed in Table 4-1, are further described in this chapter.

RISK FACTORS

Age, demographics, reproductive history, and lifestyle are risk factors for ovarian cancer. The risk of developing ovarian cancer increases as a woman gets older. Before age 30, women have a remote risk of developing ovarian cancer — even in hereditary cancer families. Then ovarian cancer incidence rates steadily rise between age 30 and 50, continuing to increase at a slower rate after age 50 (NCI, 2003c; Dolinsky, 2002, Barnes et al., 2002).

Nulliparity increases the risk. Among the general population, parity decreases the risk of ovarian cancer by 45%, compared to the risk of nulliparous women. After a woman has her first pregnancy, subsequent pregnancies appear to decrease ovarian cancer risk by 15% (NCI, 2003c; NIH, 2002).

In addition to pregnancy, lactation and the use of oral contraceptives have been associated with a protective effect against ovarian cancer. Estimates show that the risk of developing ovarian cancer is 40-60% less in women who use oral contraceptives, even if they stopped using them 10-30 years earlier (O'Rourke & Mahon, 2003). In addition, women who undergo a bilateral tubal ligation or hysterectomy have been shown to reduce their risk of developing ovarian cancer.

Unfortunately, the most striking risk factors for ovarian cancer are linked to heredity and/or genetic syndromes that are out of the woman's control. (See Risk Factors: Family Inheritance/Predisposition in this chapter.) A woman with a personal history of breast or colon cancer is at increased risk to develop ovarian cancer 3-4 times that of the general population (O'Rourke & Mahon, 2003).

Studies are investigating whether a diet high in animal fats leads to ovarian cancer. Some evidence suggests such a link (O'Rourke & Mahon, 2003). As with other cancers, researchers suggest that pursuing a diet rich in fruits and vegetables may have a small effect in preventing some cancers. Studies also advance the idea that supplementation with

TABLE 4-1: RISK FACTORS FOR OVARIAN CANCER

Age – incidence rises between age 30 and 50. Highest incidence is in women in their 70s.

Demographic – More prevalent in industrialized countries (Sweden, United States). Japanese women have low incidence rate until they move to an industrialized country, then the incidence rate matches that of the host country.

Reproductive – risk increases if the woman has had no children, started menarche early, or has late menopause. Risk decreases for those who have been pregnant, had breast fed their children, use or have used oral contraceptives.

Surgical History – risk decreases for those who have had bilateral tubal ligation and hysterectomy.

Predictive Models: Likelihood of a BRCA1 or BRCA2 Mutation (see Table 4-2)

(NCI, 2003c, NCI, 2003d)

vitamins A, C, and E may decrease a cancer risk, but no definitive guidelines have emerged.

(NOTE: No evidence has shown that the use of talc leads to the development of ovarian cancer.) (O'Rourke & Mahon, 2003.)

Risk Factors: Family Inheritance/ Predisposition

Studies of different genetic syndromes suggest that certain women are susceptible to a specific cancer syndrome. When a cancer predisposition can be passed from generation to generation, this is called a pattern of autosomal dominant inheritance. (NOTE: To have a cancer predisposition, a person inherits the predisposition from either the father or mother.) (NCI, 2003a; Barnes et al., 2002).

In ovarian cancer, studies have identified the BRCA1 or BRCA2 mutations as being associated with ovarian cancer. (Table 4-2 summarizes the BRCA1 and BRCA2 mutations.) Other syndromes associated with ovarian cancer include li-Fraumeni syndrome (due to p53 mutations) and Cowden syndrome (due to PTEN mutations, basal cell nevus (Gorlin) syndrome, multiple endocrine neoplasia type 1 (MEN1), and hereditary nonpolyposis colon cancer (HNPCC). (See Chapter 7, Colorectal Cancer In Women.) Mutations in each of these genes produce different clinical phenotypes of characteristic malignancies and occasional nonmalignant abnormalities (NCI, 2003a; NIH, 2002).

On average, women with inherited ovarian cancer are usually diagnosed at an earlier age (average age 59) (Ericksson & Frazier, 2000).

These factors are key to autosomal dominant predisposition, when related to cancer inheritance for ovarian cancer

- When a parent carries an autosomal dominant genetic predisposition, each child has a 50% chance of inheriting the predisposition.

TABLE 4-2: BRCA1 AND BRCA2 MUTATIONS IN OVARIAN CANCERS

Personal characteristics associated with an increased likelihood of a *BRCA1* or *BRCA2* mutation include:
- Breast cancer diagnosed at an early age
- Bilateral breast cancer
- A history of both breast and ovarian cancer
- The presence of breast cancer in one or more male family members.

Family history characteristics associated with an increased likelihood of carrying *BRCA1* or *BRCA2* mutation include:
- Multiple cases of breast cancer in the family
- Both breast and ovarian cancer in the family
- One or more family members with two primary cancers
- Ashkenazi Jewish background.

(NCI, 2003a)

- An autosomal dominant predisposition typically occurs at an earlier age than sporadically for those at risk for cancer.

- Most known mutations that increase breast cancer risk also appear to increase the ovarian cancer risk and may also increase the risk of other cancers for males and females.

- Two or more primary cancers may occur in a single individual. These could be multiple primary cancers of the same type (such as bilateral breast cancer) or primary cancer of different types (such as breast and ovarian cancer).

- No data exists on the impact of lactation or hormone replacement therapy on women who have an inherited risk of getting ovarian cancer.

- For a woman with BRCA1 or BRCA2 mutations, selected data demonstrates that ovarian cancer risk declines if the woman has had a tubal ligation.

- Data is inconclusive about the impact of oral contraceptive use in women who have a BRCA1 high-risk mutation or at inherited risk for getting ovarian cancer.

- For women at inherited risk of ovarian cancer, data suggests that prophylactic oophorectomy may decrease their ovarian cancer risk. Even after oophorectomy however, the peritoneum appears to remain at risk for the development of a müllerian-type adenocarcinoma. Postoophorectomy, fallopian tube cancers may also develop

(NCI, 2003a).

Studies have shown that the single greatest risk factor of ovarian cancer is a family history — especially a first-degree relative with the disease (mother, daughter, or sister) (NCI, 2003a). For a woman with a first-degree relative with ovarian cancer, the calculated risk translates to approximately a 5% lifetime probability of a woman developing ovarian cancer. For a woman with a second-degree relative (grandmother, aunt), the risk is 7.2% (NCI, 2003a; NIH, 2002).

The lifetime risk for developing ovarian cancer in patients harboring germ-line mutations in BRCA1 substantially increases over the general population (NCI, 2003a; NIH, 2002). Data suggests that the majority of women with a BRCA1 mutation probably have family members with a history of ovarian and/or breast cancer. Worth noting is that in these studies reporting data, the women may have been more vigilant and inclined to participate in cancer screening programs that led to earlier detection (NCI, 2003a; NIH, 2002).

For patients at increased risk of developing ovarian cancer — especially due to genetic heritage, prophylactic oophorectomy may be considered after age 35, if childbearing is complete. However, the certain benefit of prophylactic oophorectomy has not yet been established. A small percentage of women may develop a primary peritoneal carcinoma, similar in appearance to ovarian cancer, after prophylactic oophorectomy (NIH, 2002; Barnes et al., 2002).

Of special significance for increased risk are Ashkenazi Jews of Eastern European ancestry. These women have been found to carry the BRCA1 and BRCA2 mutations at a higher rate than the general population, thereby increasing their risk of developing ovarian cancer. (The risk is estimated to be that 1 in 40 Ashkenazi Jews carry the mutations and thus are at increased risk.) (O'Rourke & Mahon, 2003).

SCREENING

To date, no effective approaches to ovarian cancer screening have emerged.

For women of average risk (age and demographics), they should seek a yearly bimanual rectovaginal exam (pelvic examination). For women with hereditary cancer syndrome, further tests should accompany a thorough annual pelvic examination. Table 4-3 reviews such tests.

The most common reason for a physician to suspect ovarian cancer is if he or she feels a mass during a pelvic examination. When a pelvic mass is found in either a postmenopausal woman, or a young girl or teenager that hasn't yet begun menstruating, then the female patient needs to undergo a surgical laparotomy to make the final diagnosis. Chances are extremely high that a pelvic mass in a young girl or teenager that hasn't begun menstruating is cancerous (usually a germ cell ovarian cancer). However, only 5% of masses felt on pelvic examination in menstruating women are malignancies. Certain characteristics of the mass — solid, irregular, or fixed — make it more or less likely to be a cancer (NIH, 2002; Dolinsky, 2002).

If the mass is small, has holes (is cystic), is in only one ovary, is freely movable, and has regular contours, then it is unlikely to be a cancer. Follow-up of these masses is by clinical exam. In most cases these masses are ovarian cysts and will disappear on their own. However, if these masses persist or enlarge, further surgical exploration is warranted. And if a mass persists with the woman showing signs of fluid collecting in the abdomen, laporotomy follows.

CA-125 Testing

The CA-125 glycoprotein is shed from damaged ovary cells, and is often elevated in ovarian cancer. Unfortunately, an elevated CA-125 is found in other diseases besides ovarian cancer, since it can also shed from the surface of the fallopian tubes, cervix, the endometrium, peritoneum, pleura, pericardium and bronchus. CA-125 is > 35 U/ml in 80% of patients with advanced stage epithelial ovarian cancer. In early stage cancer, CA-125 level detects the cancer only 50% of the time (O'Rourke & Mahon, 2003).

Yet, completely healthy women can have elevated CA-125 levels. The elevations can be due to pregnancy, pelvic inflammatory disease, endometriosis, and fibroids. Moreover, CA-125 levels can fluctuate over the woman's menstrual cycle. Therefore, elevated levels of CA-125 may be checked at least every 6 months. If the CA-125 trend drastically rises over time, the woman can be at risk for ovarian cancer.

Trending upward CA-125 levels should prompt further workup, which can include surgery (NCI, 2003d; NIH, 2002).

Other Markers

The molecular marker p53, a tumor suppressor gene found to mutate in about 50% of human malignancies, has also been studied as a prognostic factor for ovarian cancer (Davison, 2001). One estimate has the p53 gene to be mutated or lost in 75% of ovarian cancers (Eriksson & Frazier, 2000). The mutated p53 allows uncontrolled growth of damaged cells and does not stop cell death. Therefore, an increase in mutant p53 staining has correlated with advanced stages of ovarian cancer and a decreased length of survival (Davison, 2001). Clinical use of p53 is not yet prevalent.

Another area of investigation of markers is the overexpression of human epidermal growth factor receptor-2/neu. The HER-2/neu gene (erb-2) is found on chromosome 17q. Studies have shown that advanced ovarian cancers have shown to over express HER-2/neu. These studies are similar in findings to those done in aggressive breast cancers. (See Breast Cancer, Chapter 2.)

Screening — Optimal Combination of Tests

Women who carry genetic markers that increase their tendency to develop ovarian cancer should follow an aggressive schedule for screening and follow-up. Screening can include a thorough pelvic examination with further evaluation through ultrasound. Pelvic examinations have limitations, because developing ovarian masses may be too deep to palpate. Therefore, repeat pelvic exams —

every 1-2 months for suspicious masses — are recommended.

Some women who face increased risk of developing ovarian cancer may consider a prophylactic oophorectomy, which removes the woman's ovaries before they become diseased. Still this procedure does not eliminate the woman's chances of developing ovarian cancer. Such a decision should be preceded by genetic testing and counseling (Barnes et al., 2002; NCI, 2003d; Martin, 2000).

Standards for routine screening of at risk women remains a dilemma. To establish a more effective and specific means of screening, clinicians have combined the use of CA-125 testing with ultrasound. Large studies continue to examine the most effective approach and threshold for diagnosis. The cost of the widespread use of ultrasonography and CA-125 testing is high. Adding to that, follow-up with subsequent surgical evaluation is expensive, especially with an inexact record of false-positive test results (Barnes et al., 2002, NCI, 2003d). And surgery, ultimately, may have been unnecessary if there was benign disease.

Research continues toward developing effective ovarian cancer screening tools. Ideally a simple blood test or Papanicolaou (Pap) test equivalent for ovarian cancer is needed.

In reference to emerging blood tests or Pap test equivalents, the focus of these studies is on the blood markers lysophosphatidic acid (LPA) (activated platelets during coagulation, which have been shown to elevate in women with ovarian cancer), epidermal growth factor and the erb-1 receptor (thought to be at lower levels in ovarian cancer patients) and osteopontin, a protein that over expresses in ovarian cancer (O'Rourke and Mahon, 2003). No methods have been shown yet to be clinically valuable.

DIAGNOSIS, TREATMENT, AND PROGNOSIS

Because ovarian cancer is typically diagnosed in more advanced stages, treatment includes multiple modalities.

To properly treat ovarian cancer, the tumor needs to be staged based on data gathered during the diagnostic phase. Staging leads to decisions about goals of treatment — cure, control, or palliation. Table 4-3 reviews typical diagnostic tests and work up and Table 4-4 reviews staging criteria for ovarian cancer. With ovarian cancer, diagnostic procedures become treatment strategies since staging of the cancer occurs during surgery — and treatment (excising the tumor) may occur then.

TABLE 4-3: DIAGNOSTIC TESTS AND WORK UP FOR OVARIAN CANCER

- Surgery
- Transvaginal ultrasound
- CA-125 testing
- CT and MRI of the pelvis and localized lymph nodes.
- Bone scan (for bony pain)
- Colonoscopy
- Barium enema
- Chest x-Ray
- Mammogram

(NCI, 2003e)

Based on the cell of origin established through an initial laparotomy, treatment decisions follow. Because ovarian cancer is a complicated and aggressive disease, a team of physicians may be involved in the woman's care — gynecological surgeon, medical oncology, and radiation oncologist.

Several factors lead to a favorable prognosis. Among them are younger age, good performance status, cell type other than mucinous and clear cell, earlier stage, well-differentiated tumor, smaller disease volume prior to any surgical debulking,

TABLE 4-4: STAGING CRITERIA FOR OVARIAN CANCER

Stage I

Stage I ovarian cancer is growth limited to the ovaries.

Stage IA: growth limited to one ovary; no ascites. No tumor on the external surface; capsule intact.

Stage IB: growth limited to both ovaries; no ascites. No tumor on the external surfaces; capsules intact.

Stage IC: tumor either stage IA or IB, but with tumor on the surface of one or both ovaries; or with capsule ruptured; or with ascites present containing malignant cells or with positive peritoneal washings.

Stage II

Stage II ovarian cancer is growth involving one or both ovaries with pelvic extension.

Stage IIA: extension and/or metastases to the uterus and/or tubes

Stage IIB: extension to other pelvic tissues

Stage IIC: tumor either stage IIA or stage IIB, but with tumor on the surface of one or both ovaries; or with capsule(s) ruptured; or with ascites present containing malignant cells or with positive peritoneal washings

Different criteria for allotting cases to stages IC and IIC have an impact on diagnosis. In order to evaluate this impact, it would be of value to know if rupture of the capsule was (1) spontaneous or (2) caused by the surgeon, and if the source of malignant cells detected was (1) peritoneal washings or (2) ascites.

Stage III

Stage III ovarian cancer is tumor involving one or both ovaries with peritoneal implants outside the pelvis and/or positive retroperitoneal or inguinal nodes. Superficial liver metastasis equals stage III. Tumor is limited to the true pelvis but with histologically verified malignant extension to the small bowel or omentum.

Stage IIIA: tumor grossly limited to the true pelvis with negative nodes but with histologically confirmed microscopic seeding of abdominal peritoneal surfaces

Stage IIIB: tumor of one or both ovaries with histologically confirmed implants of abdominal peritoneal surfaces, none exceeding 2 centimeters in diameter; nodes negative

Stage IIIC: abdominal implants greater than 2 centimeters in diameter and/or positive retroperitoneal or inguinal nodes

Stage IV

Stage IV ovarian cancer is growth involving one or both ovaries with distant metastasis. If pleural effusion is present, there must be positive cytologic test results to allot a case to stage IV. Parenchymal liver metastasis equals stage IV. (NCI-Tx)

(Shepherd, 1989; AJCC, 2002).

absence of ascites, and smaller residual tumor following primary cytoreductive surgery.

Surgery

An approach to surgery called debulking attempts to eliminate the ovarian tumor and tumor cells and improve the blood supply to tissue.

Specialty gynecologic surgeons should perform ovarian cancer surgery and procedures. During surgery, samples of the mass and surrounding tissue can be biopsied and analyzed (Dolinsky, 2002).

Ovarian cancer cells usually spread by shedding locally into the peritoneal cavity. Then they attach or penetrate the peritoneum, invading the bowel and bladder. Therefore, surgery includes inspection and biopsies of suspicious lesions of the ovaries, diaphragm, paracolic gutters, mesentery, and bowel, pelvic side walls, and omentum.

The incidence of positive nodes at primary surgery has been reported as high as 24% in patients with stage I disease, 50% in patient with stage II disease, 74% in patients with stage III disease, and 73% in patients with stage IV disease (NCI, 2003e; NIH, 2002). Tumor cells may also block the lymphatic drainage system of the peritoneum. This is why women presenting with advanced symptoms may have developed ascites.

Generally, women with ovarian cancer will have a hysterectomy (removal of the uterus) and bilateral salpingo-oophorectomy (removal of both ovaries and fallopian tubes) as part of their operation because there is always a risk of microscopic disease in both of the ovaries and the uterus. The surgeon may also remove the omentum (the thin tissue covering the stomach and large intestine) and lymph nodes in the abdomen.

The only circumstance in which a woman may not have this entire operation is if she has a very early stage cancer (Stage IA) that on biopsy looks favorable under the microscope (Grade 1). (This is often the case with germ cell ovarian tumors.) Delaying a more aggressive surgery — if the disease is in Stage 1 — is appropriate if the woman is still of child-bearing age and wants to have children. Once her childbearing is complete, a full operation is recommended (NCI, 2003e; NIH, 2002).

After the woman undergoes treatment (surgery and chemotherapy, for example) and achieves a clinical response, a second-look laparotomy may be performed. The merit of second-look surgery is controversial because some believe that this step does not change survival. Still, a second-look surgery clarifies the next steps in treatment if a recurrence is suspected. (Eriksson & Frazier,

2000). A laparoscopy is sometimes used as a second-look procedure, because it uses technologically improved instruments, which are noninvasive, and allows improved technique.

If the cancer recurs, a second debulking procedure — usually a year after the first surgery — is recommended. Surgery has also been used when palliating symptoms in patients with advanced disease.

With more effective methods to monitor disease, such as blood testing, imaging, second-look surgery is not as common. But with some patients — particularly patients with no signs of a recurrence during follow-up imaging and laboratory testing — second-look surgery is still appropriate (NIH, 2002).

Chemotherapy

After surgery, the risk of recurrence is high due to microscopic cancer cells that may remain or the high stage of the malignancy. Therefore, chemotherapy protocols have been developed as a component of treatment. The most common combination chemotherapies that treat epithelial ovarian cancer are based with paclitaxel and either cisplatin or carboplatin.

Other protocols include gemcitabine and doxorubicin, and various combinations or dosages of those drugs (NCI, 2003e; NIH, 2002; Otto, 2001).

The following are issues being studied in clinical trials related to the chemotherapy treatment of ovarian cancer:

- For recurrent ovarian cancer — choice of drug, dose, timing of chemotherapy, and chemotherapy combinations.

- For recurrent ovarian cancer — advantage of intraperitoneal administration.

- For patients refractory to platinum-based regimens — alternate chemotherapies, such as ifosfamide, 5-FU, leucovorin, etoposide, liposomal doxorubicin, and topotecan.

- With advancing disease — advantage of surgical debulking after courses of chemotherapy on quality of life.

- For length of remission and survival after chemotherapy — tumor-infiltrating lymphocyte measurements as a predictor.

At the time of diagnosis, CA-125 has no prognostic significance when measured. For patients with stage III or stage IV disease, CA-125 levels highly correlate with survival when measured one month after the third course of chemotherapy (NCI, 2003e; Martin, 2000). For patients whose elevated CA-125 normalizes with chemotherapy, more than one subsequent elevated CA-125 is highly predictive of active disease, but this does not mandate immediate therapy (NCI, 2003e; NIH, 2000; Martin, 2000).

Hormone Therapy

Hormone therapy is sometimes used as an alternative to second- or third-line chemotherapy, when the patient cannot tolerate further chemotherapy. It is used for short-term control for a period of time with advanced stages of tumor.

Radiation Therapy

Radiation therapy as treatment for ovarian cancer is rare. In some early stage cases, radiation therapy follows surgery to debulk the disease. In advanced cancers, it can help stop bleeding or palliate pain. Radiation is usually avoided so that it does not affect portions of the bowel and pelvis (Dolinsky, 2002).

Radioisotopes (radioactive phosphorus), when used, have been an option to treat Stage I or Stage II disease (Eriksson & Frazier, 2000).

Complications from Ovarian Cancer

Women treated for ovarian cancer may face additional complications, stemming from their treatments (surgery and chemotherapy) or the cancer itself. These complications can include ascites, bowel obstruction, pain, pleural effusion, and malnutrition. Nursing interventions to address these complications are highlighted in Nursing Diagnoses, Appendix III.

Gene Therapy

Gene therapy holds promise in the prevention and treatment of ovarian cancer but no clinical applications are in use yet. It is hoped to provide a means to identify women at high risk of developing ovarian cancer and to provide adjuvant treatment, similar to adjuvant chemotherapy.

SUMMARY

Ovarian cancer remains one of the deadliest gynecological cancers because it typically presents at more advanced stages. Women at risk for ovarian cancer are usually older and can have a personal or family history of cancer. A woman at risk also may be obese and have never been pregnant. Few effective screening methods exist for women at high risk. Vague symptoms that women present to clinicians are worsening pain and bloating. When possible ovarian cancer is the focus, a workup consists of laporatomy with subsequent trending of CA-125 levels. Standard treatments focus on surgery with adjuvant chemotherapy to eliminate micrometastasis. Areas of study include better screening and diagnostic tools and targeted therapies that can boost the effectiveness of multimodality therapy.

CASE STUDY: OVARIAN CANCER

ML is a 55-year-old Caucasian woman, who presents to her primary care physician with mild abdominal bloating for the past 5 months. On examination, her clinician palpated a medium-size mass on her left ovary.

On ultrasound, the mass was measured at approximately 6 cm x 2.5 cm. (A normal ovary measures 2 cm x 3 cm.) A tubular cystic interface appeared to surround the ovary. The cyst borders appeared irregular. The Doppler examination showed large tortuous vessels within the left ovary. The right ovary was of normal size with no irregularities. In addition to the ovarian tissue measurements, the ultrasound report indicated that the area was suspicious for malignancy.

One week after her pelvic examination, ML had an exploratory laparotomy. During the procedure (and with informed consent before she was anesthetized), ML's surgeon performed a total abdominal hysterectomy, bilateral salpingo-oophorectomy, and lymph node biopsy. Pathologic results indicated Stage IIIC epithelial ovarian cancer based on abdominal metastasis and positive lymph nodes.

After surgery, ML had periods of bleeding and bowel obstruction in the small intestine. (She reported progressing symptoms of cramping, colicky abdominal pain, bloating, and gas.) The obstruction was decompressed with an NG tube, bowel rest, and accompanying analgesics and antiemetics. The nurses caring for ML monitored for signs of infection, worsening symptoms, diet, and comfort.

Following her surgery, ML was treated with 3 courses of chemotherapy. The agents — paclitaxel and cisplatin — were given intraperitoneally. Course doses were aggressive and ML required the administration of granulocyte colony stimulating factor (G-CSF) to increase her neutrophil count. Adverse effects from her treatment were diarrhea, insomnia, nausea and vomiting, and sensory-motor deficits.

After her 3rd course of chemotherapy, ML underwent second-look surgery. No evidence of disease was noted. Maintenance therapy began, which included IV doses of paclitaxel and cisplatin. ML had a follow-up appointment every 4 months, which

included lab oratory tests, a chest x-ray, and an abdominal computed tomograhy (CT) scan.

At 16 months after ovarian cancer was diagnosed, repeat studies showed that her ovarian cancer returned and that the cancer had spread to her lungs and liver.

ML opted to forego further treatment and have her care managed by a community hospice. Palliative care included pain management and interventions that optimized her quality of life for the final 4 months.

Additional Information:

ML's medical history is remarkable for breast cancer (stage II, left breast) when she was age 45. Her breast cancer treatments were lumpectomy, followed by radiation therapy and adjuvant chemotherapy. Because she was estrogen receptor positive (ER+), she was also prescribed tamoxifen and took the medication until she was age 50. In the last 2 years, it was determined from genetic testing that ML had the BRCA1 or BRCA2 genetic factors.

Before diagnosis, ML was 20 lb overweight. She had been diagnosed with hypertension. Her father was a diabetic and died at the age of 78.

Before her ovarian cancer was diagnosed, ML dutifully had yearly follow-up physical examinations with her physician with CBE, mammograms, and pelvic examinations. For the past 5 years, her pelvic and breast checks have been unremarkable.

She is divorced, the mother of two daughters, ages 21 and 25, and the grandmother of a 1-year-old grandson. As a new mother, she breast-fed both of her daughters until they were age 6 months. She started menstruation at age 12. Menopause was induced at age 46, when she received her chemotherapy for breast cancer.

She was also a 20/pack year smoker. (ML quit smoking when she was diagnosed with breast cancer.)

From the time she was diagnosed, ML attempted to use complementary and alternative medicines (CAMs) to help her keep a sense of control and help with adverse effects. She got massages every 2 weeks and treated herself occasionally to aromatherapy to help her with her anxiety and nausea.

Throughout her illness and treatment, she was able to journal and practice meditation, which strengthened her spiritually. She was also a member of a cancer support group, which met biweekly at a local community center.

EXAM QUESTIONS

CHAPTER 4
Questions 24-33

24. The majority of ovarian cancer patients

    a. are cured.

    b. relapse.

    c. are younger than age 50.

    d. are treated with surgery only.

25. When ovarian cancer is detected as regional disease, the survival rate at 5 years, survival is about

    a. 50%.

    b. 60%.

    c. 70%.

    d. 80%.

26. The purpose of the ovaries is to produce

    a. eggs and estrogen.

    b. eggs and to produce only progesterone.

    c. only eggs.

    d. eggs, estrogen and progesterone.

27. The following factors increase the risk for ovarian cancer. The woman

    a. is childless, had an early menarche, and is age 55.

    b. had a tubal ligation, had a late menarche, and is age 65.

    c. had a *BRCA1* mutation, is Japanese, and is age 40.

    d. had three children, had a late menarche, and is age 50.

28. Early signs of ovarian cancer are

    a. productive cough.

    b. headache.

    c. pronounced thirst.

    d. generally nonspecific.

29. Among methods to detect ovarian cancer, the physician

    a. evalutes a guiac test.

    b. tests for CA-125 and determines if it is elevated.

    c. orders a bronchoscopy.

    d. evaluates the most recent Pap test.

30. A diagnostic workup of ovarian cancer can include

    a. magnetic resonance imaging, transvaginal ultrasound, and surgery.

    b. bone scan, iron levels, surgery.

    c. brain scan, gastric lavage, and surgery.

    d. oophorectomy, mammography, and sentinel node biopsy.

31. When a woman carries an autosomal dominant predisposition related to ovarian cancer

    a. a parent carries an autosomal dominant genetic predisposition and each child has a 25% chance of inheriting the predisposition.

    b. the cancers typically occur at later age than in sporadic cases.

    c. most known mutations that increase breast cancer risk also appear to increase the risk of ovarian cancer.

    d. only one primary cancer can occur.

32. Advanced stage ovarian cancer is

    a. treated with surgery alone.

    b. typically the stage that women are first diagnosed.

    c. resistant to all chemotherapy regimens.

    d. treated only with radiation.

33. The most common combination chemotherapy agents used to treat epithelial ovarian cancer are

    a. paclitaxel and cisplatin.

    b. carboplatin and 5-FU.

    c. cisplatin and prednisone.

    d. adriamycin® and methotrexate.

REFERENCES

American Cancer Society (ACS). (2003). *Cancer Facts & Figures 2003*. Atlanta: Author.

American Joint Commission on Cancer (AJCC). (2002). Gynecological Sites: Ovary. *AJCC Cancer Staging Handbook* (6th ed.), (pp. 307). New York: Springer-Verlag.

Barnes, M.B., Grizzle, W.E., Grubbs, C.J., & Partridge, E.E. (2002). Paradigms for primary prevention of ovarian carcinoma. *CA Cancer Journal for Clinicians, 52*:216-225.

Davison, D. (2001). Ovarian cancer. In *Predictive and Prognostic Information in the Diagnosis and Treatment of Cancer* (pp. 21-25). Pittsburgh: Oncology Nursing Society.

Dolinsky, C. (2002). Ovarian Cancer: The Basics. Oncolink, University of Pennsylvania Cancer Center. Retrieved February 20, 2003, from http://www.oncolink.com/types/article.cfm?c=6&s=19&ss=766&id=8589

Jemal, A., Murray, T., Samuels, A., Ghafoor, A., Ward, E., & Thun, M.J. (2002). Cancer statistics, 2002. *CA Cancer Journal for Clinicians, 52*(1);23-47.

Martin, V. (2000). Ovarian cancer. In C.H. Yarbro, M.H. Frogge, M. Goodman, & S.L. Groenwald (Eds.), *Cancer Nursing: Principles and Practice* (5th ed.), (pp. 1371-1399). Sudbury, MA: Jones & Bartlett Publishers.

National Cancer Institute (NCI). (2003a). *Genetics of Breast and Ovarian Cancer*. CancerNet (PDQ®) Web sites for health professionals. Retrieved March 1, 2003, from http://www.nci.nih.gov/cancerinfo/pdq/genetics/breast-and-ovarian

National Cancer Institute (NCI). (2003b). *Gynecological Cancers: Ovary: U.S. Racial/Ethnic Cancer Patterns*. Retrieved March 1, 2003, from http://www.cancer.gov/templates/doc.aspx?viewid=658A5E47-80B1-4DEC-9646-1DF6AD45577E

National Cancer Institute (NCI). (2003c). *Ovarian Cancer: Prevention*. CancerNet (PDQ®) web sites for health professionals. Retrieved March 1, 2003, from http://www.nci.nih.gov/cancerinfo/pdq/prevention/ovarian/healthprofessional

National Cancer Institute (NCI). (2003d). *Ovarian Cancer: Screening*. CancerNet (PDQ®) Web sites for health professionals. Retrieved March 1, 2003, from http://www.nci.nih.gov/cancerinfo/pdq/screening/ovarian/healthprofessional/#Section_1

National Cancer Institute (NCI). (2003e). *Ovarian Epithelial Cancer: Treatment*. CancerNet (PDQ®) Web sites for health professionals. Retrieved March 1, 2003, from http://www.nci.nih.gov/cancerinfo/pdq/treatment/ovarianepithelial/healthprofessional

National Institutes of Health (NIH). (2002). *What You Need To Know About™ Ovarian Cancer*. (NIH, Publication #00-1561.) Bethesda, MD: NIH.

Nolte, S., & Walczak, J. (2000). Screening and prevention of gynecologic malignancies. In G. J. Moore-Higgs (Ed.), *Women and Cancer* (2nd ed.), (p. 16). Sudbury, MA: Jones & Bartlett Publishers.

O'Rourke, J., & Mahon, S. (2003). A comprehensive look at the early detection of ovarian cancer. *Clinical Journal of Oncology Nursing, 7*(1): 41-47.

Otto, S. (2001). Gynecologic cancers. In S. Otto (Ed.), *Oncology Nursing* (4th ed.), (pp. 248-284). St. Louis, MO: Mosby, Inc.

Shepherd, J.H. (1989). Revised FIGO staging for gynecological cancer. *British Journal of Obstetrics and Gynecology, Aug. 96*(8): 889-892.

CHAPTER 5

CERVICAL CANCER

CHAPTER OBJECTIVE

After completing this chapter on cervical cancer, the reader will be able to discuss the disease's epidemiology, risk factors, prevention and detection strategies, common staging schemas, and treatments.

LEARNING OBJECTIVES

After studying this chapter, the reader will be able to

1. recognize the main risk factors for cervical cancer.

2. identify human papilloma viruses (HPVs) associated with cervical cancer.

3. identify terms that describe cervical cancer cells as they become abnormal.

4. list classification systems used in the interpretation of Papanicolaou (Pap) tests.

5. describe techniques used to evaluate abnormal cervical cells.

6. identify treatment options for Stage 1 disease.

7. recognize chemotherapy agents used in protocols to treat cervical cancer.

INTRODUCTION

Cervical cancer is one of the malignancies where medicine has made inroads, based on preven-tion and treatment successes. In practice, those successes are because of better and more widely used detection methods. (See Pap Test in this chapter). Experts estimate that because of widespread and consistent use of the Pap test, mortality rates have declined 40% in the last 3+ years.) (ACS, 2003; NCI, 2003a). Early treatment and surveillance of women at risk also has affected cervical cancer statistics.

EPIDEMIOLOGY

In 2003, an estimated 12,200 cases of new cervical cancers and 4,100 cases of cervical cancer deaths occurred in the United States (ACS, 2003). Moreover, mortality rates over time for cervical cancer are 50-80% lower than incidence rates. During the last 50 years in the United States, cervical cancer mortality rates have decreased by 70%. Cervical cancer — once considered a highly deadly disease — has now dropped to 13 on the list of cancers that kill women in the United States (ACS, 2003).

In the United States today, 78% of cervical cancers are diagnosed at an early (in situ) stage. When cervical cancer is at a preinvasive stage, the survival rate for women is nearly 89% at 1 year postdiagnosis and 71% at the 5-year mark (ACS, 2003). Before the 1970s, 75-80% of cervical cancers in the United States were at an advanced stage (invasive) when diagnosed (NCI, 2003a). When the cancer presents regionally, women survive at 5 years at an average rate of 51%; when it presents distantly, 15% (ACS, 2003; NCI 2003c).

Despite these positive statistics in the United States, epidemiological data about rates in other countries has not improved. Worldwide cervical cancer is the most common type of cancer among women, largely because the Pap test is not universally used (ACS, 2003).

Racial differences are apparent, related to cervical cancer incidence and mortality. The incidence rate for cervical cancer in White women is less than that for Black women — 13.6 per 100,000 versus 8.1 per 100,000. The highest (ethnic) incidence rates for cervical cancer are for Vietnamese women — 43 per 100,000; the lowest are for Japanese women — 5.8 per 100,000. For women from native Alaska and for Korean and Hispanic women, the rate is 15 per 100,000 (ACS, 2003; NCI, 2003e).

THE CERVIX, CANCER, AND RISK FACTORS

The cervix is the lower, narrow part of the uterus. (The uterus is the sac, which holds a developing embryo). From this section of the uterus, the cervix is a canal that opens into the vagina, which leads to the outside of the woman's body. Figure 5-1 highlights these areas of the woman's anatomy.

FIGURE 5-1: ANATOMY

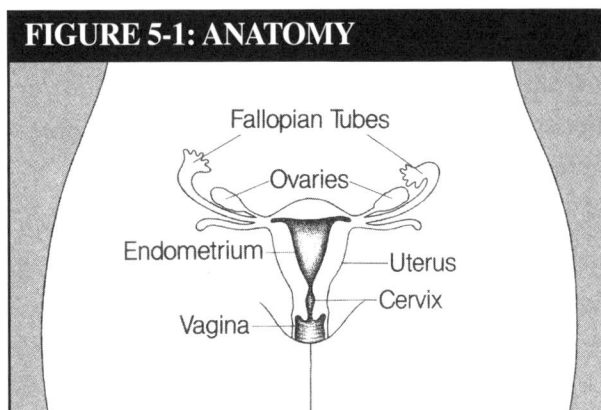

This illustration shows areas of a woman's reproductive system.

Note. From National Institutes of Health (NIH). (2002). *What You Need To Know About™ Cancer of the Cervix.* (NIH, Publication #85-2047.) Bethesda, MD: NIH.

Risk Factors

The exact etiology of cervical cancer is not yet identified. However, studies suggest that cervical cancer is caused by repeated, chronic injury to the cervical cells (NCI, 2003b; Lamb, 2000a). This type of cell injury can occur because of sexual intercourse at an early age, women who have sex with multiple male partners, women who have sex with male partners who themselves have had multiple sex partners, HPV infection, and smoking. Because the risk increases with high risk sexual behavior, unprotected sex can also be considered a risk factor.

In addition, cervical cancer can be more aggressive in younger women (teens to age 40). Therefore when cervical cancer is diagnosed in younger patients, they can have a poorer prognosis. Also, the disease is more prevalent in women of color and in lower socioeconomic groups. Although many reasons for this disparity may exist, among the reasons suggested for the difference are limited access to health care and deficient screening efforts (NCI, 2003f; Klemm, 2000; Walczak, 2000a). Table 5-1 summarizes risk factors for cervical cancer.

TABLE 5-1: RISK FACTORS FOR CERVICAL CANCER

- Sexual activity (at early age, multiple sex partners)
- Sexually transmitted disease
- Human papilloma virus infection
- Smoking
- Low socioeconomic status
- Risk increases with immuncompromise or HIV+

The herpes simplex virus type 2 (HSV-2) is associated with developing cervical cancer. Either the virus causes cervical cancer itself or the virus is associated with multiple sex partners that the woman may have. Another possible identified cause is HPV, which can cause infection and may lead to malignancy. The high-risk types of HPV known to be associated with the development of cervical cancer are types 16, 18, 31, 33, and 35 (NCI, 2003d).

There is a growing body of knowledge about cervical cancer and human immunodeficiency virus (HIV) infection and acquired immunodeficiency syndrome (AIDS). If there is a link, it is most likely the result of both opportunistic malignancies from immunosuppression and infections from the viruses HPV and HSV-2 (NCI, 2003d; Klemm, 2000).

Another risk factor being studied is a variant of the gene for tumor suppressor protein p53, a protein that is integral in keeping tumor cells from growing. Women who carry two copies of that variant have been identified as being at seven times higher risk for developing cervical cancer compared to women who carry only one variant (NCI, 2003f; NIH, 2002).

Another focus of cervical cancer risk or protection is that of exogenous estrogens. To date, replacement estrogen (hormone replacement therapy) has not been shown to increase a woman's risk of developing cervical cancer. In fact, the risk may decrease with use of exogenous estrogen (NCI, 2003b; Dolinsky, 2002; Lamb, 2000a). Because of that, the exact role of estrogen in the development of cervical cancer is unclear.

Human Papillomaviruses (HPVs)

Benign tumors are not cancerous; they do not spread and do not threaten the woman's life. They can usually be removed and, in most cases, they do not come back. Polyps, cysts, and genital warts are types of benign growths of the cervix.

HPV is a term that describes a group of more than 100 types of viruses, which cause the growth of warts or papillomas (benign tumors). One of the risk factors for cervical cancer is HPVs because some benign growths prompted by HPV have been shown to progress to cancerous tumors.

HPVs can cause benign tumors to grow on the hands and feet. The HPVs that cause mouth and genital-area warts and growths are from a different strain of virus — HPV-6 and HPV-11. These warts are identified as condylomata acuminatum. Usually these HPVs are low-risk virus for the development of cervical cancer.

High-risk HPVs increase the chance that mild abnormalities will progress to more severe abnormalities or cervical cancer. (HPVs associated with certain types of cancer of the cervix, anus, vulva, vagina, and penis include types 16, 18, 31, 33, 35, 39, 45, 51, 52, 56, 58, 59, 68, and 69) (NCI, 2003d). Growths that develop from these high-risk HPVs are nearly invisible and appear flat in comparison to other low-risk HPV-caused warts.

Only a small percentage of women with HPV-caused cervical abnormalities will develop cervical cancer. Therefore experts speculate that a combination of high-risk factors — along with high-risk HPV exposure — ultimately can lead to a woman developing cervical cancer (NCI, 2003d; Walczak, 2000a; Klemm, 2000). This theory is based on patterns of cervical cancer with women exposed to specific HPVs.

The puzzle of cervical cancer and HPVs remains unsolved. After sexual exposure to a person with HPV, the recipient's warts may appear several weeks, months, or years later — or never may appear. To make detection of cervical cancer more difficult, typically people with HPV infections are asymptomatic (NCI, 2003d).

BENIGN TUMOR TREATMENTS

Clinicians use several treatment strategies to eliminate benign tumors. These tumors are on the surface of the epithelial tissue, called SILs (squamous intraepithelial lesions). They include

- Low-grade SIL — These cells are early in the process of changing in size, shape, and number on the surface of the cervix.

• High-grade SIL — These cells are a large number of precancerous cells

(NCI, 2003c; NIH, 2002; Klemm, 2000).

Treatment of SILs and warts includes cryo-surgery (freezing the tissue to destroy the wart), laser treatment (destroying the wart with high-intensity light), LEEP (loop electrosurgical excision procedure — the removal of tissue using a hot wire loop), and standard surgery (NCI, 2003c; Walczak, 2000a). (The Diagnosis and Treatment section in this chapter further describes these procedures.)

Chemical treatments for SILs include applying podophyllin, bichloroacetic acid, and trichloroacetic acid. Podofilox (podophyllotoxin) can be applied topically either as a liquid or a gel to external genital warts. Imiquimod cream has also been approved to treat external warts. Also, fluorouracil cream (5-FU cream) is a treatment. To boost the immune system response to the warts, interferon alpha may be added to a treatment regimen (NCI, 2003c; Benjamin & Echols, 2002).

Research studies to identify or treat HPVs include the development of vaccines. Studies are also evaluating the role of specific proteins produced by HPV (E5, E6, E7), which provide cell growth regulation in relation to human protein p53. Strategies target ways to interrupt the process triggered by HPV infection that leads to abnormal cell development and/or cancer (NCI, 2003c; NIH, 2002).

The NCI-sponsored trial called the ASCUS/LSIL Triage Study (ALTS). (The letters ASCUS/LSIL stand for atypical squamous cells of undetermined significance, and low-grade squamous intraepithelial lesion.) Results from the study, which began in 1996 and were published in 2001, suggest that positive HPV results in women with atypical squamous cells of undetermined significance flags them for treatment of early cervical cell abnormalities (NCI, 2003c; NCI, 2003f).

SIGNS AND SYMPTOMS

Table 5-2 reviews the signs and symptoms of cervical cancer. Although women may not report any symptoms before they are diagnosed, typically women first report pain or abnormal bleeding. Clinicians hearing about these symptoms from their patients should look further for their cause and be suspicious for cervical disease.

TABLE 5-2: SIGNS AND SYMPTOMS OF CERVICAL CANCER
• Early stage cervical cancer can be asymptomatic.
• Later stages may include these signs and symptoms
– Abnormal bleeding (including bleeding after sexual intercourse, in between periods, heavier/longer lasting menstrual bleeding, or bleeding after menopause)
– Abnormal vaginal discharge (may be foul smelling)
– Pelvic or back pain
– Pain on urination
– Blood in the stool or urine
Note. From Dolinsky, C. (2002). *Cervical Cancer: The Basics.* University of Pennsylvania Cancer Center. Retrieved March 1, 2002, from http://www.oncolink.com/types/article.cfm?c=6&s=17&ss=129&id=8226

PREINVASIVE CERVICAL CONDITIONS

The process of benign cervical cells changing to cancerous cells can be subtle, as reviewed earlier. Cells on the surface of the cervix sometimes appear abnormal but are not cancerous. The abnormality is believed to be the first step in the development of cells slowly becoming cancerous. Therefore, abnormal cell changes are sometimes called precancerous.

Premalignant changes of epithelial cells are referred to as dysplasia. The term cervical intraepithelial neoplasia (CIN) describes many intraepithelial changes that can occur before cells become invasive cervical cancer cells. Preinvasive disease (intraepithelial neoplasia) does not penetrate the basement membrane (stroma) as does invasive disease.

Four degrees of classification grade the level of CIN. They are

- CIN I (mild dysplasia; involvement of < 1/3 thickness of epithelium)
- CIN II (moderate dysplasia; 1/3-2/3 thickness of epithelium)
- CIN III (severe dysplasia)
- Carcinoma in situ (full thickness involvement of the surface area)

(Solomon, Davey, Kurman, Moriarty, O'Connor, Prey, et al., 2002).

Mild dysplasia and CINI typically occur in younger women — age 25-35. Each year, an estimated 1.2 million women are diagnosed with SIL or CIN changes (NCI, 2003a; Solomon et al., 2002).

When high-grade SILs invade deeper layers of the cervix, becoming severe dysplasia (CIN 2 or 3) or carcinoma in situ, they can become invasive and spread. These lesions are more often identified in women age 30-40. Ultimately when cervical cancer cells spread to other tissues or organs, the condition is invasive cervical cancer. Invasive cervical cancer is most often seen in women older than age 40 (NCI, 2003a; Solomon et al., 2002; NIH, 2002).

ASSESSMENT AND WORKUP OF CIN

CIN occurs mainly in young women, peaking when they are in their early 30s. (Spinelli, 2000). Usually these women have been sexually active, starting intercourse within 5 years of being diagnosed with CIN. In addition to early sexual activity, another CIN risk factor are females exposed to diethylstilbestrol (DES), an agent given to pregnant women in the 1940s and 1950s to pre-

vent premature births or abortion. Exposure increases the risk of squamous cell tumor development, although clarity on the level of increased risk is not known (Spinelli, 2000).

To determine early stage dysplasia, a history and clinical assessment includes

- Age at first intercourse
- Number of past and present sexual partners
- Contraceptive history
- History of sexually transmitted diseases
- History of HIV or immunosuppression
- In utero DES exposure
- History of cigarette smoking
- Pap smear history and treatment of abnormalities
- History of cancer therapy (surgery, chemotherapy, radiation)

(Spinelli, 2000).

Treatment strategies for CIN can range from observation to ablative therapies (see Benign Cancer Treatments) such as electrocautery, cryotherapy, laser vaporization, excisional therapies, and hysterectomy.

If properly managed, dysplasias are nearly 100% curable. A small proportion of mild dysplasias (CIN I or low-grade SIL) will regress without treatment. However for now, clinicians do not have methods to distinguish between dysplastic areas that will either remain benign or those that will become malignant (NCI, 2003a; Solomon et al., 2002).

CERVICAL CANCER

Studies show that 30–70% of untreated patients with in situ cervical cancer will develop invasive carcinoma over a period of 10–12 years (NCI, 2003c; NIH, 2002). However, in about 10% of those patients, lesions can progress from in situ to invasive in a period of less than 1 year (NCI, 2002b; Benjamin & Echols, 2002).

Cervical cancer cells are usually squamous cell in origin. As with other malignant tumors, cervical cancer cells can invade and damage tissues and organs near the tumor and can break away from a malignant tumor and move through the lymphatics. Typical areas of spread are to the woman's rectum, bladder, bones of the spine, and lungs (NIH, 2002; Walczak, 2000a; Klemm, 2000).

SCREENING

Recommendations to screen for cervical cancer are listed in Table 5-3. Pelvic examination and the Pap test are the primary screening tools for cervical cancer.

Some level of controversy exists as to what age women can stop the Pap test as a viable screening strategy. Canadian screening guidelines recommend that women age 60 and older no longer need to have a Pap test if their previous tests have been satisfactory with no atypia noted (Nolte & Walczak, 2000). The American Cancer Society has recommended that Pap tests are no longer necessary for women age 65 and older. Now standard screening limits based on age are more often replaced with that judgment deferred to the clinicians taking care of the patient (Nolte & Walczak, 2000).

An additional area of controversy is the screening intervals in older women (such as more frequently than every 6-12 months), based on transit time of CIN to invasive cancer (Nolte & Walczak, 2000).

Other areas of research look at the merit of methods to augment Pap testing — or replace it (based on improved accuracy). Cost, time, and accuracy limit the viability of widespread screening to replace Pap testing, such as colposcopy, cervicography, self-administered cervical cancer screening, and automated cytology (Nolte & Walczak, 2000).

TABLE 5-3: CERVICAL CANCER SCREENING GUIDELINES

- Cervical cancer screening should begin approximately 3 years after a woman begins having sexual intercourse, but no later than age 21.

- Experts recommend waiting approximately 3 years following the initiation of sexual activity because transient HPV infections and cervical cell changes that are not significant are common and it takes years for a significant abnormality or cancer to develop. Cervical cancer is extremely rare in women under age 25.

- Women should have a Papanicolaou (Pap) test at least once every 3 years.

- Women age 65–70 who have had at least three normal Pap tests and no abnormal Pap tests in the last 10 years may decide, upon consultation with their health care provider, to stop cervical cancer screening.

- Women who have had a total hysterectomy (removal of the uterus and cervix) do not need to undergo cervical cancer screening, unless the surgery was done as a treatment for cervical precancer or cancer.

- Women should seek expert medical advice about when they should begin screening, how often they should be screened, and when they can discontinue cervical screenings, especially if they are at a higher than average risk of cervical cancer due to factors such as HIV infection.

(NCI, 2003b; NCI, 2003f)

Nursing Role in Screening

Although cervical cancer is potentially preventable because the time between preinvasive and invasive stages usually is long and screening methods are effective, the rate of cancer deaths due to cervical cancer is high. Therefore, patient education — toward improving primary and secondary prevention — is a key area of nursing influence. Key populations to target for preventive information are adolescents, women testing positive for HIV, and women with multiple sex partners. In addition to information about cervical cancer and safer sex practices, nurses can emphasize the importance to reduce risk factors that are thought to contribute to cervical dysplasia and tumor development. Among those risks are cigarette smoking (Nolte & Walczak, 2000).

Pap Test

The Pap test (also called a Pap smear) collects cells from the cervix during the pelvic examination to be analyzed for abnormal cell changes, thus providing an early means of detecting precancerous conditions. During the pelvic examination, the clinician also checks the woman's uterus, vagina, ovaries, fallopian tubes, bladder, and rectum, and notes any abnormality in their shape or size.

The Pap test was introduced as a cervical cancer screening test in 1943 by Dr. George Papanicolaou. In the United States, about 55 million Pap tests are performed each year with approximately 3.5 million (6%) reported as abnormal and requiring medical followup (NCI, 2003a; Benjamin & Echols, 2002). Annual Pap testing has been estimated to reduce mortality in women from cervical cancer from 4/1,000 to 4/10,000 — a difference of almost 90% (Spinelli, 2000).

Table 5-4 further summarizes terms used to describe cells analyzed from the Pap test.

For women at higher risk for developing cervical cancer, more frequent screening than the timetable included in the guideline is recommended. (For example for women with symptomatic HIV infection or CD4 cell counts <200/mm^3, Pap test screening is recommended every 6 months. After HIV infection is diagnosed, a Pap test is recommended twice during the first year, then annually.) (NCI, 2003f; Benjamin & Echols, 2002).

TABLE 5-4: PAP TEST TERMS, FOLLOW-UP, AND TESTING STRATEGIES

Pap Test Result	Abbreviation	Also Known As	Tests and Treatments May Include
Atypical squamous cells–undetermined signficance	ASC–US		HPV testing repeat Pap test Colposcopy and biopsy Estrogen cream
Atypical squamous cells–cannot exclude HSIL	ASC–H		Colposcopy and biopsy
Atypical glandular cells	AGC		Colposcopy and biopsy and/or endocervical curettage
Endocervical adenocarcinoma in situ	AIS		Colposcopy and biopsy and/or endocervical curettage
Low-grade squamous intraepithelial lesion	LSIL	Mild dysplasia or cervical intraepithelial neoplasia–1 (CIN–1)	Colposcopy and biopsy
High-grade squamous intraepithelial lesion	HSIL	Moderate dysplasia, Severe dysplasia, CIN–2, CIN–3, or Carcinoma in situ (CIS)	Colposcopy and biopsy and/or endocervical curettage, further treatment with LEEP, cryotherapy, laser therapy, conization, or hysterectomy

(NCI, 2003a; Solomon et al., 2002)

The Pap test is one of the most successful strategies developed for screening a specific cancer. Nevertheless, the test continues to have sensitivity issues, which clinicians need to anticipate.

Pap Test Technique

The patient has a responsibility in allowing the clinician to provide an adequate Pap smear. A Pap test appointment should be scheduled preferably in the first half of the menstrual cycle — before ovulation but after completion of menses (10-20 days after the first day of menses). Ideally the Pap test should not be given at menses or if the woman is experiencing any bleeding because the presence of blood interferes with accurate interpretation (NCI, 2003a).

For 2–3 days before the Pap test, women should be instructed to avoid coitus, tampon use, douching, or intravaginal medication use.

An optimal Pap test requires sampling of the entire transformation zone (T-zone) of the cervix, including epithelium from the endocervical canal as well as epithelium from the inner cervix (ectocervix). The sample is taken with a small, narrow brush or saline-moistened cotton-tipped applicator. The brush has been shown to be more effective in obtaining endocervical cells (NCI, 2003a). The clinician is advised to spread the cells uniformly over the slide, then rapidly affix the cells with an aerosol fixative to prevent air-drying artifacts (Benjamin & Echols, 2002; NCI, 2003a; Walczak, 2000a).

Due to poor sampling technique, inadequate analysis, and patient factors, the rate of smear failure for invasive cancer has been reported at 24–50% (Walczak, 2000). Numerous demonstrations of cervical smear failure in the presence of precancerous lesions have also been reported (NCI, 2003a; Walczak, 2000a). Therefore, meticulous technique is the goal to reduce false-negative results. For example, to avoid contamination of the cell sample, the clinician should remove excess cervical mucus with a dry, cotton-tipped applicator and avoid using lubricants (NCI, 2003a).

Interpretation

Scales to interpret Pap tests have evolved in their precision. Currently, the Bethesda System offers the most clarity in reporting cytologic results between the clinician and pathologist. The Bethesda system offers a way to correlate colposcopic, cytologic, and histologic data (Solomon et al., 2002; Spinelli, 2000). Previous systems included the original Papanicolaou classification — using I-V classes — and the CIN (cervical intraepithelial neoplasia) system. Table 5-5 lists features of the various systems.

The Bethesda system includes three main categories: (1) a statement of specimen adequacy, (2) a general categorization of normal or abnormal, and (3) descriptive diagnoses. Epithelial cell abnormalities are divided into low- and high-grade groups. The Bethesda System also provides a means to evaluate hormonal state, infection, reactive and reparative changes, and glandular cell components (Solomon et al., 2002; NCI, 2003a). Table 5-6 summarizes Bethesda System terms.

Interpretation methods and accuracy of results have been shown to improve with these strategies: rescreening 10% of all negative smears, making sure the sample has enough cells for a proper evaluation, regulated workload for cytotechnologists to prevent "fatigue" error (mandatory in California only), competency examination (mandatory in New York State only) and continuing education programs (NCI, 2003a).

One new method — liquid-based thin-layer slide preparation — has been shown to improve the collection technique and subsequent interpretation of Pap smear cells, especially when screening for abnormal cells. Cervical cells are collected with a brush or other collection instrument. The instrument is rinsed in a vial of liquid preservative. The vial is sent to a laboratory, where an automated thin-layer slide device prepares the slide for viewing.

Another method that may improve the accuracy of Pap tests is computer automated readings. This

TABLE 5-5: PAP TEST CLASSIFICATIONS OF ABNORMALITIES

Description	CIN Grading	Bethesda System (1)	Class (outdated)
Normal	Normal	Normal	Class I
Atypia Reactive or Neoplastic	Atypical squamous cells	ASCUS (2)	Class II
HPV	HPV	Low-Grade SIL (3)	Class II
Atypia with HPV	Atypia, "condylomatous atypia" and "koilocytic atypia"	Low-Grade SIL	Class II
Mild Dysplasia	CIN I	Low-Grade SIL	Class III
Moderate Dysplasia	CIN II	High-Grade SIL	Class III
Severe Dysplasia	CIN III	High-Grade SIL	Class III
Carcinoma in situ	CIS	High-Grade SIL	Class IV
Invasive Cancer	Invasive Cancer	Invasive Cancer	Class V

ASCUS: Atypical squamous or glandular cells of undetermined significance should be qualified further, if possible, as to whether a reactive or neoplastic process is favored.

SIL: Squamous intraepithelial lesion.

(Benjamin, 2002; NCI, 2003a; Solomon, 2002; Dolinksy, 2002; Klemm, 2000; Spinelli, 2000)

TABLE 5-6: CATEGORIES OF CELL ABNORMALITIES BASED ON THE BETHESDA SYSTEM

No cell abnormalities – negative for intraepithelial lesion or malignancy.

ASC – atypical squamous cells. Squamous cells are the thin flat cells that form the surface of the cervix. The Bethesda System divides this category into two groups:

ASC–US – atypical squamous cells of undetermined significance. The squamous cells do not appear completely normal, but doctors are uncertain about what the cell changes mean. Sometimes the changes are related to HPV infection. ACS–US are considered mild abnormalities.

ASC–H – atypical squamous cells cannot exclude a high-grade squamous intraepithelial lesion. The cells do not appear normal, but doctors are uncertain about what the cell changes mean. ASC–H may be at higher risk of being precancerous.

AGC – atypical glandular cells. Glandular cells are mucus-producing cells found in the endocervical canal (opening in the center of the cervix) or in the lining of the uterus. The glandular cells do not appear normal, but doctors are uncertain about what the cell changes mean.

AIS – endocervical adenocarcinoma in situ. Precancerous cells are found in the glandular tissue.

LSIL – low-grade squamous intraepithelial lesion. Low-grade means there are early changes in the size and shape of cells. The word lesion refers to an area of abnormal tissue. Intraepithelial refers to the layer of cells that forms the surface of the cervix.

LSILs are considered mild abnormalities caused by HPV infection.

HSIL – high-grade squamous intraepithelial lesion. High-grade means that there are more marked changes in the size and shape of the abnormal (precancerous) cells, meaning that the cells look very different from normal cells. HSILs are more severe abnormalities and have a higher likelihood of progressing to invasive cancer.

(NCI, 2003a; Solomon, 2002)

technology uses a microscope that conveys a cellular image to a computer, which analyzes the image for the presence of abnormal cells.

Inflammation often results in mildly abnormal Pap tests. Table 5-7 reviews some of the causes of inflammation. When cervical inflammation is treated and cleared, the tissue repairs itself. Then in several months, a repeat Pap test often will be normal (Dolinsky, 2002).

TABLE 5-7: CAUSES OF INFLAMED CERVICAL TISSUE (affecting the results of a Pap smear)
• Viruses, especially herpes infections and condyloma cuminata (warts)
• Yeast or monilia infections
• Trichomonas infections
• Pregnancy, miscarriage, or abortion
• Chemicals (for example, medications)
• Hormonal changes
(NCI, 2002d; Dolinksy, 2002; Klemm, 2000)

Diagnosis and Treatment

If the Pap test shows an ambiguous or minor abnormality, the clinician may repeat the test to determine the need for further follow-up. Often cervical cell changes will go away without treatment. Sometimes, clinicians will recommend that women apply estrogen cream since certain cell changes are caused by low hormone levels (NCI, 2003c).

If the Pap test shows a finding of ASC–H, LSIL, or HSIL, the clinician may perform a colposcopy. This procedure involves the use of an instrument similar to a microscope (called a colposcope) to examine the vagina and the cervix. The colposcope does not enter the body. During a colposcopy, the clinician coats the cervix with a dilute vinegar solution that causes abnormal areas to turn white. During the procedure (called the Shiller test), the clinician can biopsy the tissue.

Another procedure to evaluate abnormal cells is endocervical curettage (ECC). This test involves scraping cells from inside the endocervical canal with a small spoon-shaped tool called a curette, then sending the tissue sample for evaluation.

These biopsy procedures may cause some bleeding or other watery discharge, but the area should heal quickly. Women also often experience some pain — similar to menstrual cramping.

If under laboratory analysis the abnormal tissue cells are considered at high risk to becoming invasive cancer, further treatment options are needed. Many of these techniques (or a combination of these) can be done in the physician's office or on an out-patient basis. In addition to providing a way to biopsy abnormal tissues, these techniques can also remove the abnormal tissue areas:

• LEEP (loop electrosurgical excision procedure) — surgery that uses an electrical current transmitted through a thin wire loop, which acts as a knife.

• Cryotherapy or cryosurgery — technique destroys abnormal tissue by freezing it.

• Cauterization — burning the tissue.

• Laser therapy — technique that uses a narrow beam of intense light to destroy or remove abnormal cells.

• Conization — technique that removes a cone-shaped piece of tissue using a knife, a laser, or the LEEP technique. Conization sampling allows a view of the tissue beneath the surface of the cervix. It can also be a treatment to remove precancerous lesions.

• Simple hysterectomy — removal of the uterus and cervix. If abnormal cells are found inside the opening of the cervix, this is a surgical option (Childbearing years are complete.) (NIH, 2002).

• Dilation & curettage (D & C) — this method scrapes cells from the endometrium and the cervix, in an attempt to isolate sampling in the suspicious area (NCI, 2003c; Solomon et al., 2002).

Further treatment decisions are based on staging criteria (Tables 5-8 and 5-9 review the AJCC and FIGO staging systems.) After a woman is diagnosed and treated for invasive cervical cancer, follow-up is recommended for 8-10 years. (NCI, 2003c; AJCC 2002).

SURGERY

For early stage cervical cancer, surgery is the treatment of choice. Surgeries can be simple hysterectomies coupled with lymphadenectomies (removal of lymph nodes in the pelvis). Depending on the amount of disease, tissues may be removed around the uterus, as well as part of the vagina and the fallopian tubes (NCI, 2003c; NIH, 2002).

Sometimes for young women, the ovaries can be salvaged, so that they do not go through menopause at an early age. In some cases, clinicians decide to proceed with radiation therapy or chemotherapy to initially debulk the diseased area before surgery. A pelvic exenteration is reserved for recurrent cervical cancers. (A pelvic exenteration is a drastic surgery, removing the uterus, cervix, fallopian tubes, ovaries, vagina, bladder, rectum, and part of the colon.) (NCI 2003c; NIH, 2002).

Surgery advantages over radiation therapy include shorter treatment time, preserving the function of the ovaries and limited sexual dysfunction. Surgery can also be the more appropriate treatment if the patient had previous radiation therapy, has inflammatory bowel or pelvic disease, or is pregnant (Lamb, 2000a).

The surgical technique — or extent of the excision — depends on the patient's risk of lymph node metastasis or recurrence. Simple hysterectomy is for regional disease or for women who want to preserve their ability to have a child. Radical hysterec-

tomy (removal of the uterus, upper third of the vagina, the uterosacral uterovesical ligaments, and pelvic nodes) is for disease confined to the cervix. In radical hysterectomy, the ovaries are preserved.

Complications of radical hysterectomy can include infection, pulmonary embolism, small-bowel obstruction, and lymphedema of the lower extremities (Lamb, 2000a).

RADIOTHERAPY

Radiation therapy is an extremely effective treatment option for cervical cancer. Surgery and radiation have been studied as equivalent treatments for early stage cervical cancers. Radiation therapy can be a treatment for early-stage disease or for advanced stage disease. It can be targeted at the main malignant area as well as the lymph nodes. The advantage of radiation therapy is that the woman can avoid surgery if she is too ill or at too high of a risk for surgical anesthesia.

External beam radiation therapy and internal sourced radiation therapy are treatments for cervical cancer. External beam radiation therapy protocols have the woman receiving treatments 5 days a week over 6-8 weeks. The treatment takes just a few minutes and it is painless. With all cervical cancers above stage IB, external beam radiation is combined with internal brachytherapy, which boosts the radiation dose to the tumor site. Brachytherapy (also called intracavitary irradiation) can spare normal tissues (NCI, 2003c; NIH, 2002).

The brachytherapy vehicle that delivers the treatment is a hollow, metal tube with two egg-shaped cartridges. The tube is inserted into the vagina. Then a small low dose radiation (LDR) radioactive source is placed in the tube and cartridges. Typically the LDR source remains in the woman for a few days while she is in the hospital.

Another type of brachytherapy, called high dose rate (HDR) brachytherapy, uses more powerful

TABLE 5-8: CERVICAL CANCER STAGING

TNM definitions

(The definitions of the T categories correspond to the several stages accepted by FIGO.)

Primary tumor (T)

TX: Primary tumor cannot be assessed

T0: No evidence of primary tumor

Tis: Carcinoma in situ

T1/I: Cervical carcinoma confined to uterus (extension to corpus should be disregarded)

T1a/IA: Invasive carcinoma diagnosed only by microscopy. All macroscopically visible lesions — even with superficial invasion — are T1b/IB. Stromal invasion with a maximal depth of 5 mm measured from the base of the epithelium and a horizontal spread of 7 mm or less. Vascular space involvement, venous or lymphatic, does not affect classification.

T1a1/Ia1: Measured stromal invasion 3 mm or less in depth and 7 mm or less in horizontal spread

T1a2/IA2: Measured stromal invasion more than 3 mm and not more than 5 mm with a horizontal spread 7 mm or less

T1b/IB: Clinically visible lesion confined to the cervix or microscopic lesion greater than T1a2/IA2

T1b1/IB1: Clinically visible lesion 4 cm or less in greatest dimension

T1b2/IB2: Clinically visible lesion more than 4 cm in greatest dimension

T2/II: Cervical carcinoma invades beyond uterus but not to pelvic wall or to the lower third of the vagina

T2a/IIa: Tumor without parametrial involvement

T2b/IIb: Tumor with parametrial involvement

T3/III: Tumor extends to the pelvic wall and/or involves the lower third of the vagina, and/or causes hydronephrosis or nonfunctioning kidney

T3a/IIIA: Tumor involves lower third of the vagina, no extension to pelvic wall

T3b/IIIB: Tumor extends to pelvic wall and/or causes hydronephrosis or nonfunctioning kidney

T4/IVA: Tumor invades mucosa of the bladder or rectum, and/or extends beyond true pelvis (bullous edema is not sufficient to classify a tumor as T4)

M1/IVB: Distant metastasis

Regional lymph nodes (N)

NX: Regional lymph nodes cannot be assessed

N0: No regional lymph node metastasis

N1: Regional lymph node metastasis

Distant metastasis (M)

MX: Distant metastasis cannot be assessed

M0: No distant metastasis

M1: Distant metastasis

AJCC stage groupings

Stage 0

Stage 0 is carcinoma in situ, intraepithelial carcinoma. There is no stromal invasion.

Tis, N0, M0

Stage IA1

T1a1, N0, M0

Stage IA2

T1a2, N0, M0

Stage IB1

T1b1, N0, M0

Stage IB2

T1b2, N0, M0

Stage IIA

T2a, N0, M0

Stage IIB

T2b, N0, M0

Stage IIIA

T3a, N0, M0

Stage IIIB

T1, N1, M0

T2, N1, M0

T3a, N1, M0

T3b, Any N, M0

Stage IVA

T4, Any N, M0

Stage IVB

Any T, Any N, M1

Note. From American Joint Committee on Cancer's (AJCC) TNM classification, 2002.

TABLE 5-9: STAGING – FIGO (simplified version)

- Stage IA - microscopic cancer confined to the uterus
- Stage IB - cancer visible by the naked eye confined to the uterus
- Stage II - cervical cancer invading beyond the uterus but not to the pelvic wall or lower one-third of the vagina
- Stage III - cervical cancer invading to the pelvic wall and/or lower one-third of the vagina and/or causing a non-functioning kidney
- Stage IVA - cervical cancer that invades the bladder or rectum, or extends beyond the pelvis
- Stage IVB - distant metastases

Note. From Shepherd, J.H. (1989). Revised FIGO staging for gynecological cancer. *British Journal of Obstetrics and Gynecology, Aug.* 96(8): 889-92.

sources that only remain in the woman for a few minutes. Studies are mixed on whether HDR has benefits over LDR (NCI, 2003c).

Acute and delayed radiation complications that require management can include effects on the bowel and bladder (cramping, diarrhea, dysuria, occasional bleeding, fistula formation, perforation, and vaginal stenosis). Complications increase with higher doses of radiation. Treatment for these conditions can include bowel rest, diet changes, and surgical interventions. Appendix III reviews common nursing diagnoses and interventions for patients undergoing radiation therapy.

Strategies when preventing vaginal stenosis focus on healing tissue trauma and optimizing the vaginal tissue's ability to stretch. Vaginal dilator regimens can help.

Radiation can also be a treatment to palliate symptoms and can combine with chemotherapy in treatment protocols.

CHEMOTHERAPY

Chemotherapy can be used as adjuvant treatment in cervical cancer to reduce the risk of recurrence from microscopic tumor cells but its role is limited.

Mostly all patients who are in good medical condition and receiving radiation for stage IIA or higher cervical cancer will be offered chemotherapy in addition to their radiation. Studies have shown that adding chemotherapy to radiation decreases mortality from cervical cancer (NCI, 2003c; NIH, 2002).

The most common chemotherapy regimens include cisplatin, 5-FU, hydroxyurea, ifosfamide, and paclitaxel (Dolinsky, 2002; NCI, 2002b). Tumors are more receptive to chemotherapy if tissue has not been radiated. Because cervical tissue is more sensitive to radiotherapy, radiation therapy usually precedes any chemotherapy-based treatment protocols. Thus inirradiated cervical lesions that present for chemotherapy treatment are rare. (Lamb, 2000a).

Cervical cancer has not been shown to respond to hormone treatment.

RECURRENT CERVICAL CANCER

About one third of patients with invasive cervical cancer will recur. About two thirds of those who recur will present with the disease within 2 years after initial treatment (Lamb, 2000). Recurrent disease typically presents as unexplained weight loss, excessive unilateral leg edema, pelvic, thigh or buttock, pain and vaginal discharge.

Patients with recurrent disease have limited effective options. More surgery may be elected such as pelvic exenteration. Additional radiation therapy may be necessary.

SUMMARY

Cervical cancer morbidity has decreased because of widely used detection methods, specifically the Pap smear. Women at risk are usually younger with risk factors of active or unprotected sexual activity, and exposure to HPV or other viruses. Morbidity and mortality related to cervical cancer can be traced to clinician vigilance in detecting and treating benign cervical tumors and those in early stages of cervical cancer. Once diagnosed, patients are usually treated with excision procedures or surgery. Radiation therapy (external and internal) also plays a role in effective treatment protocols.

CASE STUDY: CERVICAL CANCER

JN is a 37-year-old Vietnamese woman, who has not had regular annual pelvic examinations. At the community clinic, JN reports symptoms of abnormal postcoital bleeding for the past year. She also complains of urinary urgency. Her nurse practitioner performs a pelvic examination and Papanicolaou (Pap) test. On examination, her clinician notes lesions in the perineal area that are suspicious for human papilloma virus (HPV).

Her Pap test was sent to a local laboratory. The Pap results came back noting HPV and dysplasia. On follow-up colposcopy, additional punch biopsies were taken with results showing CIN II (based on Bethesda staging criteria, high-grade SIL).

JN's risk factors include multiple sex partners in her teens and 20s. She is married but she and her husband are now separated. Her husband still returns to have intercourse with her when he is home from his deployments with the Navy.

To treat her CIN, JN returned to the clinic for a cryosurgical procedure to remove the cervical lesions. Postprocedure, she had some abdominal cramping and bleeding, which resolved within 48 hours. She was given Tylenol #3 to help with pain.

She was instructed to return to the clinic for a follow-up pelvic examination in 6 months. A year and a half later, JN presented at the clinic with abnormal vaginal bleeding, dysuria, and hematuria. She has also lost 10 pounds in the last 6 months. Diagnostically, JN had an additional tissue biopsy via curettage. The biopsy indicated that she now had squamous cell cancer of the cervix. Based on clinical data, chest x-ray and a computed tomography (CT) of the colon and rectum, she was staged at IIA (AJCC staging) disease.

JN was scheduled for a total abdominal hysterectomy (TAH). Postoperatively, JN experienced bleeding and pain. She also had surgical drains, which were removed on day 2 postoperatively. She was discharged from the hospital on day 3.

Postoperatively, 5 weeks later, JN underwent additional external beam radiotherapy (4,500 cGy over 5 weeks-5x/week) and intracavitary cesium radiotherapy (2 applications). Postradiation, she complained of pain and dryness in her vagina. She also showed signs of vaginitis. She was given a 10-day course of antibiotics and instructed to use a water-soluble lubrication on her perineum for comfort.

Follow-up after her surgery and radiation treatments was scheduled at 3-month intervals during the 1st year, then every 3-4 months during the 2nd year. JN was somewhat compliant with her follow-up examinations, returning to the clinic every 5-6 months. Two years after surgery, JN continued to be disease free on follow-up exam. (Follow-up exams included chest x-Ray, CBC, liver function tests, and a CT scan.)

Additional Information:

JN says that since her cancer diagnosis, her husband and she have decided to divorce. She has not seen him for the last year. She continues to work as a check-out clerk at the local warehouse store. She has said she used a diaphragm as birth control but now no longer requires birth control since her hysterectomy. She says she has had two sexual partners in the past 6 months.

On return visits to her physician, JN is reluctant to discuss any other aspects about her health (such as mammography, colonoscopy). She also has isolated herself from friends or neighbors. Her sons (ages 4 and 10) although appearing to be clean and fed, act out when they are out with her. She looks distressed and tired.

JN does admit to regularly visiting her local Vietnamese market to get ingredients for her own "health" tea, which she says will keep any future cancer away.

EXAM QUESTIONS

CHAPTER 5
Questions 34-43

34. Mortality rates for cervical cancer have declined 40% in the last 3+ years, due in large part to wider and consistent use of

    a. the Papanicolaou (Pap) test.

    b. clinical staging.

    c. hysterectomies.

    d. hormone replacement therapy.

35. A major risk factor of cervical cancer is

    a. sexual activity (at early age, multiple sex partners).

    b. colon cancer.

    c. estrogen receptor negative (ER–) status.

    d. obesity.

36. Types of human paplilloma viruses (HPV) associated with cervical cancer are

    a. HPV-11.

    b. HVP-6.

    c. HPV-16.

    d. condylomata acuminatum.

37. When cervical cells first become abnormal, they can be called

    a. malignant.

    b. squamous intraepithelial lesions (SIL).

    c. virulent.

    d. concave.

38. Abnormal Pap test results may be reported as

    a. atypical glandular cells.

    b. atypical adipose cells.

    c. atypical epithelial.

    d. atypical mucosa.

39. Carcinoma in situ of the cervix is staged as

    a. T1a.

    b. Tis.

    c. T1b.

    d. T2.

40. The Bethesda System for interpreting a Pap test includes

    a. CIN grading only.

    b. general categorization of normal or abnormal.

    c. categorization by class.

    d. no grading distinctions.

41. A technique or strategy that is thought to improve the interpretation of Pap tests is

    a. immediate refrigeration of slides.

    b. central testing.

    c. liquid-based thin-layer slide preparation.

    d. combing the smear with betadyne.

42. The treatment for a woman with Stage I cervical cancer is typically

    a. surgery.

    b. radiation.

    c. chemotherapy.

    d. ointment.

43. Chemotherapy agents used as a treatment for cervical cancer include

    a. methotrexate and cyclophosphamide.

    b. adriamycin and arabinocide.

    c. cisplatin, 5-FU, hydroxyurea.

    d. BCNU and cisplatin.

REFERENCES

American Cancer Society. (2002). *Cancer Facts and Figures 2002.* Atlanta: Author.

American Joint Commission on Cancer (AJCC). (2002). Cervix Uteri. *AJCC Cancer Staging Handbook* (6th ed.), (pp. 223). New York: Springer-Verlag.

Benjamin, I., & Echols, L. (2002). *The Pap test: Cervical Changes and Health Care.* University of Pennsylvania Cancer Center. Retrieved March 1, 2003, from http://www.oncolink.com/types/article.cfm?c=6&s=17&ss=131&id=6027

Dolinksy, C. (2002). *Cervical Cancer: The Basics.* University of Pennsylvania Cancer Center. Retrieved March 1, 2003, from http://www.oncolink.com/types/article.cfm?c=6&s=17&ss=129&id=8226

Klemm, P. (2000). Cervical cancer. In C.H. Yarbro, M.H. Frogge, M. Goodman & S.L. Groenwald (Eds.), *Cancer Nursing: Principles and Practice* (5th ed.), (pp. 1097-1116). Sudbury, MA: Jones & Bartlett Publishers.

Lamb, M. (2000a). Invasive cancer of the cervix. In G. J. Moore-Higgs (Ed.), *Women and Cancer.* (2nd ed.), (pp. 82-112). Sudbury, MA: Jones & Bartlett Publishers.

Lamb, M. (2000b). Cervical cancer invasive etiology. In *Women and Cancer: A Gynecologic Oncology Nursing Perspective.* CancerSource. Retrieved March 1, 2003, from http://www.cancersourcemd.com

NANDA. (2001). *Nursing Diagnoses: Definitions and Classification, 2001-2003.* Philadelphia: North American Nursing Diagnosis Association.

National Cancer Institute (NCI). (2001). *Digest Page: The ALTS Cervical Cancer Screening Trial.* Retrieved March 1, 2003, from http://www.cancer.gov/clinicaltrials/digestpage/ALTS

National Cancer Institute (NCI). (2003a). *Cancer Facts: The Pap Test: Questions and Answers.* Retrieved March 1, 2003, from http://cis.nci.nih.gov/fact/5_16.htm

National Cancer Institute (NCI). (2003b). *Cervical Cancer: Prevention.* CancerNet (PDQ®) Web sites for health professionals. Retrieved March 1, 2003, from http://www.cancer.gov/cancerinfo/pdq/prevention/cervical/healthprofessional

National Cancer Institute (NCI). (2003c). *Cervical Cancer Treatment.* CancerNet (PDQ®) Web sites for health professionals. Retrieved March 1, 2003, from http://www.cancer.gov/cancerinfo/pdq/treatment/cervical/healthprofessional

National Cancer Institute (NCI). (2003d). *Cancer Facts: Human Papillomaviruses and Cancer.* Retrieved March 1, 2003, from http://cis.nci.nih.gov/fact/3_20.htm

National Cancer Institute (NCI). (2003e). *Gynecological Cancers: Cervix Uteri Cancer: U.S. Racial/Ethnic Cancer Patterns* Retrieved March 1, 2003, from http://www.cancer.gov/statistics/cancertype/cervix-uteri-racial-ethnic

National Cancer Institute (NCI). (2003f). *Task Force Announces New Cervical Cancer Screening Guidelines.* Retrieved March 1, 2003, from http://www.cancer.gov/newscenter/pressreleases/cervicalscreen

National Institutes of Health (NIH). (2002). *What You Need To Know About™ Cancer of the Cervix.* (NIH, Publication #95-2047.) Bethesda, MD: NIH.

Nolte, S., & Walczak, J. (2000). Screening and prevention of gynecologic malignancies. In G.J. Moore-Higgs (Ed.), *Women and Cancer* (2nd ed.), (pp. 16, 18-25). Sudbury, MA: Jones & Bartlett Publishers.

Shepherd, J.H. (1989). Revised FIGO staging for gynecological cancer. *British Journal of Obstetrics and Gynecology, Aug. 96*(8): 889-92.

Solomon, D., Davey, D., Kurman, R., Moriarty, A., O'Connor, D., Prey, M., et al. (2002). The 2001 Bethesda system: Terminology for reporting results of cervical cytology. *Journal of the American Medical Association, 287*(16):2114-2119.

Spinelli, A. (2000). Preinvasive disease of the cervix, vulva and vagina. In G.J. Moore-Higgs (Ed.), *Women and Cancer* (2nd ed.), (pp. 50-81). Sudbury, MA: Jones & Bartlett Publishers.

Walczak, J. (2000a). Cervical cancer risk factors. In *Women and Cancer: A Gynecologic Oncology Nursing Perspective.* CancerSource. Retrieved March 1, 2003, from http://www.cancersource md.com

Walczak, J. (2000b). Cervical screening methods. In *Women and Cancer: A Gynecologic Oncology Nursing Perspective.* CancerSource. Retrieved March 1, 2003, from http://www. cancersourcemed.com

CHAPTER 6

LUNG CANCER IN WOMEN

CHAPTER OBJECTIVE

After completing this chapter, the reader will be able to discuss the epidemiology, risk factors, prevention and detection strategies, and main treatments for lung cancer in women.

LEARNING OBJECTIVES

After studying this chapter, the reader will be able to

1. recognize the main risk factors.

2. identify the main symptoms.

3. describe two strategies to help women quit smoking.

4. describe prognostic indicators used in the diagnosis of lung cancer.

5. cite the main modalities for the treatment of lung cancer.

6. recognize chemotherapy agents used to treat lung cancer.

INTRODUCTION

A review of cancer in women typically focuses on the gender-specific cancers unique to women. Yet, the most prevalent cancer in women is lung cancer, a cancer that continues to scorn prevention efforts and spurn the hope promised by new treatments. Lung cancer accounts for 25% of all cancer deaths in women (CDC, 2002).

Unfortunately, the history of lung cancer has not changed much in the last 20 years. What is renewed are some approaches to treatment — the multidisciplinary approach to care, society's success in showing how deadly tobacco use can be, and promising novel targeted therapies that have modestly extended still too-short survival rates. This chapter provides a brief review of the well-known challenges of lung cancer and the rays of hope associated with early detection and more strategic treatments.

EPIDEMIOLOGY

In 2003, lung cancer in the United States was expected to kill an estimated 157,200 men and women combined, largely due to smoking. Because statistical data gathering began early in the last century, the rates of incidence and mortality for men and women has increased significantly. Rises were first noted in men, and later in women. Figure 6-1 shows the rise over time. Lung cancer now accounts for 14% of new cancer cases and 28% of all cancer deaths each year in the United States (ACS, 2003). Figures 6-2 and 6-3 compare lung cancer incidence and mortality rates with other cancers.

In women, death rates for lung cancer surpassed those for breast cancer starting in 1987. Lung cancer is now the leading cause of cancer

FIGURE 6-1: GROWTH IN LUNG CANCER

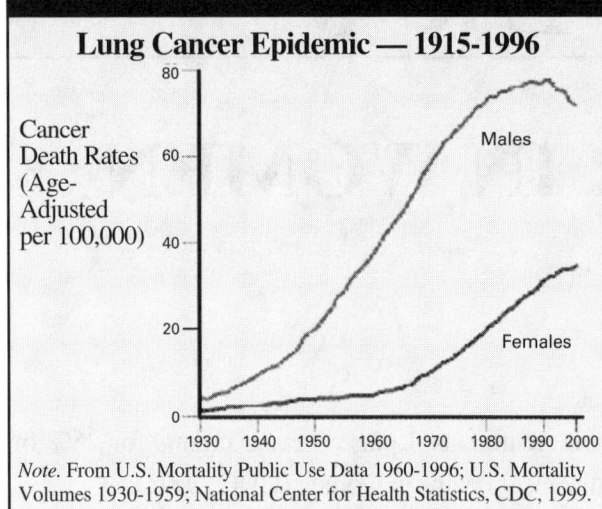

Lung Cancer Epidemic — 1915-1996

Cancer Death Rates (Age-Adjusted per 100,000)

Note. From U.S. Mortality Public Use Data 1960-1996; U.S. Mortality Volumes 1930-1959; National Center for Health Statistics, CDC, 1999.

deaths in both genders. In 2002, there were an estimated 68,800 deaths among United States women due to lung cancer, compared to 39,800 due to breast cancer (NCI, 2002). At 5 years, the overall survival rate for those diagnosed with lung cancer at any stage is 5-10% (NCI, 2003a).

Only 15% of lung cancers are detected early enough for any chance of successful treatment (Aberle & McLeskey, 2003).

FIGURE 6-2: LUNG CANCER INCIDENCE COMPARED TO OTHER CANCERS

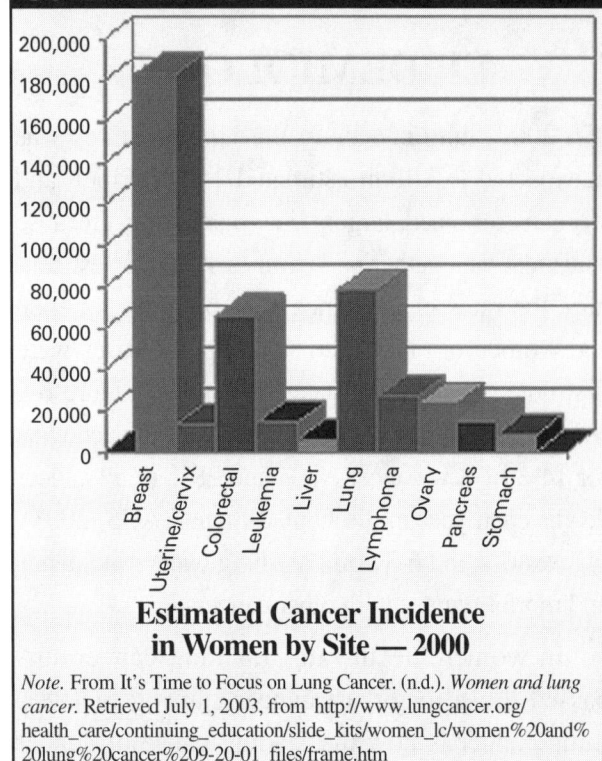

Estimated Cancer Incidence in Women by Site — 2000

Note. From It's Time to Focus on Lung Cancer. (n.d.). *Women and lung cancer.* Retrieved July 1, 2003, from http://www.lungcancer.org/health_care/continuing_education/slide_kits/women_lc/women%20and%20lung%20cancer%209-20-01_files/frame.htm

MYTHS

Several myths related to lung cancer and tobacco are worth clarifying:

Myth: Men and women are equally susceptible to the effects of lung carcinogens found in tobacco smoke.

Fact: Research suggests that women may have a greater susceptibility to these carcinogens than men.

Recent epidemiologic data suggests that women may be more susceptible to the effects of tobacco smoke than are men. Studies have shown that women who are exposed to tobacco smoke, whether active or passive, are at greater risk for developing lung cancer than are men (NCTFK, 2001a).

One study suggests that the gastrin-releasing peptide receptor (GRPR) gene is expressed more often in women than in men, even without tobacco smoke. It does appear to express earlier in women who are exposed to tobacco smoke (NCTFK, 2001a).

FIGURE 6-3: LUNG CANCER DEATHS COMPARED TO OTHER CANCERS

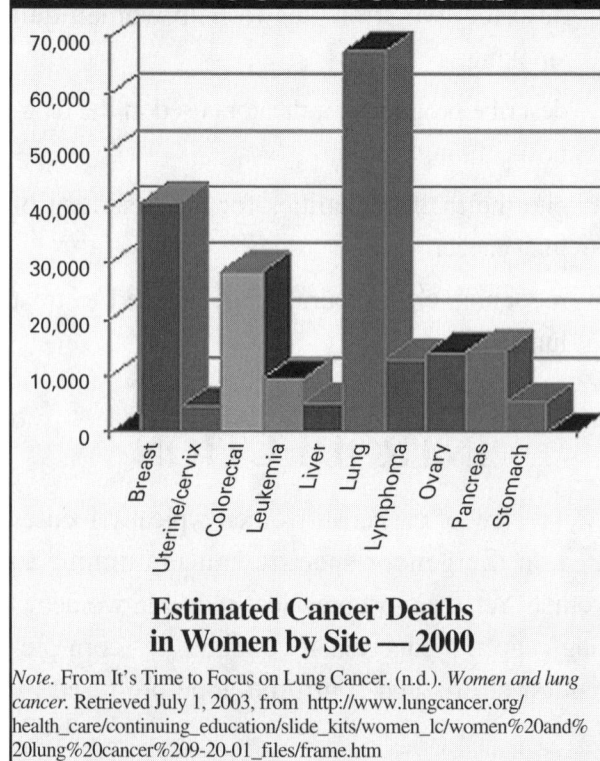

Estimated Cancer Deaths in Women by Site — 2000

Note. From It's Time to Focus on Lung Cancer. (n.d.). *Women and lung cancer.* Retrieved July 1, 2003, from http://www.lungcancer.org/health_care/continuing_education/slide_kits/women_lc/women%20and%20lung%20cancer%209-20-01_files/frame.htm

Myth: Lung cancer is a man's disease.

Fact: Despite the incidence of lung cancer in men leveling off, the incidence in women is rising, especially in younger women.

Female smokers — age 35 and older — are 12 times more likely to die prematurely from lung cancer and 10.5 times more likely to die from emphysema or chronic bronchitis than nonsmoking females. Figure 6-4 breaks down lung cancer compared to other diseases in women (NCTFK, 2001a).

Myth: All heavy smokers get lung cancer.

Fact: Only 5-10% of heavy smokers develop lung cancer.

Despite logical conclusions, not all heavy smokers develop lung cancer. Therefore, the molecular and genetic basis of the disease truly provides the key to lung cancer carcinogenesis (Aberle & McLeskey, 2003).

FIGURE 6-4: WOMEN – LUNG ILLNESSES

Women, Tobacco, & Lung Cancer

Each year, more than 150,000 women die from illnesses related to smoking.

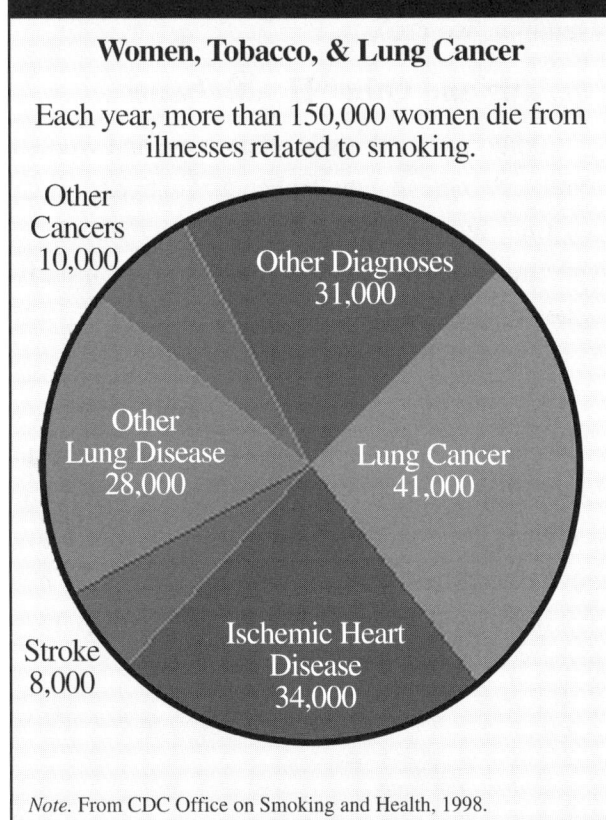

Other Cancers 10,000

Other Diagnoses 31,000

Other Lung Disease 28,000

Lung Cancer 41,000

Stroke 8,000

Ischemic Heart Disease 34,000

Note. From CDC Office on Smoking and Health, 1998.

RISK FACTORS: SMOKING

Cigarette smoking is the dominant cause of lung cancer and therefore its main risk factor. Although cigarette smoking and exposure to tobacco are not absolute causes of lung cancer, 90% of lung cancers can be linked to the patient's tobacco exposure.

The risk of getting lung cancer due to smoking increases with these factors

• the age at which smoking began

• how long the person has smoked

• the number of cigarettes smoked per day

• how deeply the smoker inhales.

Studies report that approximately 50% of those who smoke and want to quit have difficulty quitting because of the addictive nature of tobacco and nicotine products (Cooley, 2003). The Surgeon General's Report on Nicotine Addiction in 1988 was the first study that provided conclusive evidence: Cigarettes and other types of tobacco are addictive. The report underscored the fact that willpower alone could not eliminate smoking as a public health threat (Cooley, 2003).

Nicotine creates a physical dependence. Nicotine receptors in the brain become saturated with exposure, creating an increased tolerance to more nicotine. Studies have suggested that a person's genetics may increase the risk of tobacco dependence (Cooley, 2003). These early studies may lead to ways to target those more susceptible to nicotine and smoking behaviors, so that early treatment or cessation interventions are effective.

Smoking behavior is also linked with psychological and social factors. Among those factors are people prone to anxiety and depression. Once again, methods to establish ways to target interventions are being studied. With women, social support has been established as a method to help them quit smoking (Cooley, 2003).

Once diagnosed, many of those with lung cancer continue to smoke because their tobacco addiction is well entrenched. Studies show that with acute illness, most lung cancer patients make attempts to quit (Cooley, 2003). Nursing support to help patients quit is an important focus of care. Table 6-1 highlights some well-known strategies to help patients quit smoking.

Teenagers and Smoking

The overall decline in adult smoking has prompted the tobacco industry to recruit almost 1 million new smokers a year, most of them children and adolescents. Tobacco advertising targets younger smokers, luring them to begin a lifelong addiction before they truly understand the long-term consequences (NCTFK, 2001b).

More than 5 million smokers under age 18 alive today will eventually die from smoking. According to the Centers for Disease Control and Prevention (CDC) in 1999, 34.8% of all high school students reported using some type of tobacco product (NCTFK, 2001a; CDC, 2000b).

The average teenage smoker begins smoking by age 14 and becomes a daily smoker by age 18 (NCTFK, 2001a; CDC, 2000b). Studies show that a person who does not begin smoking as a child or adolescent is not likely to begin as an adult (NCTFK, 2001a). Adolescents with lower levels of school achievement are more likely than their peers to use tobacco (NCTFK, 2001a).

Women and Smoking

According to the CDC Office on Smoking and Health, about 23 million adult women and at least 1.5 million adolescent girls smoke cigarettes, despite what they know about death, disease, and addiction caused by smoking (CDC, 2002).

Overall smoking prevalence among women age 18 and older has decreased from 34% in 1965 to 24.7% in 1997. However, the earlier trend toward a reduction in smoking by women has leveled off. Currently, it's estimated that 23% of all American women smoke. Female smokers typically take up smoking during adolescence, usually before their senior year in high school, often in middle school or junior high. The earlier a young woman begins smoking, the more likely she is to become a heavy smoker as an adult (CDC, 2002, NCTFK, 2001c).

With young girls, the temptation to smoke is more striking. Many girls as young as those in the third and fourth grades are already concerned about their weight and body image, and many have already been on diets by the time they enter junior high school. Smoking is perceived as a means to lose weight and look sophisticated, which is a big concern of young women struggling with self esteem and feeling like they belong.

Girls who have been aggressive, self-confident, athletic, or who have excelled in school (particularly in math or science) may begin to get messages that these behaviors are not "feminine." (CDC, 2002; NCTFK, 2001a). Cigarette advertisements targeting women depict sexy, attractive, traditionally feminine women.

Smoking and Other Health Issues

Additional health risks of smoking and women are related to pregnancy, oral contraceptive use, and menstrual function. Much that is known about the exposure of smoke to nonsmokers is from early studies of passive smoke on wives and girlfriends who lived with male smokers.

The prevalence of smoking during pregnancy has declined steadily in the past few years. But data shows that a substantial number of pregnant women resume smoking after they deliver. Only about one third of these women were still not smoking a year after their child was born (CDC, 2002).

TABLE 6-1: EXCERPTS — WAYS TO QUIT SMOKING

Preparing Yourself for Quitting

Decide positively that you want to quit.

List all the reasons you want to quit.

Develop strong personal reasons, in addition to your health and obligations to others for quitting. For example, think of all the time you waste taking cigarette breaks, rushing out to buy a pack, or hunting for a light.

Begin to condition yourself physically: Start a modest exercise program by drinking more fluids, getting plenty of rest, and avoiding fatigue.

Set a target date for quitting — perhaps a special day such as your birthday, your anniversary, or the Great American Smokeout.

Knowing What to Expect

Have realistic expectations.

Understand that withdrawal symptoms are temporary. They usually last only 1-2 weeks.

Know that most relapses occur in the 1st week after quitting, when withdrawal symptoms are strongest, and your body is still dependent on nicotine.

Mobilize all your personal resources — willpower, family, friends, and the tips — to get you through this critical period successfully.

Know that most other relapses occur in the first 3 months after quitting, when situational triggers — such as a particularly stressful event — occur unexpectedly.

Realize that most successful ex-smokers quit for good only after several attempts.

Involving Someone Else

Ask your friend or spouse to quit with you.

Tell your family and friends that you're quitting and when.

Quitting tips

Switch brands.

Smoke only half of each cigarette.

Decide beforehand how many cigarettes you'll smoke during the day.

Change your eating habits to help you cut down.

Reach for a glass of juice instead of a cigarette for a "pick-me-up."

Don't empty your ashtrays.

Make Smoking Inconvenient; stop buying cigarettes by the carton. Stop carrying cigarettes with you at home or at work.

Making Smoking Unpleasant

Smoke only under circumstances that aren't especially pleasurable for you. If you like to smoke with others, smoke alone.

Collect all your cigarette butts in one large glass container as a visual reminder of the filth made by smoking.

Avoiding Temptation

For the first 1-3 weeks, avoid situations you strongly associate with the pleasurable aspects of smoking,

Limit your socializing to healthful, outdoor activities or situations where smoking is not allowed.

Keep oral substitutes handy. Try carrots, pickles, sunflower seeds, apples, celery, raisins, or sugarless gum instead of a cigarette.

Take 10 deep breaths and hold the last one while lighting a match.

Never allow yourself to think that "one won't hurt" — it will.

Finding New Habits

Change your habits to make smoking difficult — such as swimming, jogging, or playing tennis or handball.

Do things that require you to use your hands.

Find activities that you enjoy — without the need to smoke.

Using Medication and Pharmacology methods

Nicotine replacement treatments (NRT): gum, patch, nasal spray, inhaler.

Bupropion (antidepressant)

(NCI, 2003a; Cooley, 2003)

FIGURE 6-5: CANCER DEATHS INTERNATIONALLY

Female Death Rates From Lung Cancer — A Global Perspective

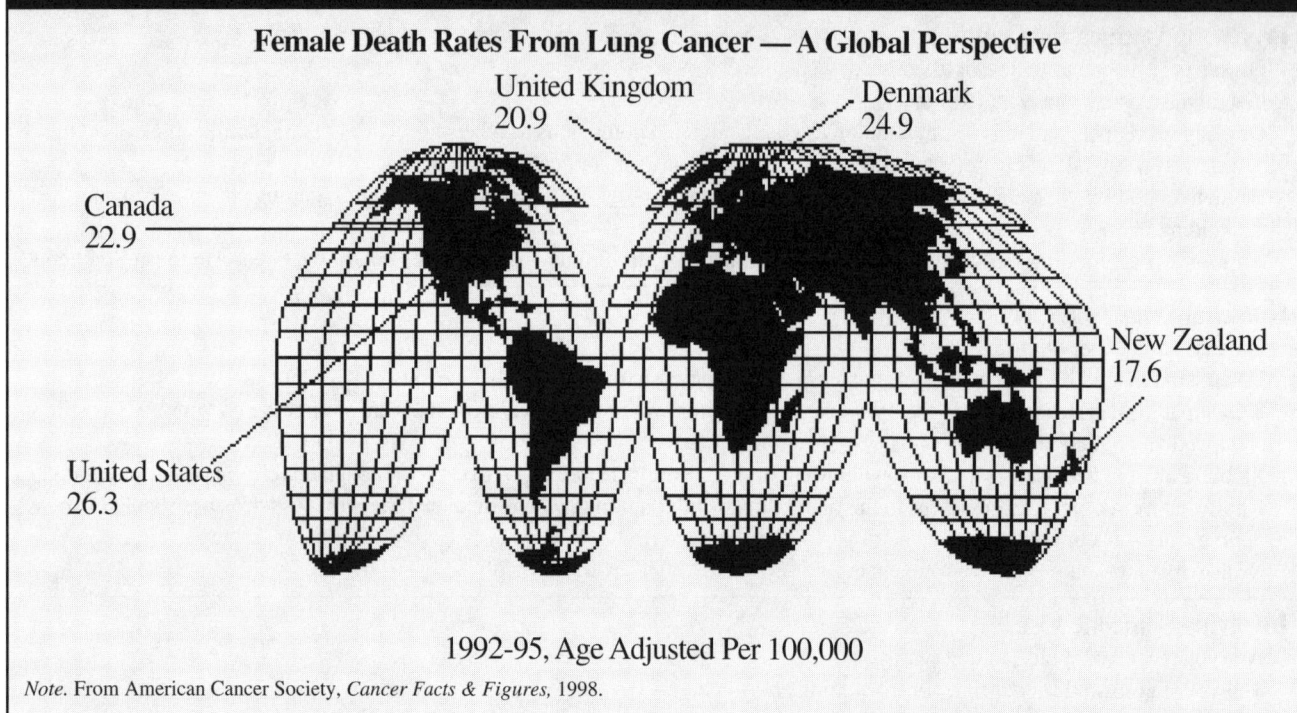

United Kingdom
20.9

Denmark
24.9

Canada
22.9

New Zealand
17.6

United States
26.3

1992-95, Age Adjusted Per 100,000

Note. From American Cancer Society, *Cancer Facts & Figures*, 1998.

Tobacco in the World

Tobacco companies increasingly look toward previously untapped markets abroad. So it is not surprising that the tobacco epidemic is pandemic, now spanning the globe. How widespread is depicted in Figure 6-5, which shows the death rate in women due to lung cancer.

OTHER RISK FACTORS

Table 6-2 lists other risk factors of lung cancer. Most lung cancers develop from environmental exposures — carcinogens, viruses, and chemicals. Of note are the risks associated with exposure to asbestos, air pollutants, and radon. Table 6-3 provides a self-administered lung cancer profile, to assess the risk of lung cancer.

LUNG CANCER

The lungs exchange oxygen and carbon dioxide in the blood, serving as a major clearing house of the circulatory and respiratory system. Figure 6-6 shows the anatomy of the lungs. Air passes through the nose or mouth into the lungs through the trachea or windpipe. The trachea divides into two tubes called bronchi and into ever smaller tubules called

TABLE 6-2: LUNG CANCER RISKS

- Smoking cigarettes, cigars, and pipes
- Exposure to environmental tobacco smoke (secondhand smoke)
- Exposure to radon, the radioactive gas that occurs naturally in soil and rocks.
- Exposure to asbestos, naturally occurring minerals used in shipbuilding, asbestos mining and manufacturing, insulation work, and brake repair.
- Exposure to pollution and certain air pollutants, such as by-products of the combustion of diesel, and other fossil fuels, such as coal, coke, and soot. Also, uranium, nickel, arsenic, and cadmium aluminum
- Lung diseases and tuberculosis
- Personal history and previous lung cancer

Note. From National Cancer Institute (NCI). (2003a). *Lung Cancer. Prevention.* CancerNet (PDQ®) web sites for health professionals. Retrieved March 1, 2003, from http://www.nci.nih.gov/cancerinfo/pdq/prevention/lung/healthprofessional/#Section_1

TABLE 6-3: LUNG CANCER PROFILE

	If yes, circle risk points
I smoke	
• 25 or more cigarettes/day	+50
• 15-24 cigarettes/day	+25
• 14 or fewer cigarettes/day	+10
I have smoked one or more cigars/day for the past year.	+5
I eat 3 or more servings of vegetables/day.	-5
My brother, sister, or parent has lung cancer.	+10
I have lived with a smoker most of my life.	+5
I have lived in or near a large city for at least 10 years of my life.	+5
I worked in the production of asbestos with asbestos insulation products without adequate respiratory protections for	
• 5-20 years	+25
• more than 20 years	+50
I worked with the following compounds without adequate protection — radon, cadmium, chromium, beryllium, aluminum, silica, sulfuric acid mist, Bis (chloromethyl) ether, or chloromethyl methyl ether or coke	
• for 5-20 years	+10
• more than 20 years	+25
I eat 3 or more servings of fruit/day.	-5
TOTAL Score	

Risk Chart

Score	Risk
< 0	Very much below average
0-6	Much below average
7-10	Below average
11-12	Average
13-21	Above average
22-53	Much above average
54 or higher	Very much above average

Note. From It's Time to Focus on Lung Cancer. (n.d.). *Women and lung cancer.* Retrieved March 1, 2003, from http://www.lungcancer.org/health_care/
continuing_education/slide_kits/women_lc/women%20and%20lung%20cancer%209-20-01_files/frame.htm

FIGURE 6-6: ANATOMY OF A LUNG

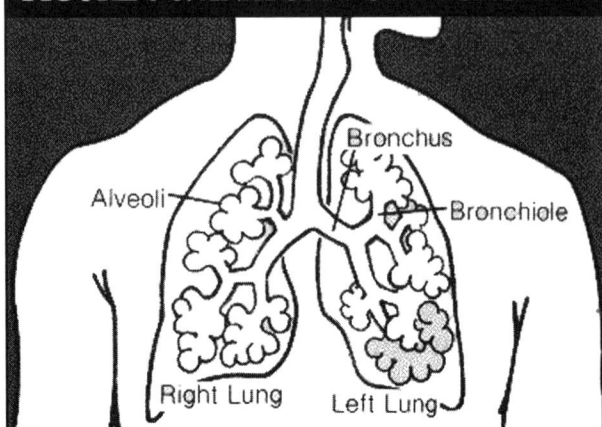

Note. From National Institutes of Health (NIH). (2002).*What You Need To Know About™ Cancer of the Lung.* (NIH, Publication #99-1553). Bethesda, MD: NIH.

bronchioles. The exchange of oxygen and carbon dioxide passes through the walls of the alveoli, the microscopic air sacs within the lobes of the lung. The right lung has three sections or lobes and the left lung has two lobes.

There are 12 different cell types of lung cancer, which are listed in Table 6-4. The two most common cell types are non-small cell lung cancer (NSCLC) and small cell lung cancer (SCLC). Cell types are determined by their cellular make-up and how the cells grow and spread. NSCLC is more common than SCLC. Generally, it grows and spreads more slowly than SCLC. The three main types of non-small cell lung cancer are: squamous cell carcinoma (also called epidermoid carcinoma), adenocarcinoma, and large cell carcinoma.

Squamous cell lung cancer was once the most prevalent cell type, but its incidence has declined over the past 30 years. This decline is thought to be because smokers are more likely to use filtered cigarettes, increasing the volume that they inhale. The deep inhaling is more likely to lead to adenocarcinoma (40-50% of lung cancer) (Cooley, 2003).

Adenocarcinoma is the most common lung cancer of nonsmokers and of women. Adenocarcinomas arise peripherally — from the mucosa or alveolar surface. These tumors tend to form glands and produce mucin. Early on, these tumor cells invade lymphatics and blood vessels. They also quickly spread distantly (Ross, 2003).

TABLE 6-4: HISTOPATHOLOGIC CELL TYPES, BRONCHOGENIC, AND LUNG CARCINOMAS

Types	Variations
Small Cell Carinoma	Oat Cell Intermediate Type Combined Oat Cell
Large Cell Carcinoma	Giant Cell Carcinoma Variant Clear Cell Carcinoma Variant
Adenosquamous Carcinoma	
Bronchial Gland Carcinoma	Adenoid Cystic Carcinoma Mucoepidermoid Carcinoma
Adenocarcinoma	Acinar Adenocarcinoma Papillary Adenocarcinoma Brochioloalveolar Carcinoma Solid Carcinoma with Mucus Formation
Squamous Cell Carcinoma (epidermoid)	Spindle Cell Variant
Carcinoid	

Note. From Hass, M. (2003). Controversies in detection and screenings. In M. Hass, *Contemporary issues in lung cancer: A nursing perspective* (pp. 24-29). Sudbury, MA: Jones & Bartlett Publishers.

Small cell lung cancer (SCLC) is less common than NSCLC. It accounts for 15-20% of all lung cancers and occurs in women 10-30% of the time. It arises from the large central airways.

SCLC presents in sheets of small cells accompanied by small areas of cytoplasm that are round or oval. When diagnosed, about 30% of SCLC is contained. However, most cases of SCLC quickly grow and spread to other organs of the body.

Genetic Carcinogenesis

Lung cancer cells arise from bronchial epithelial cells. No single mutation has been determined to cause lung cancer, but researchers are making small steps in understanding the mechanisms of the different cells types of lung cancer. Among the areas of study are genetic mutations, specifically protooncogenes and tumor suppressor genes.

Protooncogenes are key players in how cells proliferate and differentiate. When these encoded proteins are damaged or mutate, cell growth has no control. These changes happen on a molecular level and amplify in their overexpression, ultimately damaging genes that lead to cellular proliferation (Ross, 2003). Of interest in particular to lung cancer are the protooncogene family of tyrosine kinase protooncogenes (including erbB-1, erbB-2 [also known as HER-2/neu]). The erbB-2 is expressed in up to one-third of NSCLC (Ross, 2003). The tyrosine kinase receptor KIT has been found in many SCLCs. Another tyrosine kinase receptor RAS has been found to mutate in adenocarcinoma (Ross, 2003).

When expressed, tumor suppressor genes allow normal cell growth. When they mutate, cell growth goes unchallenged and allow malignancies to develop. Areas of interest in relation to lung cancer are the tumor suppressor gene TP53. TP53 has been shown to abnormally express in SCLC and NSCLC. Another tumor suppressor gene, cyclin D1, has been shown to mutate in both SCLC and NSCLC. A step in the pathway of p16-cycline D1-CDK4 retinoblas-

toma — a key cell cycle regulator — has been shown to become abnormal in most SCLCs and some NSCLC. Other tumor suppressor genes being studied for their involvement in lung cancer are TSG101 and DMBT1 (located at specific chromosome locations). Other areas of inquiry are the chromosome locations on the gene maps themselves (Ross, 2003).

In addition to genetic and molecular research, other areas explored for their influence on lung cancer are the cell's cellular adhesion properties and their inherent mechanism to start or stop programmed death (apoptosis) (Ross, 2003).

PREVENTION AND DETECTION STRATEGIES

If a woman stops smoking, her risk of dying of lung cancer decreases. The threshold for reducing risk is notable when the woman has not smoked for at least 10 years. We know this because of the lowered incidence rates of lung cancer in recent years with men when cigarette smoking cessation programs became effective (NCI, 2003a).

As has been shown with men, the mortality rate for female lung cancer has declined if the person is younger than age 60. This change prompts a marked slowing of the mortality rate. Previously, overall lung cancer mortality rates among women showed a steep increase.

In 1996 in an effort to help nicotine-dependent patients and health care providers, the Agency for Health Care Policy and Research released clinical smoking-cessation guidelines. Highlights of these guidelines follow:

- Clinicians must document the tobacco-use status of every patient.

- Every patient using tobacco should be offered one or more of the available effective smoking cessation treatments.

- Every patient using tobacco should be provided

with at least one of the available effective brief cessation interventions.

- One or more of the three treatment elements identified as being particularly effective should be included in smoking-cessation treatment

    - nicotine-replacement, for example, nicotine patches, gum

    - social support from nurse in the form of encouragement and assistance

    - skills training and problem solving (cessation and abstinence techniques)

(NCI, 2003a).

SIGNS AND SYMPTOMS

The signs and symptoms of early lung cancer can be vague with patients not seeking help until their cancer is advanced. Symptoms — cough, shortness of breath — can be similar to bronchial infections that patients can regularly get. These masked lung cancer symptoms are especially familiar to smokers, who are used to living with these symptoms.

These are the common signs and symptoms of lung cancer

- persistent cough that worsens over time

- constant chest pain

- coughing up blood

- shortness of breath, wheezing, or hoarseness

- repeated complications from pneumonia or bronchitis

- neck and face swelling

- loss of appetite or weight loss

- fatigue

(NCI, 2002).

Patients delay seeking help for symptoms, either because they deny the problem is serious or believe the symptoms will pass.

DIAGNOSIS AND STAGING

In diagnosing lung cancer, the health care team completes a history and physical, smoking history and family history of cancer. Diagnostic tests can include a chest x-ray, sputum cytology, computed tomography (CT) scan, positron emission tomography (PET) scan, magnetic resonance imaging (MRI), and bronchoscopies (a fine-needle aspiration using image-guided technology). Other diagnostic tests are thoracentesis (fluid removed from the area surrounding the lung), and thoracotomy (major surgery through the chest wall). Table 6-5 further specifies the type of test for biopsies for lung cells and tissue. Staging for lung cancer is listed in Table 6-6.

TABLE 6-5: DIAGNOSTIC TESTS (for biopsy)	
SPUTUM CYTOLOGY:	Noninvasive; low-tech
BRONCHOSCOPY (FOB):	Assesses airway Indication: all central tumors; surgical candidate
TRANSTHORACIC FINE NEEDLE ASPIRATION (FNA):	Chest x-ray or CT guided Indication: peripheral lesions; 15% F (-)
MEDIASTINOSCOPY:	Assess mediastinal nodes Indication: surgical candidates
VIDEO-ASSISTED THORACOSCOPY (VATS):	Less invasive than thoracotomy Indication: small, visible, peripheral lesions

Note. From It's Time to Focus on Lung Cancer. (n.d.). *Women and lung cancer.* Retrieved March 1, 2003, from http://www.lungcancer.org/health_care/ continuing_education/slide_kits/women_lc/women%20and%20lung%20cancer%209-20-01_files/frame.htm

TABLE 6-6: REVISED INTERNATIONAL SYSTEM FOR STAGING LUNG CANCER

Primary tumor (T)	AJCC stage groupings
• TX: Primary tumor cannot be assessed, or tumor proven by the presence of malignant cells in sputum or bronchial washings but not visualized by imaging or bronchoscopy	**Occult carcinoma** • TX, N0, M0
• T0: No evidence of primary tumor	**Stage 0** • Tis, N0, M0
• Tis: Carcinoma in situ	**Stage IA** • T1, N0, M0
• T1: A tumor that is 3 cm or less in greatest dimension, surrounded by lung or visceral pleura, and without bronchoscopic evidence of invasion more proximal than the lobar bronchus (in other words, not in the main bronchus). (Note: The uncommon superficial tumor of any size with its invasive component limited to the bronchial wall, which may extend proximal to the main bronchus, is also classified as T1.)	**Stage IB** • T2, N0, M0

• T2: A tumor with any of the following features of size or extent:
  * More than 3 cm in greatest dimension
  * Involves the main bronchus, 2 cm or more distal to the carina
  * Invades the visceral pleura
  * Associated with atelectasis or obstructive pneumonitis that extends to the hilar region but does not involve the entire lung
	Stage IIA
	• T1, N1, M0
	Stage IIB
	• T2, N1, M0
	• T3, N0, M0

• T3: A tumor of any size that directly invades any of the following: chestwall (including superior sulcus tumors), diaphragm, mediastinal pleura, parietal pericardium; or tumor in the main bronchus less than 2 cm distal to the carina but without involvement of the carina; or associated atelectasis or obstructive pneumonitis of the entire lung.	**Stage IIIA** • T1, N2, M0 • T2, N2, M0 • T3, N1, M0 • T3, N2, M0
• T4: A tumor of any size that invades any of the following: mediastinum, heart, great vessels, trachea, esophagus, vertebral body, carina; or separate tumor nodules in the same lobe; or tumor with a malignant pleural effusion.	**Stage IIIB** • Any T, N3, M0 • T4, any N, M0
Regional lymph nodes (N) • NX: Regional lymph nodes cannot be assessed	**Stage IV** • Any T, any N, M1
• N0: No regional lymph node metastasis	
• N1: Metastasis to ipsilateral peribronchial and/or ipsilateral hilar lymph nodes, and intrapulmonary nodes including involvement by direct extension of the primary tumor	
• N2: Metastasis to ipsilateral mediastinal and/or subcarinal lymph node(s)	
• N3: Metastasis to contralateral mediastinal, contralateral hilar, ipsilateral or contralateral scalene, or supraclavicular lymph node(s)	
Distant Metastasis (M) • MX: Distant metastasis cannot be assessed	
• M0: No distant metastasis	
• M1: Distant metastasis present. *(Note: M1 includes separate tumor nodule(s) in a different lobe [ipsilateral or contralateral].)*	

Specify sites according to the following notations:

BRA = brain	EYE = eye	HEP = hepatic
LYM = lymph nodes	MAR = bone marrow	OSS = osseous
OTH = other	OVR = ovary	PER = peritoneal
PLE = pleura	PUL = pulmonary	SKI = skin

Note. From American Joint Commission on Cancer (AJCC). (2002). Gynecological Sites: Ovary. *AJCC Cancer Staging Handbook* (6th ed.), (pp. 307). New York: Springer-Verlag.

PROGNOSIS

The prognosis of a patient diagnosed with NSCLC is determined by

- stage (extent of disease)
- performance status (see Table 6-7)
- weight loss
- gender

(NCI, 2003b).

TABLE 6-7: PERFORMANCE STATUS

0. Minimal symptoms; fully functional
1. Symptomatic; able to carry out all ordinary tasks
2. ≤ 50% waking hours in bed
3. 50% waking hours in bed
4. Bedridden; often moribund

Note. From It's Time to Focus on Lung Cancer. (n.d.). *Women and lung cancer.* Retrieved March 1, 2003, from http://www.lung cancer.org/health_care/continuing_education/slide_kits/women_lc/women%20and%20lung%20cancer%209-20-01_files/frame.htm

For patients with operable NSCLC disease, prognosis is adversely influenced by the presence of pulmonary symptoms, large tumor size (>3 centimeters), and presence of the erbB-2 oncoprotein. Other adverse prognostic factors for some patients with NSCLC include mutation of the K-ras gene, vascular invasion, and increased numbers of blood vessels in the tumor specimen (NCI, 2003b).

For NSCLC patients, 25% are diagnosed at Stage I or II, 35% are diagnosed at stage III, and 40% of patients are diagnosed at Stage IV (Foxella & Waxman, 2001). The cure rate for NSCLC at Stage I disease is 70-80%. At stage II, the cure rate is 40-50% (Fosella & Waxman, 2001).

Staging of SCLC is typically reported as limited stage (cancer is confined to the lung and lymph nodes in the chest) or extensive stage (cancer has metastasized, usually to the brain, liver, or bone.)

Without treatment, the median survival for patients with SCLC — from diagnosis to death — is only 2-4 months. At the time of diagnosis, approxi-mately 30% of SCLC patients will have tumor confined to the hemithorax of origin, the mediastinum, or the supraclavicular lymph nodes (NCI, 2003c).

TREATMENTS

Treatment depends on a number of factors, including the type of lung cancer, the size, location and extent of the tumor, and the patient's general health. Many different treatments and combinations of treatments may be used to control lung cancer, and/or to improve quality of life by reducing symptoms.

Surgery

The cornerstone of lung cancer treatment is resecting the malignancy and isolating it from further spread. Various surgical techniques and approaches are used. During surgery, lymph nodes are harvested and biopsied to establish clear staging of the tumor. Thoracic surgical treatment strategies include

- Lobectomy — removal of a single lobe. Lobectomy is a standard surgical resection, used in Stage I disease.
- Sleeve resection — approach for tumors that protrude into the main bronchus. Area of lobe and bronchus are resected, then bronchial reanastomosis preserves uninvolved lobes, allowing for adequate margins around the tumor.
- Segmentectomy — segment(s) of are lung removed
- Pneumonectomy — removal of an entire lung. Some tumors are inoperable because of their size or location. For patients whose tumor has spread (Stage III and IV), some patients with good performance status, women, and patients with distant metastases confined to a single site appear to live longer than others.

Unfortunately for SCLC, the tumors have often spread to near or distant locations at the time of diagnosis, which make the tumor more difficult to treat with surgery. Therefore the standard treatments for SCLC are radiation therapy and chemotherapy.

Radiation Therapy

For early stages of NSCLC, radiation therapy can be added to surgery as treatment. Radiation therapy is a treatment of choice when the tumor is unresectable. In NSCLC, it is used in adjuvant treatment postoperatively (N1 or N2) and can precede surgery to aide in tumor debulking.

Secondary primary tumors often develop after treatment of the primary lung cancer. In early stage disease, adjuvant radiation therapy after surgery is targeted to the mediastinal lymph nodes.

Radiation therapy also provides a means to palliate symptoms of advanced disease such as dyspnea, pain, and oncologic emergencies such as superior vena cava syndrome or spinal cord compression.

For SCLC in limited stage, radiation treatment is concurrent with chemotherapy, typically cisplatin or carboplatin and VP-16 (etoposide).

NSCLC: Treatment of Stage III and Stage IV Disease

In the last decade, the use of systemic chemotherapy with surgery and radiation therapy is one of the most important advances in the treatment of NSCLC for Stage III disease. Chemotherapy can precede radiation or be given concurrently.

For NSCLC Stage IV disease, treatment is chemotherapy. Cisplatin-based chemotherapy has been associated with short-term palliation of symptoms and a small survival advantage. Currently no single chemotherapy regimen benefits patients (NCI, 2003b).

Chemotherapies targeted for NSCLC include paclitaxel (Taxol®), docetaxel (Taxotere®), topotecan, irinotecan, vinorelbine, and gemcitabine (NCI, 2003b). More active agents against lung cancer have been available in the last 5 years (Fosella & Waxman, 2001). Table 6-8 lists older and newer agents used in adjuvant and advanced stages for lung cancer.

TABLE 6-8: NSCLC/SCLC CHEMOTHERAPY AGENTS
OLD (pre-1990)
Cisplatin
Etoposide
Vinblastine
Ifosfamide
Mitomycin-C
NEW (post-1990)
Paclitaxel
Docetaxel
Gemcitabine
Vinorelbine
Irinotecan

About one third of patients who receive chemotherapy for Stage IV NSCLC show a response to therapy. Another third show stabilization of disease that allows them some modest survival benefit and better symptom management (Fosella & Waxman, 2001).

Because treatment is not satisfactory for almost all patients with NSCLC (with the possible exception of a subset of patients with Stage I (T1, N0, M0), some patients consider enrolling in clinical trials.

Protocols fall into classifications of 1st-line therapies (patient has received no chemotherapy before), 2nd-line therapies (chemotherapy protocols tried before), and 3rd-line therapies (two different chemotherapy protocols tried before). To date, no therapy has proven superior to another in clinical trials (Thomas, 2003).

‹›8‹›‹‹›8‹›

SCLC and Chemotherapy

Because SCLC tends to be more widely disseminated at the time of diagnosis, aggressive chemotherapy is the standard treatment.

Treatments being studied for SCLC include the timing of thoracic radiation therapy (for patients with limited stage disease) and studies of multimodality therapies.

A study that compared the combination of dose-intensive cisplatin, vincristine, doxorubicin, and etoposide with standard doses of cyclophosphamide, doxorubicin, vincristine/etoposide, and cisplatin (CAV/EP) found that the more dose intensive regimens produce a higher response rate. These more intense regimens increase treatment-related complications and adverse effects. So far, progression-free or overall survival was not significant (NCI, 2003c).

COMPLICATIONS

Complications specific to the treatment of lung cancer or the effects of spreading disease include pain, pleural effusions, anxiety, depression, and sleep disturbance. (See Appendix III, Selected Nursing Diagnoses). In addition to these complications, nurses also need to help patients with lung cancer manage their fatigue, pain, loss of appetite, diarrhea, mucositis, and weight loss.

Based on preliminary research, of special distress to women with lung cancer are dyspnea, coughing, and wheezing (Chernecky, 2003).

SUMMARY

The incidence and death rates for lung cancer are daunting, especially because the rate of smoking in young people rises. Lung cancer in women is especially disturbing because some data indicates that women have particular susceptibilities to tobacco. Patients continue to ignore the signs

and symptoms of lung cancer, delaying treatments that could be much more effective when lung cancer is diagnosed early. Effective treatment is still based on surgery with some modest inroads when radiation and chemotherapy are added. New chemotherapy agents are being used in clinical trials, with the most effective results indicated with aggressive dosing balanced by coordinated symptom management. Among one of the common complications of lung cancer disease and treatment is dyspnea.

CASE STUDY: LUNG CANCER

TM is a 59-year-old Black woman, who has been a homemaker and part-time secretary for a manufacturing plant. She has been a 30/pack year smoker, attempting to quit at least twice for approximately 10 years. She says she now has about 5 cigarettes/week.

She visits her primary care physician (PCP) because of a persistent cough (x 2 months), which keeps her up at night. Occasionally she sees blood in phlegm from her cough. She has tried to quit smoking again in the past 6 weeks, using Nicoderm® patches and keeping in contact with a friend, who also is trying to quit smoking.

Her PCP has ordered a chest x-ray. He also started TM on a round of antibiotics, because she has had bronchial infections before. During the office visit, auscultation of TM's right lobe (middle) was muffled. The PCP also took a sputum sample and ordered laboratory tests including CBC and a standard metabolic panel.

Results from the chest x-ray showed an opaque area in the right center of her chest. The following week, TM was scheduled for a CT guided needle biopsy. Results came back as non-small cell lung cancer (NSCLC) (adenocarcinoma).

TM's breathing status continued to worsen with more dyspnea and swelling in her neck area. (Of concern was the possibility of a superior vena cava syndrome and developing pleural effusions.) Therefore, a lobectomy was scheduled within a few days.

The thoracic surgeon removed the right lobe and sampled lymph nodes. Staging indicated that TM's adenocarcinoma is Stage IIIB, T2, N2, N0. TM was referred to a medical oncologist for further treatment. Three courses of adjuvant chemotherapy began — cisplatin and paclitaxel (every 21 days). Because of severe neutropenia and fatigue, TM delayed the 2nd course of chemotherapy for approximately 6 weeks.

With the latest chemotherapy treatment, she had a repeat chest x-ray, which showed the mass back in her lung and appearing as large as before her surgery. As a 2nd line treatment, she is enrolled in a Phase II clinical trial, which will look at the doses for gemcitabine, days 1-8, 15 with carboplatin on day 1.

Additional Information

Her health history is remarkable for two negative breast tissue FNAs in the past 10 years, when she detected small masses in her left breast. She is slightly overweight and takes medication for hypertension. But in the last 3 months, she has lost 15 lb.

She is 42 years married to her husband, a truck driver, who plans to retire in 2 more years. She has two daughters and three sons, who no longer live with her. TM started menopause at age 50. She keeps annual physical examination appointments and has a yearly mammogram. At age 55, she had a sigmoidoscopy.

With her advancing disease, TM complains of dyspnea and profound fatigue. She has quit her job and receives continual O2 from a nasal cannula. Her husband has cut down on his hours away from home. One of her daughters who lives in the area helps TM with her housekeeping and groceries.

TM, a lifelong Baptist, has found comfort in reading the Bible and listening to inspirational tapes, which her pastor and fellow church members send to her. She says her outlook is "sunny," but she states that she knows her good days are limited. Each week she finds herself staying in bed to rest longer. Her appetite has diminished and she gets about 4 hours of fitful sleep a night.

TM has developed a trust with her PCP's nurse and looks toward her for help with her symptom management (dyspnea, fatigue, no appetite) and guidance on what is next in the progression of her illness. TM has said she wants to face the reality of her lung cancer but wants to spare her husband and children the stress of her illness. Her condition is deteriorating and her energy to make decisions is waning. TM had expressed previously to the nurse that she was profoundly sad about her condition and found herself feeling defiant against her faith and family.

EXAM QUESTIONS

CHAPTER 6
Questions 44-49

44. In addition to smoking, additional risk factors for lung cancer are

    a. high-fat diet, sedentary lifestyle, and exposure to second-hand smoke.

    b. exposure to second-hand smoke, air pollution, and radon.

    c. a previous history of colon, lung, or breast cancer.

    d. a well-defined genetic mutation, coupled with a history of tuberculosis.

45. The main signs and symptoms of lung cancer include

    a. a persistent cough that worsens over time, shortness of breath, and nausea.

    b. constant chest pain, especially radiating up the left arm; a persistent cough that worsens over time.

    c. shortness of breath, a persistent cough that worsens over time, bloody sputum.

    d. back pain, weight loss, insomnia.

46. An effective strategy to quit smoking is

    a. drinking protein drinks.

    b. nicotine patches.

    c. carbohydrate intake.

    d. extended periods of coughing.

47. NSCLC is

    a. more common than SCLC.

    b. spreads more quickly than SCLC.

    c. treated with chemotherapy in its early stages.

    d. has a better prognosis in elderly patients.

48. Still the main way to treat NSCLC (Stage II) is

    a. surgery.

    b. 5-fluorouracil (5-FU).

    c. immunotherapy.

    d. steroids.

49. The agent that is the base for many lung cancer chemotherapy protocols is

    a. Decadron.

    b. cisplatin.

    c. 5-fluorouracil (5-FU).

    d. Adriamycin.

REFERENCES

Aberle, M.F., & McLeskey, S.W. (2003). Biology of lung cancer with implications for new therapies. *Oncology Nursing Forum, 30*(2):273-278.

American Cancer Society. (2003). *Cancer facts & figures 2003.* Atlanta: Author.

American Joint Commission on Cancer (AJCC). (2002). Gynecological Sites: Ovary. *AJCC Cancer Staging Handbook* (6th ed.), (pp. 307). New York: Springer-Verlag.

Centers for Disease Control and Prevention (CDC) (2002). "Women and smoking: A report of the surgeon general" *MMWR Recommendations and Reports, 51*:RR-12.

Centers for Disease Control and Prevention (CDC) (2000a). "Cigarette smoking among adults — United States, 1998," *Morbidity and Mortality Weekly Report (MMWR), 49,* (39).

Centers for Disease Control and Prevention (CDC) (2000b). "Youth risk behavior surveillance — United States, 1999," *Morbidity and Mortality Weekly Report (MMWR), 49,* (SS-5. 2).

Chernecky, C. (2003). Challenges of conducting research in women with lung cancer. In M. Hass, *Contemporary issues in lung cancer: A nursing perspective* (pp. 271-280). Sudbury, MA: Jones & Bartlett Publishers.

Cooley, M.E. (2003). Understanding and treating tobacco dependence in adults with lung cancer. In M. Hass, *Contemporary issues in lung cancer: A nursing perspective* (pp. 271-280). Sudbury, MA: Jones & Bartlett Publishers.

Fossella, F.V., & Waxman, E. (2001). *Living your life with lung cancer.* Melville, NY: PRR, Inc.

Hass, M. (2003). Controversies in detection and screening. In M. Hass, *Contemporary issues in lung cancer: A nursing perspective* (pp. 24-29). Sudbury, MA: Jones & Bartlett Publishers.

National Cancer Institute (NCI). (2003a). *Lung Cancer. Prevention.* CancerNet (PDQ®) Web sites for health professionals. Retrieved March 1, 2003, from http://www.nci.nih.gov/cancerinfo/pdq/prevention/lung/healthprofessional/#Section_1

National Cancer Institute (NCI). (2003b). *Non-small lung cancer: Treatment.* CancerNet (PDQ®) Web sites for health professionals. Retrieved March 1, 2003, from http://www.nci.nih.gov/cancerinfo/pdq/treatment/non-small-cell-lung/healthprofessional

National Cancer Institute (NCI). (2003c). *Small cell lung cancer: Treatment.* CancerNet (PDQ®) Web sites for health professionals. Retrieved March 1, 2003, from http://www.nci.nih.gov/cancerinfo/pdq/treatment/small-cell-lung/healthprofessional

National Cancer Institute (NCI). (2002). *What You Need to Know About Lung Cancer.* NIH Publication No. 99-1553. Retrieved March 8, 2004, from http://www.nci.nih.gov/cancerinfo/wyntk/lung#6

National Center for Tobacco-Free Kids (NCTFK) (2001a). Research and facts. *Background: women & girls.* Retrieved July 1, 2003, from http://www.tobaccofreekids.org/research/factsheets/index.php?CategoryID=24

National Center for Tobacco-Free Kids (NCTFK) (2001b). Research and facts. *Tobacco industry targeting of women and children.* Retrieved July 1, 2003, from http://www.tobacco freekids.org/research/factsheets/index.php? CategoryID=24

National Center for Tobacco-Free Kids (NCTFK) (2001c). Research and facts. *Women & girls and tobacco.* Retrieved July 1, 2003, from http://www.tobaccofreekids.org/research/ factsheets/index.php?CategoryID=24

National Institutes of Health (NIH). (2002). *What you need to know about™ cancer of the lung.* (NIH, Publication #99-1553.) Bethesda, MD: NIH.

Ross, J. (2003). Biology of lung cancer. In M. Hass, *Contemporary issues in lung cancer: A nursing perspective* (pp. 11-23). Sudbury, MA: Jones & Bartlett Publishers.

Thomas, M. (2003). Advances in chemotherapy. In M. Hass, *Contemporary issues in lung cancer: A nursing perspective* (pp. 49-82). Sudbury, MA: Jones & Bartlett Publishers.

It's Time to Focus on Lung Cancer. (n.d.). *Women and lung cancer.* Retrieved March 1, 2003, from http://www.lungcancer.org/health_care/ continuing_education/slide_kits/women_lc/ women%20and%20lung%20cancer%209-20-01_files/frame.htm

CHAPTER 7

COLORECTAL CANCER
IN WOMEN

CHAPTER OBJECTIVE

After completing this chapter, the reader will be able to discuss, the epidemiology, risk factors, prevention and detection strategies, and main treatments of colorectal cancer in women.

LEARNING OBJECTIVES

After studying this chapter the reader will be able to

1. recognize main risk factors of colorectal cancer.

2. identify main symptoms of colorectal cancer.

3. list detection methods to determine early stage colorectal cancer.

4. list a method for staging colorectal cancer.

5. cite the main modalities for the treatment of colorectal cancer.

6. recognize adjuvant chemotherapy agents used to treat colorectal cancer.

7. identify elements of a teaching plan for a new ostomy patient.

INTRODUCTION

This chapter provides an overview about colorectal cancer, with an emphasis on the disease in women.

Colorectal cancer remains one of the major challenges in prevention and treatment of the major cancers. With colorectal cancer, the tools to prevent and detect this cancer in its earlier stages are well known, but the public's recognition of symptoms and the desire to seek regular, thorough follow-ups, are major barriers.

Myths about colorectal cancer continue — it is only a disease of elderly patients (it is not), that only men get it (women are equal in incidence rates), that it is a disease of Caucasians (colorectal incidence covers all races and ethnic groups), and that there is little that can be done to prevent the disease (see Prevention in this chapter.) With so many myths about colorectal cancer in circulation, educating patients with correct information should be a constant focus for nurses in clinical practice.

EPIDEMIOLOGY

In 2003, new cases of colorectal cancer were estimated at 147,500. Between 1985 and 1995 in the United States, colorectal cancer incidence rates declined by 1.8% per year. The rates then stabilized again during 1995-1999. The slight decrease about 10 years ago has been attributed to better public and professional awareness of colorectal cancer, somewhat better dietary habits, and screening efforts that emphasized early polyp removal (Berg, 2003).

In 2003, death from colorectal cancer was estimated at 57,100. Over the past 15 years in the

United States, the mortality rate for both men and women declined by 1.7% per year (see Figure 7-1). In the United States the overall 5-year survival rate for colorectal cancer is 62.1%. About 6% of Americans are expected to develop the disease within their lifetime (NCI, 2003a).

The morbidity rate of colon cancer — although improving because of surgical technique (wider margins), better supportive care and more accurate staging — remains dismal for those without health insurance. Those diagnosed with colorectal cancer without health insurance have a 64% higher mortality rate than those with health insurance (Reuters, 2000).

Although incidence of colorectal cancer has declined somewhat in men and women, the rate of decline in African Americans (men and women) has not. Both incidence and mortality rates are highest for African Americans. African Americans more often present with metastatic disease than those from other ethnic groups. Table 7-1 shows percentage incidence and mortality rates for colorectal cancer as to race and ethnicity, women and men.

These higher rates, as delineated by race and ethnic group, are thought to be because of genetic makeup, tumor pathology, comorbid conditions, and potential differences in treatment (Berg, 2003).

Worldwide, colorectal cancer is more prevalent in industrialized countries. Those areas with the highest incidence are in Eastern and Western Europe, the Scandinavian countries, New Zealand, Australia, Canada, and the United States (Jemal et al., 2002).

FIGURE 7-1: MOST RECENT AGE-ADJUSTED CANCER INCIDENCE AND DEATH RATES BY SEX

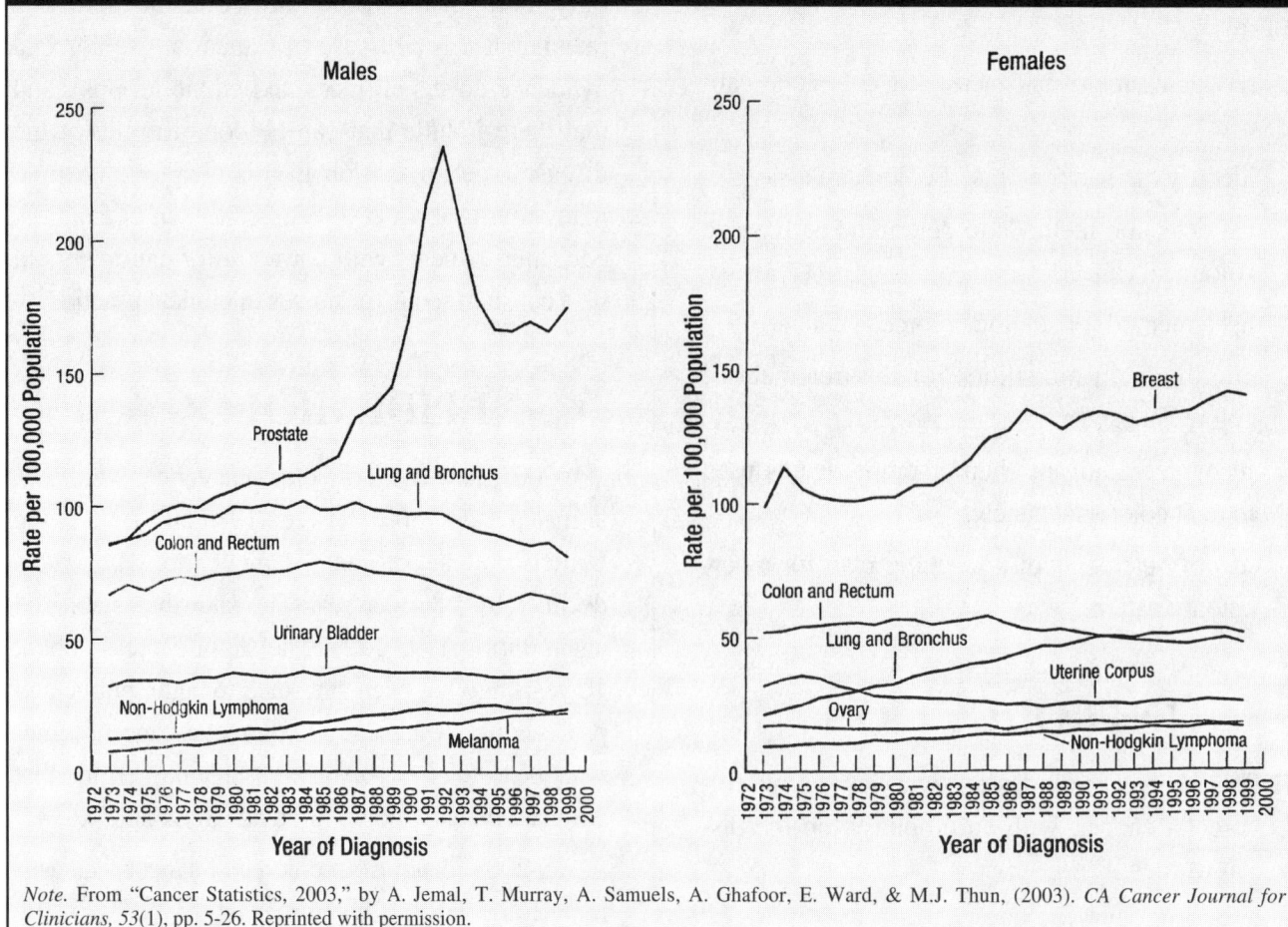

Note. From "Cancer Statistics, 2003," by A. Jemal, T. Murray, A. Samuels, A. Ghafoor, E. Ward, & M.J. Thun, (2003). *CA Cancer Journal for Clinicians, 53*(1), pp. 5-26. Reprinted with permission.

TABLE 7-1: RACE AND ETHNICITY — INCIDENCE AND MORTALITY

Incidence and Mortality Rates, United States 1990-1997

Racial/ Ethnic Group	Incidence (%)	Mortality (%)
White women	36.3	13.9
White men	51.4	20.6
African American women	44.7	19.6
African American men	57.7	27.3
Asian/Pacific Islander women	31.0	8.9
Asian/Pacific Islander men	47.3	12.9
American Indian women	24.6	8.9
American Indian men	33.5	11.9
Hispanic women	23.2	8.0
Hispanic men	35.2	13.0

Note. From "Cancer Statistics, 2002," by A. Jemal, A. Thomas, T. Murray, & M.J. Thun, (2002). *CA Cancer Journal for Clinincians,* 52(1):23-47.

Based on data gathered about cancer in women internationally, colorectal cancer has the 3rd highest incidence. In the United States it is the 2nd leading cause of death in men and women. Most frequently, colorectal cancer is diagnosed when people are older than age 50; 90% of colorectal cancer patients are > 50 (Berg, 2003). The highest incidence rate for colorectal cancer is between the ages of 65-74.

Colorectal Cancer and Women

The incidence rate for colorectal cancer in the two genders is similar (see Figure 7-2). Colorectal cancer accounts for 12% of all new cancer cases in women; in women, colon cancer is more common than rectal cancer. For women

in 2002, approximately 57,300 new cases of colon cancer occurred (compared to 50,000 new cases for men). In 2002, there were 18,400 new cases of rectal cancer in women (compared to 22,600 cases for men). A woman has a cumulative lifetime risk of getting colorectal cancer of 1 in 18 (Jemal et al., 2002).

FIGURE 7-2: LEADING CANCER CASES (ESTIMATED) FOR FEMALES, 2003

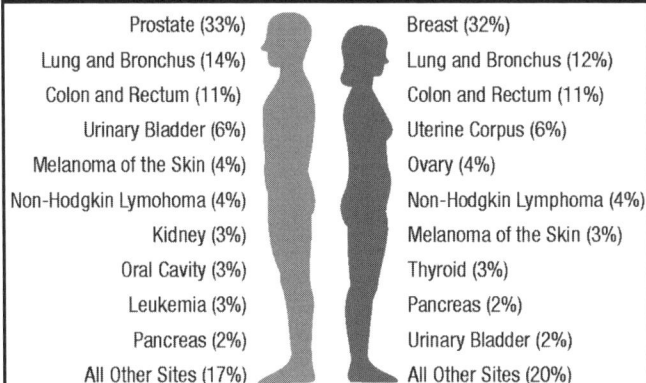

Prostate (33%)	Breast (32%)
Lung and Bronchus (14%)	Lung and Bronchus (12%)
Colon and Rectum (11%)	Colon and Rectum (11%)
Urinary Bladder (6%)	Uterine Corpus (6%)
Melanoma of the Skin (4%)	Ovary (4%)
Non-Hodgkin Lymohoma (4%)	Non-Hodgkin Lymphoma (4%)
Kidney (3%)	Melanoma of the Skin (3%)
Oral Cavity (3%)	Thyroid (3%)
Leukemia (3%)	Pancreas (2%)
Pancreas (2%)	Urinary Bladder (2%)
All Other Sites (17%)	All Other Sites (20%)

Excludes basal and squamous cell skin cancers and in situ carcinomas except urinary bladder.
Note: Percentages may not total 100 percent due to rounding.

Note. From "Cancer Statistics, 2003," by A. Jemal, T. Murray, A. Samuels, A. Ghafoor, E. Ward, & M.J. Thun, (2003). *CA Cancer Journal for Clinincians,* 53:5-26.

COLORECTAL CANCER

The colon is the first 6 feet of the large intestine. The rectum is the last 8-10 inches. Together they serve as a long muscular tube that stores and then transports waste products from the body (see Figure 7-3).

When found early with the disease localized to the bowel, colorectal cancer is highly treatable and cure rates are high. Those with local disease have a 90% 5-year survival rate. Those with regional disease have a 65% survival rate. Those with metastatic disease have an 8% survival rate (Jemal et al., 2002).

Proximal tumors are more common (Greenlee et al., 2000). When found early, surgery is the treatment of choice. Surgery cures about 50% of those diagnosed with colorectal cancer. However, when colorectal tumor cells have penetrated the bowel wall or spread to nodes, treatments are less effective.

FIGURE 7-3: COLON ANATOMY

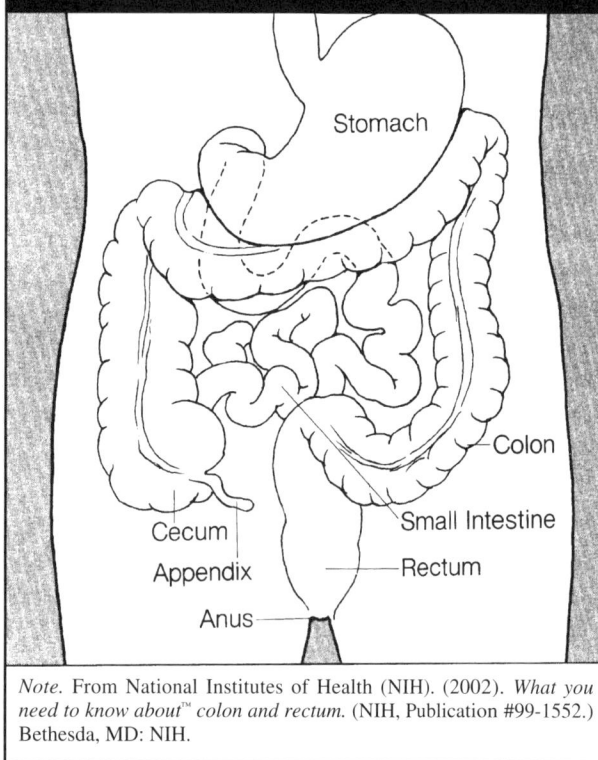

Stomach

Colon

Cecum

Small Intestine

Appendix

Rectum

Anus

Note. From National Institutes of Health (NIH). (2002). *What you need to know about™ colon and rectum.* (NIH, Publication #99-1552.) Bethesda, MD: NIH.

Prognostic markers when staging colorectal cancer include bowel obstruction and perforation and pretreatment blood levels of carcinoembryonic antigen (CEA). (But these markers have been shown to have a level of false positives.) (NCI, 2003a). Additional prognostic factors under study include genetic predisposition and susceptibility of some people to development of adenomas, polyps or early stage forms of colorectal tumors (NCI, 2003a).

Genetic Origins

Genetic changes are thought to cause colorectal cancer. Among them are tumor suppressor genes, prompted by initial mutations of adenomatous polyposis coli (APC). These changes lead to hyperproliferation of the epithelial tissue in the colon's lining.

Another mutation is the DCC gene, found in 80% of colorectal cancers. When this gene is deleted, benign adenomas develop. Another mutation is the p53 mutation, which appears to contribute to inappropriate progression of normal cell development through the cell cycle.

Oncogenes associated with colon cancer are C-Myc gene amplification and the Ras oncogene, found in one half of all carcinomas and larger adenomas (Goldberg, 2000). Mismatch repair genes contribute to the instability of the cells.

RISK FACTORS

Table 7-2 reviews risk factors for colorectal cancer. Although a disease of aging (median age at diagnosis is 67), colorectal cancer increases in those older than age 50. When diagnosed at a younger age, colorectal cancer presents at a more advanced stage; but those > 80 years old at diagnosis, can present with earlier stage disease. After treatment, survival is somewhat better for younger patients, thought to be due to adjuvant treatment regimens more often targeted to relatively younger patients (Berg, 2003).

Approximately one quarter of those who are diagnosed with colorectal cancer are from high risk groups. Those groups include

- Personal history of colorectal cancer, polyps, Crohn's disease, ulcerative colitis, or adenomas

- Hereditary conditions, such as familial polyposis, hereditary nonpolyposis colon cancer (HNPCC) Lynch Syndrome Variants I and II, and ulcerative colitis

- First-degree family history of colorectal cancer or adenomas

- Personal history of ovarian, endometrial, or breast cancer (NCI, 2003b)

- Diet high in animal fat and processed meat, low in fruits and vegetables

- Sedentary lifestyle

- Age (more common in people > 50; rare in people < 30)

The following sections further describe the areas that can increase colorectal cancer risk.

TABLE 7-2: CRITERIA IDENTIFYING HEREDITARY RISK FOR COLORECTAL CANCER

Amsterdam Criteria-II

(1-2-3 Rule)

• 1 or more family members with colorectal cancer diagnosed before age 50 AND

• 2 or more generations affected by colorectal cancer AND

• 3 or more relatives with verified HNPCC-associated cancer (colorectal, endometrial, small bowel, ureter, or renal cancers), one of which must be a first-degree relative of the other two members.

Bethesda Criteria

(only one criteria needed)

1. Individuals whose families meet the Amsterdam Criteria

2. Individuals with two HNPCC-related cancers — colonic and associated extracolonic

3. Individuals with colorectal cancer plus a first degree-relative with CRC and/or HNPCC-related associated extracolonic cancer, and/or colorectal adenoma (diagnosed before age 40); one of the cancers must have been diagnosed before age 45.

4. Individuals with colorectal cancer or endometiral cancer diagnosed before age 45.

5. Individuals with a right-sided colorectal cancer (undifferentiated or poorly differentiated pattern) diagnosed before age 45.

6. Individuals with a signet-ring cell colorectal cancer, diagnosed before age 45.

7. Individuals diagnosed before the age of 40 with colorectal adenomas.

Note. From Berg, D. (2003). *Pocket guide to colorectal cancer.* Sudbury, MA: Jones & Bartlett Publishers.

Polyps

Polyps are precursors to colorectal cancers. They are most common as people age — approximately 30% of individuals in their 50s produce polyps. About 50% of individuals in their 70s produce polyps (Dadoly, 2000).

Approximately 70% of polyps are adenomatous with malignant potential. Nevertheless, most polyps do not become cancerous. (Only 5% become malignant.) (Goldberg, 2000). Most polyps are pedunculated (stalked or tubular) rather than flat or a combination stalked/flat. Polyps that develop into cancerous cells develop over several years, starting by growing larger, then forming an adenoma that can become carcinoma in situ.

Polyps that are more likely to become cancerous are a higher grade and severely dysplastic. Patients who develop more than one polyp increase

the likelihood 5-7 times that they will develop a malignancy (Goldberg, 2000). When detected, the smaller the polyp, the less likely that it will become malignant. For those who undergo regular polypectomy for recurring polyps, the incidence of developing colorectal cancer decreases by 90% (Goldberg, 2000).

Personal and Family History

Inherited genetic factors and previous cancers increase the risk for some patients. Those who were previously diagnosed with colon cancer are at higher risk. Women with breast, endometrial, and ovarian cancer are at higher risk to develop colorectal cancers. (See Chapters 2, 3, and 4.) People with a family history of colon cancer are at increased risk.

For example, colon cancer risk increases in women who have been diagnosed with ovarian cancer. In turn, colon cancer increases the risk of a woman developing ovarian cancer, especially in women before age 50 (O'Rourke & Mahon, 2003). Most women with ovarian cancer will not survive long enough to develop colon cancer. These risks may be based on hormonal and nutrition interactions and their relationship to HNPCC syndrome.

Family History

A family history of colorectal cancer involving a first-degree relative increases the risk of developing colon cancer 2-3 fold. The risk is higher when the relative was diagnosed before age 60 or if there are many family members that were diagnosed with colorectal cancer.

The genetic syndromes, HNPCC and Familial Adenomatous Polyposis (FAP), increase the risk 70% and 100% respectively (Greenlee et al., 2000). These syndromes create a condition whereby family members develop polyps that advance to adenomas and possible malignancies.

HNPCC is an inherited autosomal dominant syndrome. It accounts for 5% of colorectal cancers (about 1 in 500) (Berg, 2003). HNPCC is also associated with breast, ovarian, endometrial, kidney, stomach, biliary tract, brain, and small intestine cancers (Berg, 2003).

Those with HNPCC can present with polyps that are scattered throughout the colon; the polyps accelerate to cancer quickly. If the syndrome develops into cancer, the mean age of diagnosis is age 44. The mean age for colorectal cancer developing in the general populations is age 68 (Berg, 2003).

The genetic origin of HNPCC is due to a change in the mismatch repair (MMR) genes. Only a few MMRs are identified so many individuals may have HNPCC but have an unknown mutation (Berg, 2003). Genetic testing is recommended for those with a three-generation family history of colorectal cancer, a first-degree relative with HNPCC and criteria established by the Amsterdam Criteria-II and Bethesda Criteria (Table 7-2).

FAP syndrome accounts for only 1% of those diagnosed with colorectal cancer. Polyps develop early — on average when the individual is younger than age 25. By age 35, those with FAP develop polyps 90% of the time (Berg, 2003). The adenamatous polyposis coli (APC) gene predisposes those to FAP. If colorectal cancer develops, the average age at diagnosis is age 42 (range age 34-43). (Standard management is total colectomy with reconstruction of ileal pouch and anal anastomosis.)

Those with inflammatory bowel disease (ulcerative colitis and Crohn's disease) increase their risk 30-fold for colorectal cancer. The risk increases with each decade (3% at 10 years; 30% at 30 years after diagnosis.) A history of Crohn's disease increases the risk of colorectal cancer about 1-2 times (Ellenhorn et al., 2002).

Other Lifestyle Risk Factors

For those without a genetic predisposition, there are no specific and unique risks for colorectal cancer. But together, many risk factors can put an individual at risk (NCI, 2003a).

High-Fat Diet

Epidemiologic, experimental (animal), and clinical investigations suggest that diets high in total fat (saturated and monounsaturated), protein, calories, alcohol, and meat (both red and white), and low in calcium and folate (vegetables), are associated with an increased incidence of colorectal cancer. The risk is 2-2.5 times higher for those who follow a high-fat diet compared to those with low-fat diets (NCI, 2002).

Colon cancer rates have been shown to be high in populations with high total fat intake and are lower in those populations where people consume less fat. This means that Western countries — with high-fat diets — have been shown to have more colorectal cancer (NCI, 2002).

Cigarette Smoking

Cigarette smoking is associated with an increased tendency to form adenomas and develop colorectal cancer. Those who have smoked for less than 20 years are 3 times more likely to have small adenomas; those who smoke > 20 years are 2.5 times at risk to develop large adenomas (Goldberg, 2000).

In 1997, it was estimated that 12% of colorectal cancer deaths in the U.S. population were from smoking. A large population-based cohort study of Swedish twins found that heavy smoking of 35 or more years was associated with nearly 3 times an increased risk of developing colon cancer. Another large population-based case-controlled study indicates that those who smoke now or within the last 10 years can develop colon cancer. A 50% increase in risk was associated with smoking more than a pack a day compared to never smoking (NCI, 2003b).

Other Lifestyle Risks

Research studies also focus on the effects of an increased risk for colorectal cancer with alcohol consumption and obesity. Other studies are looking at the possibility of reducing risk with aspirin and nonsteroidal anti-inflammatory drugs (NSAIDs) and hormone replacement therapy (HRT). No definitive conclusions have emerged from these studies.

SYMPTOMS

Colon cancer can be asymptomatic until the tumor is well advanced. Signs and symptoms of colorectal cancer are

- rectal bleeding
- blood in the stool
- abdominal cramping or pain
- change in bowel habits lasting more than a few days
- narrowing of the stool
- fatigue
- urge to defecate after defecating.

Colorectal cancer develops from a polyp that grows and becomes malignant. Tumor cells spread through the colon wall to regional then distant sites. Areas where colon tumors initially develop are in the left colon (descending, sigmoid, and rectal areas): 56%; right colon (cecum and ascending colon): 34%; transverse colon: 10%.

Individuals have been known to ignore symptoms because they were thought to be caused by a hemorrhoid or irritable bowel syndrome, other intestinal upsets, or food poisoning.

SCREENING AND DETECTION

Common screening methods for colorectal cancer include

- Digital Rectal Examination (DRE) — The DRE should be performed with other tests. Fewer than 20% of rectal cancers and no colon cancers can be detected with DRE.

- Fecal Occult Blood Test (FOBT) — The FOBT is one of the earliest methods to detect early-stage colorectal cancer. The FOBT can reduce incidence by 20% and mortality by one third if repeated yearly. It is best to do the test on multiple bowel movements. Compliance is a challenge and the test has its limitations: It does not detect tumors in the rectosigmoid colon. Patients need to be instructed about dietary and medication restrictions before doing the FOBT. (Table 7-3 reviews those instructions.) Some colorectal tumors do not bleed, so the FOBT can have false negatives.

- Endoscopic visualization methods

  — Flexible sigmoidoscopy — visualizes the rectum, sigmoid, and descending colon. The rigid scope reaches to about 30 cm. The flexible scope reaches to about 60 cm, allowing better view of the lower bowel. Because 50% of colon lesions are in the

TABLE 7-3: FECAL OCCULT BLOOD TEST (FOBT) INSTRUCTIONS

• For 3 days before testing, do not ingest anti-inflammatory drugs or aspirin; vitamin C or supplements; or citrus fruits and juices.

• For 2 days before testing, do not eat red meat, turnips, or horseradish.

• Take two samples from three consecutive bowel movements.

• Place sample on testing card, then mail to laboratory immediately.

distal colon, sigmoidoscopy is 80% accurate in diagnosing tumors. Cleansing enemas must precede the test.

— Colonoscopy — Offers complete visualization of the colon, therefore it allows the most accurate method to screen for colorectal cancer. The colonoscopy can reduce incidence by 75-90% with accompanying removal of polyps and tissue for biopsy. It must be preceded by full bowel preparation with oral cathartics and laxatives. The procedure requires the patient to be premedicated with sedative.

• Double Contrast Barium Enema (DCBE) — After patient swallows barium, a radiologic examination follows. (Barium advances as far as cecum.) The examination offers evaluation only of larger lesions — a colonoscopy follows if lesions or adenomas are detected. The procedure is preceded with bowel preparation of enemas and laxatives. (False negative range for DCBE is 2-61% due to poor bowel preparation.) (Berg, 2003.)

Although these screening tools can be effective, challenges are inherent. They include

• The FOBT has a record of false-negative and false-positive results. FOBT affects the mortality rate for colorectal cancer but overall survival rate has been unchanged.

• After DCBE, 5-15% of patients will have a positive test that prompts follow-up colonoscopy. Further evaluation and excision of smaller adenomas may not be necessary because they pose a low risk of developing into colorectal cancers.

• Sigmoidoscopies have low sensitivity to adenomas. The left colon view is better than other areas of the colon.

• Colonoscopies are the most expensive screening tool ($800-1,600 per exam). Screening colonoscopies are labor intensive; waits are lengthy.

• Studies analyzing the cost and benefit of screening for those of average risk are ongoing. These analyses take into account a patient's risk factors, starting with the least expensive (and least invasive) screening tools (FOBT, barium enemas) before advancing to sigmoidoscopies and colonoscopies (Berg, 2003). Still some individuals with developing colorectal cancers are missed.

• Recommendations exist for scheduling of preventive tests, specifically the hemoccult test (yearly), the flexible sigmoidoscopy (starting at age 50, every 5 years after), and the colonoscopy (starting at age 50, every 10 years after) (Berg, 2003). In light of the cost and availability of screening, the age to stop screening is not well established. For now, screening recommendations, supported by the National Cancer Institute (NCI) and American Cancer Society (ACS), are listed in Table 7-4.

• Screening barriers are linked to insurance coverage, cost of care, and access to care. Care also can be disjointed between primary care and specialist care practices.

TABLE 7-4: COLORECTAL SCREENING

American Cancer Society Recommendations for Early Colorectal Cancer Detection, 2003

Beginning at age 50, both men and women should follow one of the five screening options below:

1. Fecal occult blood test (FOBT) every year*

2. Flexible sigmoidoscopy every 5 years

3. Fecal occult blood test every year plus flexible sigmoidoscopy every 5 years*

4. Double contrast barium enema every 5 years

5. Colonoscopy every 10 years

NOTE: Of the first three options, the American Cancer Society recommends option three, the combination of FOBT every year and flexible sigmoidoscopy every 5 years.

- Social and cultural barriers challenge any adoption of widespread screening for colorectal cancer.

PROTECTIVE STRATEGIES

Aspirin and NSAIDs inhibit cyclooxygenase (COX) that can produce prostaglandins that can protect the GI tract. Some early studies report that low-dose aspirin may be able to reduce polyps and adenomas. Further research is needed to clarify the benefits of aspirin, NSAIDs, and COX-2 inhibitors on polyp development, and patients with genetic syndrome-related colorectal cancers (Berg, 2003).

Increased physical activity and reduced sedentary lifestyle are thought to reduce the risk of colorectal cancer (although the type, amount, frequency, and level measured with changes in diet are unclear.) Physical activity and body weight reduction are associated with bowel mobility, which help reduce exposure of the colon to possible carcinogens. ACS recommendations emphasize 30-45 minutes of exercise 5 times a week to maintain healthy weight (ACS, 2002).

Data on dietary fiber protecting against colorectal cancer is inconsistent. Additional studies are needed to clarify the benefit of high-fiber, low-fat diets (Ellenhorn et al., 2002).

The protective effect of yellow and green vegetables and fruits is not yet proven (Berg, 2002). Studies about the benefits of vitamins A, C, E, and beta carotene have been inconsistent in establishing their protective effects against colorectal cancer (Berg, 2003).

Alcohol consumption, based on epidemiologic data, is linked to rectal cancer. No such association is clear with colon cancer (Berg, 2003).

HRT in postmenopausal women has been shown to reduce the incidence of colorectal cancer in women. The use of HRT is controversial, because of the risk it creates for breast and endometrial cancer. (See Chapters 2 and 3, Breast and Endometrial Cancer).

Table 7-5 reviews practical behaviors that can help prevent colorectal cancer.

STAGING AND DIAGNOSIS

If colon cancer is suspected, diagnostic tests may include

- chest x-ray
- computed tomography (CT) scan of the abdomen or pelvis
- positron emission tomography (PET) scan
- transrectal ultrasound
- blood tests (CBC, serum chemistry, and liver studies). The serum carcinoembryonic antigen (CEA) is a tumor-associated marker for cancer (normal, < 2.5 ng/mL).
- bone scan.

TABLE 7-5: SUGGESTIONS TO LIMIT RISK OF COLORECTAL CANCER

American Cancer Society Recommendations for Early Colorectal Cancer Detection

- Exercise regularly
- Stabilize weight at normal range
- Eat less red meat
- Eat more fruits and vegetables (5-6 servings/day)
- Take a multivitamin with folic acid and calcium
- Don't smoke
- Limit alcohol
- By physician recommendation, consider a daily dose of aspirin, NSAIDs or COX-2 inhibitor

Note. From National Cancer Institute (NCI). (2003b). *Colorectal Cancer: Prevention.* CancerNet (PDQ®) Web sites for health professionals. Retrieved May 1, 2003, from http://www.nci.nih.gov/cancerinfo/pdq/prevention/colo-rectal/healthprofessional/

TREATMENTS

Treatment for colorectal cancer depends on the size, location, and extent of the tumor, and on the patient's general health. Clinical staging of the tumor is the most important prognosticator. Highlights of the staging schema for colorectal cancer are listed in Table 7-6.

TABLE 7-6: COLORECTAL STAGING

Stage 0. (Found only in the innermost lining of the colon or rectum.)

Stage I. (Involves more of the inner wall of the colon or rectum.)

Stage II. (Tumor has spread outside the colon or rectum to nearby tissue, but not to the lymph nodes.)

Stage III. (Tumor has spread to nearby lymph nodes, but not to other parts of the body.)

Stage IV. (Tumor has spread to other parts of the body, especially the liver and/or lungs.)

Note. From National Cancer Institute (NCI). (2003a). *Colorectal Cancer.* CancerNet (PDQ®) Web sites for health professionals. Retrieved May 1, 2003, from http://www.nci.nih.gov/cancerinfo/pdq/treatment/colon/healthprofessional/#Section_1

Areas of metastasis include the liver, lymph nodes, peritoneal cavity, lungs, bones, and adrenal glands. At diagnosis, approximately 37% of colon cancer cells and 50-60% of rectal cancer cells have metastasized to regional lymph nodes (Jemal et al., 2003).

Surgery

Surgery is the initial treatment of choice for early stage and localized colorectal tumors. Among surgical techniques are

— polypectomy

— laparoscopic colectomy

— sentinel lymph node biopsy

— open colectomy.

In most cases for an open colectomy, the surgeon is able to reconnect the healthy portions of the colon or rectum. If that is not possible, a temporary or permanent colostomy is placed. (Some patients need a temporary colostomy to allow the lower colon or rectum to heal after surgery.)

About 15% of colorectal cancer patients require a permanent colostomy (NCI, 2003c). The most common ostomy (surgical opening to divert body waste) is the colostomy. Table 7-7 highlights management issues involved with a colostomy. (NOTE: Ileostomies provide a surgical opening to eliminate waste from the small intestine — drainage is watery.)

More complicated surgical resections are needed when the tumor has perforated the colon, invading adjacent organs. For rectal cancers, the tumor can be locally excised or resected with efforts to preserve the sphincter.

The role of sentinel lymph node mapping to stage regional nodes for rectal cancer is under clinical evaluation. (See Chapter 2, Breast Cancer, Sentinel Node Mapping.) Also being investigated is the role of laparoscopic techniques in the treatment of colon cancer.

TABLE 7-7: IMPORTANT ASPECTS OF OSTOMY MANAGEMENT
• Early participation in care is key to self-care after surgery. Teaching should begin as soon as possible before surgery.
• One-piece system placed immediately after surgery (allows healing), then appliance changed to 2-piece.
• Initial drainage after surgery is liquid with blood. Then with increased diet, discharge becomes solid. Final consistency depends on placement of stoma along the colon. Proximal portion of colon returns to normal 3-5 days postoperatively.
• Flatulence begins through stoma. Occasional venting of appliance needs to be done throughout the day.
• Appliance choice depends on location of stoma.
• Appliance fit is key to prevent fecal leakage.
• Flange (faceplates) vary in size, shape, adhesive, pre-cut, or customized.
• Skin barriers also vary.
• Pay attention to signs of infection, prompted by adhesive, appliance materials.
• Changing the appliance requires systematic cleaning, airing, and replacement of the bag. Routine schedule is encouraged.
• Adapting colostomy needs to lifestyle— Returning to physical activities, work schedule, and sexual activities creates fear and apprehension. Open discussion is essential for healthy coping.

Chemotherapy

Patients with Stage II or III rectal cancer are at high risk for local and systemic relapse. With more advanced cancers, adjuvant chemotherapy is prescribed.

Standard adjuvant therapy for colorectal cancer includes infusions of fluorouracil (5-FU) plus either levamisole or leucovorin and radiation therapy. Other chemotherapeutic agents being studied are listed in Table 7-8 along with their main adverse effects.

Adjuvant regimens have prompted an increase in the numbers of partial responses and have extended the time for progression of disease. Chemotherapy has also improved survival and quality of life for patients with more advanced disease (NCI, 2003c).

Radiation Therapy

External beam therapy attempts to eradicate cancer cells while preserving organ function in localized disease. An example of a colon cancer therapy regimen is 180 cGy for 25 fractions for a total dose of 5,000 cGy.

For rectal cancer, radiation therapy is an important treatment modality. Preoperative radiation therapy helps reduce tumor bulk and seeding, reduce adverse effects of therapy, and preserve the rectal sphincter.

Most trials of preoperative or postoperative radiation therapy alone have shown to decrease the local recurrence rate of colorectal cancer but have not shown a definite effect on survival (NCI, 2003c).

Advanced Disease

For locally advanced disease, the role of radiation therapy with chemotherapy in colon cancer is under clinical evaluation. Typical protocols combine radiation therapy and 5-FU-based chemotherapies.

Radiation therapy in advanced rectal cancer is palliative in most situations but may have greater impact when used perioperatively.

Approximately 10-20% of patients can be palliated with 5-FU. Other agents used in late-stage or refractory colorectal cancers add leucovorin. Other therapies are irinotecan (CPT-11) and oxaliplatin, alone or combined with 5-FU and leucovorin.

TABLE 7-8: SELECTED CHEMOTHERAPIES FOR COLORECTAL CANCER AND COMMON ADVERSE EFFECTS

Chemotherapy	Potential Toxicity or Adverse Effect
5-fluorouracil (5-FU)	Diarrhea, stomatitis, leukopenia
Leukovorin	Diarrhea, stomatitis, leukopenia
Irinotecan (CPT-11)	Late onset diarrhea, neutropenia, nausea, vomiting, hair loss
Capecitabine	Hand-foot syndrome, diarrhea, fatigue, abdominal pain, dermatitis, nausea, vomiting, anorexia, stomatitis
Oxaliplatin	Cold-induced peripheral sensory neuropathy, acute laryngopharyngeal dysethesia, nausea, vomiting, muscle cramping, diarrhea, stomatitis, neutropenia, anemia, thrombocytopenia, and fatigue
Cetuximab (C225)	Allergic reactions, skin reactions, asthenia, fever, nausea, and elevated liver function levels (for example, SGPT)
Thalidomide	Neurotoxicities (sedation, peripheral neuropathy, constipation) hypotension and peripheral edema
Bevacizumab	Hypersensitivity, acute hypertension, thrombosis, bleeding, and headache
Iressa	Acne-like rash, nausea, vomiting, bone pain, fatigue, and diarrhea

Metastatic Disease: Hepatic Involvement

Because half of the patients diagnosed with colorectal cancer will recur, the chance of recurrence with spread to the liver is high (Berg, 2003).

Treatment strategies for hepatic involvement include additional surgery (wedge resections or segmental hepatectomy), and/or postoperative chemotherapy, hepatic arterial infusion (which provides a higher concentration of chemotherapy to the liver), radiofrequency ablation (RFA), and cryoablation.

Surgery is the only treatment that offers a potential cure of colon cancer with liver metastasis. The 5-year survival rate with successful surgery is 30-40%. The goal is to remove tumor-invaded liver tissue while leaving enough tissue for the liver tissue to regenerate.

In a healthy liver, up to 80% — or 6-8 segments — can be removed while still leaving enough liver for the patient to survive. Two thirds of liver resections remove more than one half of the liver. It takes approximately 3 weeks for the liver to regenerate to its original size (Braccia & Heffernan, 2003).

As a means of control of liver metastasis, RFA involves an electrode inserted into the tumor via ultrasound, CT scan, or magnetic resonance imaging guided imagery. It is only effective if tumors are < 3 cm.

Another ablation treatment is cryoablation, which freezes and thaws tissue causing tumor cell death. With ultrasound guidance, a special cryoprobe is inserted into the tumor, carrying liquid nitrogen. As with RFA, the tumors need to be small for cryoablation to be effective (Braccia & Heffernan, 2003).

Clinical trials continue to evaluate the effectiveness of treatments for liver metastasis in colorectal cancer.

FOLLOW-UP CARE AFTER TREATMENT

To date, there have been no large-scale randomized trials documenting the efficacy of a standard, postoperative monitoring program. Therefore, management of patients with recurrence is challenging. No clear timeline has been established that recommends the optimal regimen and frequency of follow-up examinations.

SUMMARY

Progress continues in the detection, screening, and treatment of colorectal cancer. Women share a similar incidence and mortality rate to men for colorectal cancers. Polyp identification and removal are cornerstones in the successful early treatment of colorectal cancer. Hereditary conditions, such as familial polyposis, HNPCC, and ulcerative colitis, have been determined to be risk factors. Screening efforts include attention to signs, symptoms, genetic histories, and follow-up to find precancerous conditions early, when treatment is most effective. Surgery is the main treatment modality, although radiation therapy and chemotherapy play an important role in advanced colorectal cancers. When colorectal cancer has spread to the liver, treatment to control additional tumor spread focuses on surgery and ablative therapies.

CASE STUDY: COLORECTAL CANCER

AP is a 62-year-old Caucasian woman, who visits her physician, complaining of cramping and bloating for the past month. She notes that she believes she sees blood in her stool. She also complains of crushing fatigue, which seems to have started a few months ago.

AP worked as a waitress for many years but retired from her job several years ago. She now provides childcare for her grandchildren, while her granddaughter and daughter work.

She comments that her aunt had "cancer of the bowel." While waiting for the physician to see her, she reveals that she enjoys eating a blue-plate special with her husband of 40 years. She smoked until she was age 50, but quit with the help of a support group. She also enjoys a mixed drink twice a week.

Two years ago, her physician removed benign polyps from her colon. But because of a lapse in her insurance, she has not been to the physician for 2 years.

On digital rectal exam (DRE), her physician did not note any masses but was concerned about her symptoms because of her past polypectomies. Her physician immediately scheduled her for a colonoscopy. Based on her symptoms and history, the physician also ordered a CBC and CEA.

During AP's colonoscopy, biopsies of three lesions were taken, found in her left and sigmoid colon. The biopsy results came back as adenocarcinoma in the sigmoid colon. Her CBC indicated anemia and her CEA was 5.0 mg/nl.

A sigmoid colectomy was scheduled. In preparation for her surgery, her physician ordered a chest x-ray, CT scan of the pelvis, and bone scan. As part of surgery preparation, the procedure was reviewed with AP. Preoperative teaching about her colostomy began. She was told that depending on the spread of the cancer to regional lymph nodes, she might need postoperative chemotherapy.

Postoperatively, while she recovered in the hospital, nurses continued to teach AP how to take care of her colostomy. Because her cancer had spread to regional lymph nodes, AP was referred to a medical oncologist for adjuvant chemotherapy.

Three weeks after surgery, AP began a chemotherapy protocol which included 5-FU, leucovorin and CPT-11 (Days 1, 8, 15, 22) every 6 weeks. Adverse effects from the chemotherapy included diarrhea, stomatitis, leukopenia, which the nurses managed with antidiarrheals, good hygiene (perineum and mouth care), and monitoring for infection (AP received two courses of antibiotics).

Six months after her surgery, a repeat CT scan, bone scan, and chest x-ray were ordered. All test results were negative. Her CEA level was unchanged.

While in the hospital after her surgery and during her chemotherapy treatments, AP had been made aware that her colon cancer may be associated with a hereditary syndrome. She was encouraged to proceed with genetic counseling and encourage family members to be checked regularly for polyp formation.

Additional Information

AP continues to do well after her colectomy and adjuvant chemotherapy treatments. She returns to her physician for checks every 3-6 months. Because of stability with the final years of her husband's job (as a police dispatcher), her insurance remains intact.

AP has also worked to accept her colostomy, but grieves that she no longer can wear certain clothes and must schedule her day around her colostomy care. She states that her husband and children have been supportive since she was first diagnosed, but that she senses they distance themselves from her — either because of her appliances or because they fear her colon cancer and the seriousness of her illness.

EXAM QUESTIONS

CHAPTER 7

Questions 50-58

50. Risk factors of colorectal cancer are

    a. age (more common in people younger than age 50).

    b. low-fat, low-calorie, low-fiber diet.

    c. polyps formation or history of polyps.

    d. history of colorectal or skin cancer.

51. Genetic predisposition to colorectal cancer is associated with

    a. BRCA1.

    b. BRCA2.

    c. CA-125.

    d. HNPCC and FAP.

52. The main signs and symptoms of colorectal cancer include

    a. a change in bowel habits, diarrhea, constipation, blood in the stool.

    b. weight gain, constipation, and anxiety.

    c. specific abdominal discomfort.

    d. SOB, fatigue, loss of appetite.

53. The most accurate method to screen for colorectal cancer is

    a. colonoscopy.

    b. double contrast barium enema.

    c. fecal occult blood test (FOBT).

    d. sigmoidoscopy.

54. Beginning at age 50, the ACS recommends a flexible sigmoidoscopy every

    a. 2 years.

    b. 3 years.

    c. 4 years.

    d. 5 years.

55. When colorectal cancer has spread to nearby lymph nodes, the cancer is staged as

    a. Stage I.

    b. Stage II.

    c. Stage III.

    d. Stage IV.

56. The treatment of choice for early-stage colorectal cancer is

    a. radiation.

    b. surgery.

    c. multimodality therapy.

    d. chemotherapy.

57. An adjuvant chemotherapy regimen for colorectal cancer is

    a. Rituxan™ and interferon.

    b. Bleomycin and etoposide.

    c. 5-fluorouracil (5-FU) and leucovorin.

    d. Tamoxifen and docetaxel.

58. Teaching a colorectal patient about their ostomy care should begin

    a. as soon as possible, before surgery.

    b. the day of surgery.

    c. postoperatively day 2.

    d. 2 weeks after surgery.

REFERENCES

American Cancer Society. (2002a). Cancer Facts and Figures 2002. Atlanta: Author.

American Cancer Society. (2002b). *The Complete Guide – Nutrition and Physical Activity,* Feb. 21, 2002. Retrieved June 28, 2003, from http://www.cancer.org/eprise/main/doc-root/PED/content/PED-3-2X-Diet-and-Activity-Factors-That Affect-Risks?sitearea=PED

Berg, D. (2003). *Pocket Guide to Colorectal Cancer.* Sudbury, MA: Jones & Bartlett Publishers.

Braccia, D.P., & Heffernan, N. (2003). Surgical and ablative modalities for the treatment of colorectal cancer metastatic to the liver. *Clinical Journal of Oncology Nursing, 7*(2):178-183.

Ellenhorn, J.D., Coia, L.R, Alberts, S.R., & Hoff, P.M. (2002). Colorectal and anal cancers. In R. Pazdur, L.R. Coia, H.J., Hoskins, & L.D. Wagman (Eds.), *Cancer Management: A Multidisiplinary Approach* (6th ed.), (pp. 295-318). Melville, NY: PRR, Inc.

Dadoly, A.M. (2000). Moving into the spotlight. *Harvard Pilgrim Health Care: Your Health.* (Fall):8-12.

Goldberg, R.M. (2000). Gastrointestinal tract cancers. In D.A. Casciato & B.B. Lowitz (Eds.), *Manual of Clinical Oncology* (4th ed.), (pp. 182-194). Philadelphia: Lippincott Williams & Wilkins.

Greenlee, R.T., Murray, T., & Bolden, S. (2000). Cancer statistics, 2000. *CA Cancer Journal for Clinicians, 50*(1):7-31.

Jemal, A., Thomas, A., Murray, T., Samuels, A., Ghafoor, A., Ward, E., & Thun, M.J. (2002). Cancer statistics, 2002. *CA Cancer Journal for Clinicians, 523*(1):23-47.

Jemal, A., Murray, T., Samuels, A., Ghafoor, A., Ward, E., & Thun, M.J. (2003). Cancer statistics, 2003. *CA Cancer Journal for Clinicians, 53*(1):5-26.

National Cancer Institute (NCI). (2003a). *Colon Cancer.* CancerNet (PDQ®) Web sites for health professionals. Retrieved May 1, 2003, from http://www.nci.nih.gov/cancerinfo/pdq/treatment/colon/healthprofessional/#Section_1

National Cancer Institute (NCI). (2003b). *Colorectal Cancer: Prevention.* CancerNet (PDQ®) Web sites for health professionals. Retrieved May 1, 2003, from http://www.nci.nih.gov/cancerinfo/pdq/prevention/colo-rectal/healthprofessional/

National Cancer Institute (NCI). (2003c). *Rectal Cancer: Treatment.* CancerNet (PDQ®) Web sites for health professionals. Retrieved May 1, 2003, from http://www.nci.nih.gov/cancerinfo/pdq/treatment/rectal/healthprofessional/#Section_1

National Institutes of Health (NIH). (2002). What You Need to Know About™ *Cancer of the Colon and Rectum.* (NIH, Publication #99-1552). Retrieved May 1, 2003, from http://www.nci.nih.gov/cancerinfo/wyntk/colon-and-rectum

Reuters News. (2000). Colorectal cancer mortality higher among black and the uninsured. Retrieved May 1, 2003, from http://medscape.com/reuters/prof/2000/11/11.06/200001103epid002.html

CHAPTER 8

PSYCHOSOCIAL ISSUES

CHAPTER OBJECTIVE

After completing this chapter on psychosocial issues, the reader will be able to discuss psychosocial elements of the cancer patient's experience, including the basis for the stress response, reactions to psychosocial interventions, anxiety, depression, and the benefits of social support.

LEARNING OBJECTIVES

After studying this chapter, the reader will be able to

1. recognize the physiologic basis for stress.

2. cite stages when the cancer patient benefits from psychosocial interventions.

3. identify two examples of maladjustment disorders, which may affect cancer patients.

4. identify two symptoms of anxiety.

5. identify a short-acting benzodiazepine for anxiety.

6. identify two risk factors for depression.

7. identify a major adverse effect of antidepressants.

8. identify two risk factors for suicide.

9. describe two psychosocial interventions.

10. list two ways that patients can receive group or peer support.

INTRODUCTION

Psychosocial issues are important elements of the cancer experience for women, affecting their outlook, quality of life, and possibly their outcome. Several studies show that the psychosocial realm of the woman's experience when ill can concretely affect her experience during treatment, her feelings of well-being while in treatment and beyond. It also can frame her experience so that she approaches her illness and treatment decisions with certainty and peace (Swenson, MacLeod, Williams, Miller, & Champion, 2003; Ferrell, Smith, Juarez, & Melanon, 2003; Lacey, 2002; Kessler, 2003). Among psychosocial areas of focused study have been quality of life, hope, the search for meaning in the experience, relationship issues, and spirituality (Ferrell, 2003; Ebright & Lyon, 2002; Kessler, 2002; Barsevick, Much & Sweeney, 2000; Detmar, 2000).

In 2002, Kessler and colleagues reviewed published studies on quality of life issues for breast cancer patients. Among issues identified in these quality of life studies are psychological well-being (changes in body image and sexuality), social well-being (interpersonal and family relationship issues), and spiritual well-being (uncertainty, hope). Other studies have concurred with these findings about issues of concern to women (Ferrell et al., 2003; NCI, 2003a; Ebright & Lyon, 2002; Halstead & Hull, 2001). In 2003, Ferrell and her colleagues looked at issues with ovarian cancer patients. Additional themes that emerged for these patients included the feeling of isolation, their need for support, fear of recurrence, and further treatment. These issues challenge women and affect the ways they cope. Spirituality is also a major focus of quality of life studies.

This chapter will provide a brief overview of the biology behind stress and psychosocial issues with cancer patients. It will then focus on psychosocial distress and two common manifestations of psychosocial distress — anxiety and depression. The chapter also includes a brief review of the merits of social support and other psychosocial interventions.

STRESS

A person's response to a stressful input mobilizes a neuroendocrine response, which differs somewhat with each individual depending on the stressor, perception of the stressor, and other variables. Those variables that can affect the response are the person's mood, coping styles, and personality, as well as his or her reaction to social support (NCI, 2003c; Barsevick et al., 2000; Shell & Karish, 2001).

Researchers have identified a wide range of stressors that can induce maladaptive psychoneuroimmune responses. These stressors move along pathways that involve the hypothalamus, the pituitary gland, and the sympathetic nervous system (NCI, 2003c). Moreover, physiological responses differ depending on whether the stressor is acute or chronic in nature and the way in which the person copes or adapts to the stressor (Shell & Karish, 2001; Barsevick, 2000).

If a patient's exposure to the stressor becomes more long term, the physiological responses can change from being an acute response to one of habituation. For example, initial increased pulse and sweat rates may gradually resolve and be replaced by increased basal muscle tension. When responding to a stressor during an acute period, individuals may respond in an exaggerated way and have difficulty returning to the prestress state of relaxation. Long term, they may exhibit higher blood pressures, increased sweating, increased respiratory rates and epinephrine levels when compared to nonstressed individuals. Also, over time they may develop mood changes, such as anxiety, depression, and more serious reactions (NCI, 2003c; Winningham, 2000).

SURVIVING CANCER AND PSYCHOSOCIAL ISSUES

Some people may have more difficulty adjusting to the diagnosis of cancer than others. These variations will vary as the patient responds to the diagnosis.

Epidemiologic studies, however, suggest that at least one half of all people diagnosed with cancer will successfully adapt. Markers of successful adaptation include maintaining active involvement in daily life; reaching out for support and resources (including spiritual support); minimizing the disruptions of the illness to one's life roles, such as work, spouse, or parent; regulating the normal emotional reactions to the illness; and managing feelings of hopelessness, helplessness, worthlessness, and/or guilt (Spencer, Carver, & Price, 1998).

Assessment and Screening

As with any sound plan of care, health care professionals can better target their care and interventions with appropriate assessment. Psychosocial concerns are no exception.

The National Comprehensive Cancer Network (NCCN) has the broad goal of establishing standards of care so that all patients experiencing psychosocial distress will be accurately and routinely identified, recognized, and treated. These guidelines include recommendations for screening, triage, and initial evaluation, as well as referral and treatment guidelines for each participating profession: mental health (psychology and psychiatry), social work, palliative care, and pastoral care. Screening methods, using tools to be used by nurses or more specialized mental health professionals, provide the foundation for the patient to be properly identified and treated (NCCN, 2003).

Any assessment time with the patient should incorporate ways to communicate that exhibit trust, expertise, warmth, care, and concern. When discussing psychosocial issues with patients, choose your words wisely. Some words can suggest the stigma of serious mental illness, such as psychiatric, psychological, mental disorder, maladjustment, or mental illness. Experts recommend using less clinical words with patients — words such as distress, concerns, worries, uncertainties, or stressors from the illness or its treatment.

Here are some ways to approach issues of psychosocial distress

- The questionnaire you filled out helps us understand you as a whole person, and we want to provide the best care possible for you — physically, emotionally, socially, and spiritually.

- As you may realize, a serious illness can affect the quality of your life in many ways (emotionally, socially, work, relationships, finances, energy). There is much more to this illness than just the physical, and we want to be sure we are addressing these other dimensions of your life.

- Your concerns and worries are very understandable, given your illness and its treatment. We don't want to ignore the (emotional, social, spiritual) aspects of your experience right now. We have found that many patients benefit greatly from a chance to talk further about their concerns with a (social worker, mental health professional, palliative care specialist, or pastoral counselor), and we would like to schedule that for you (NCI, 2003c; NCI, 2002).

PSYCHOSOCIAL DISTRESS AND ADJUSTMENTS

Most cancer patients do not fit a diagnosis of a serious mental disorder requiring specialized mental health interventions (NIH, 2003c). However, they do experience a variety of emotional responses that can be addressed through a standard approach of psychosocial support and intervention (Shell & Karish, 2001).

To best care for cancer patients going through the continuum of emotional crises and psychological stress, the nurse needs to know the difference between normal adjustment responses and those that are abnormal (for example, major depressive disorder). Table 8-1 lists selected abnormal adjustments, as identified in the *Diagnostic and Statistical Manual of Mental Disorders, Text Revision* (DSM-IV-TR), 4th Edition, (APA, 2000).

Coping Theory — Stages for Cancer Patients

One cognitive model of coping theory is that the woman responds to a significant life event with responses to two questions: 1) Is the event personally significant? and 2) What personal resources can I bring to the event to help me manage it? In asking these two questions, the balance between perception and demand in dealing with the event leads to whether the patient is coping adequately with the situation and distress (NCI, 2003c; Ebright & Lyon, 2002; Barsevick et al., 2000).

Factors That Affect Coping

Many factors affect whether a patient can or is coping with the adjustment to cancer and the situation. Among these are the

- type, stage, and prognosis of the cancer,
- treatment and recovery plan from the cancer,
- patient's intrapersonal coping resources,
- patient's social support,
- developmental stage of life,

TABLE 8-1: DIAGNOSTIC CRITERIA FOR THE ADJUSTMENT DISORDERS

Criterion A. The development of emotional or behavioral symptoms in response to an identifiable stressor(s) occurring within 3 months of the onset of the stressor(s).

Criterion B. These symptoms or behaviors are clinically significant as evidenced by either of the following:

- Marked distress that is in excess of what would be expected from exposure to the stressor.
- Significant impairment in social or occupational (academic) functioning

Criterion C. The stress-related disturbance does not meet the criteria for another specific Axis I disorder and is not merely an exacerbation of a preexisting Axis I or Axis II disorder.

Criterion D. The symptoms do not represent bereavement.

Criterion E. Once the stressor (or its consequences) has terminated, the symptoms do not persist for more than an additional 6 months. Specify:

- Acute if the disturbance lasts less than 6 months.
- Chronic if the disturbance lasts for 6 months or longer.

Specific subtypes represent the predominant symptoms and include:
- with depressed mood
- with anxiety
- with mixed anxiety and depressed mood
- with disturbance of conduct
- with mixed disturbance of emotions and conduct unspecified

Source: American Psychiatric Association. (2000). *Diagnostic and Statistical Manual of Mental Disorders (DSM-IV-TR)*, 4th Edition. Washington, DC: American Psychiatric Association, 2000.

- stigma of the community (viewpoint of cancer),

- timing of the situation (initial diagnosis, treatment phase, post treatment phase, recurrence period).

In general when first diagnosed cancer patients can go through a 3-phase period — initial response (disbelief, denial, shock, numbness, forgetfulness), which can last for 5-7 days; dysphoria including depression, anxiety, insomnia, anorexia, poor concentration, inability to function, lasting for 1-2 weeks; and longer-term adaptation, when coping strategies and styles emerge, allowing the patient to process, feel understood, and develop more frequent feelings of hope and optimism. The adaptation period can last weeks to months (NCI, 2003c; Kessler, 2002; Shell & Karish, 2001). Despite identifying these phases, each patient is different. There is no best approach to response or coping.

Later during treatment, the cavalcade of responses and adjustment can be extensive. The patient mounts responses to fear, apprehension, annoyance, disruptions (in daily activities, life roles), discomforts, and the overall experience of cancer treatment (pain, nausea, fatigue) (NCI, 2003c; Kessler, 2002; Barsevick et al., 2000).

Still after treatment and when the patient is in remission, the patient can be euphoric but also ambivalent. Returning to "the way it was" before treatment is not possible. So uncertainty, anxiety, and worry may appear again, as well as a feeling of losing control. Adjusting to this period is a navigation between positive and negative emotions. The tasks of the patient — with support from the nurse — are to support those emotions and build coping strategies (Swenson et al., 2003; Barsevick et al., 2000; Shell & Karish, 2001). The patient benefits from those who can help her deal honestly with her emotions, and support an awareness of her feelings.

If the patient's cancer recurs and is destined for palliative care, the psychological distress is typically profound. There is much anguish and the patient can suffer from the effects of disease, treatment, and the existential crisis of death. Reactions can be of shock, disbelief, denial, depression, difficulty concentrating, and frequent intrusive thoughts of death, anger, feelings of isolation, and withdrawal.

In time, the patient can make adjustments and accommodations so the emotions are not as intense. Still, the psychosocial needs of these patients are paramount, requiring help with shifting expectations, maintaining hope, spiritual awakening and comfort, mending or renegotiating relationships, and quality of remaining life (NCI, 2003c; Swenson et al., 2003; Barsevick et al., 2000).

SELECTED STUDIES OF CANCER PATIENTS AND THEIR COPING

Participants in various studies about the breast cancer experience describe "going through" a common process that researchers have categorized in phases. Suggested phases are interpreting the diagnosis, confronting mortality, reprioritizing, coming to terms, moving on, and flashing back. These phases were not chronologic and women describe moving back and forth among the categories (Loerzel, 2004; CancerSource, 2000).

During these phases women describe psychosocial aspects of their experience in terms of a phenomenological experience — initial primary concerns of long-term survivors are focused on their biological survival and making the right choices about treatment, including facing mortality, managing symptoms, and prioritizing their lives in order to undergo treatment successfully.

Later, patients' psychosocial issues include focusing on living with the impact of cancer on their lives. Their concerns include managing an altered body image, maintaining relationships, managing the negative reactions of others, coping with infertility, maintaining a balance in their lives, maintaining their jobs and health insurance, and managing their fear of cancer recurrence. With increased survival time, most survivors' concerns about their biological survival became less intense (Loerzel, 2004).

Studies also identify the woman's experiences, described as the "why me" — a searching for meaning of the experience. By seeking and achieving an inward resolve, survivors appear to be better adjusted and able to integrate changes in their lifestyles, perspectives, and social world after cancer. Not all survivors are able to make these adjustments. Some of them are ambivalent about their past and future. They have a vulnerable sense of self. These feelings translate: "I am now mortal, diminished, newly stigmatized, and/or discriminated against by a social and work world." (Loerzel, 2004).

In 2003, Swenson et al., identified main themes that emerged from studying the experience of women surviving with ovarian germ cell cancer. (See Table 8-2 for highlights from the study's results.) The broad themes included celebrating illness, experiencing empathetic affirmation, mourning losses, and valuing illness. These themes indicate that the care of women during their cancer experience requires health care professionals to acknowledge the patient's experience and provide appropriate support in the form of listening, affirmation, and acknowledgment (Swenson et al., 2003).

In a study of women with recurrent breast cancer, significant impairments in physical, functional, and emotional well-being were found within 1 month after recurrence; however, a patient's self-efficacy (confidence in the ability to manage the demands of illness), social support, and family har-

TABLE 8-2: MEANING IN OVARIAN CANCER SURVIVORSHIP

Themes from research with ovarian cancer survivors:

Theme 1: On diagnosis of ovarian cancer, women experience a sense of isolation and struggle to find other women living with the disease.

Theme 2: Prediagnosis symptoms often are ignored, delaying diagnosis of ovarian cancer to its late stages. Women struggle with the question of what if they were diagnosed sooner.

Theme 3: Initially, women may avoid others with ovarian cancer to avoid confronting more advanced disease. Ultimately, these women find significant support through the sisterhood of ovarian cancer. These bonds provide a mixed blessing of opportunity to help others more recently diagnosed while creating anguish in confronting those whose disease is more advanced.

Theme 4: Women with ovarian cancer guide their own treatments, combining conventional and complementary therapies. Alternative therapies often are viewed as less toxic than conventional treatments for symptoms and are seen as offering hope for a cure. Active involvement is a means of exerting control over an uncontrollable disease. Women anxiously await new options.

Theme 5: Ovarian cancer often is an insult to femininity, evoking loss of fertility and sexuality.

Theme 6: Great anguish exists in the genetic legacy of ovarian cancer when women recall the disease of their mothers and grandmothers and fear the future for their daughters.

Theme 7: The trajectory of ovarian cancer includes aggressive, often toxic treatment. Periods of remission and recurrence create the stress and uncertainty of living with this chronic, life-threatening illness.

Theme 8: For many women, the unique experience of ovarian cancer results in a profound appreciation of life and deep meaning.

Note. From "Meaning of illness and spirituality in ovarian cancer survivors." B.R. Ferrell, S.L. Smith, G. Juarez, & C. Melancon, 2003. *Oncology Nursing Forum, 30*(2):249-258.

diness (family's internal strength and ability to manage hardship and change) had positive effects on quality of life. Conversely, more distress about physical symptoms, additional life concerns, a sense of hopelessness, and a negative perception of illness or caregiving were associated with a lower quality of life (Northouse et al., 2002).

For patients who become long-term survivors, their adjustments have the best outcomes when they are supported in their quest to make meaning of their lives, strengthen life and spiritual values, and reprioritize their situations. Those who have poorer periods of adjustment return to anger, depression, anxiety, and other emotions prompted when they were first diagnosed and treated. They, in general, have fewer social supports, economic resources, and more medical problems (NCI, 2003c; Stacey, Degrasse, & Johnston, 2002).

In general, studies of cancer survivors and healthy comparison groups have found no significant differences in measures of psychological distress, marital and sexual adjustment, social functioning, and overall psychosocial functioning. Nevertheless, cancer survivors have been shown to have anxiety about recurrence, increased sense of vulnerability, lowered sense of control, conditioned reminders of chemotherapy (smells, sights), which produce anxiety and nausea, posttraumatic stress-like symptoms, such as persistent, intrusive thoughts, recurrent imagery associated with cancer treatments, feelings of estrangement from others, and concerns about body image and sexuality (NCI, 2002; Shell & Karish, 2001; Barsevick et al., 2002).

ADJUSTMENT DISORDERS

Psychosocial adaptation to cancer is an ongoing coping process, when the patient tries to manage ongoing emotional distress, solve specific cancer-related problems, and gain mastery or control over cancer-related life events. Patients face common periods of crisis, including diagnosis, treatment (surgery, radiation, chemotherapy), posttreatment and remission, recurrence and palliative care, and survivorship. Each period requires the patients to cope and ask particular life-challenging questions. This ongoing coping process prompts particular emotions that require the patient to confront specific problems.

Those patients who can adjust can minimize the stress and distress in their lives and remain active in the tasks of daily living. They find meaning and importance in their lives (NCI, 2003c; Swenson et al., 2003). The patient finds ways to self-regulate and respond — with the support of others and resources — so not to disengage, withdraw, or become hopeless and helpless (NCI, 2003c). A predictor of the ability to cope in crisis is the way the patient has coped — and their predominant coping style — before illness (in other words, optimism, pessimism, introversion, extroversion) (NCI, 2003c; Rawl, Given, Given, Kozachik, Baron, Emsley, et al., 2002; Shell & Karish, 2001).

Prevalence

In the general population, adjustment disorders are common. Prevalence in children, adolescents, and elderly people are estimated at 2-8% (NCI, 2003c). In outpatient mental health settings, estimates of adjustment disorders are 10-30%; while in general hospital inpatients, prevalence rates have been as high as 12% of those referred for a mental health consultation.

Nearly every cancer patient's experiences have elements of an adjustment disorder, whether that is focused on the diagnosis, treatment, recurrence, or adverse effects. One study determined that more than half of the patients in a cancer center could be diagnosed with an adjustment disorder (NCI, 2003c). Yet, the presence of a true adjustment disorder is determined more by the patient's response to the identifiable stressor, and whether that response is more than what would be expected or which would significantly affect functioning (NCI, 2003c; Shell & Karish, 2001; Barsevick et al., 2000).

Among two very common adjustment disorders, which affect cancer patients, are anxiety and depression.

ANXIETY

Anxiety can be a mainstay of the woman's experience during cancer screening, diagnosis, treatment, or recurrence. It can affect the patient's behavior, contributing to depression, pain, nausea, and the patient's quality of life. Although anxiety can be part of a normal adaptation reaction to stress and trauma, it can contribute to the patient's feelings of lack of control. Therefore, interventions to alleviate anxiety are always appropriate (NCI, 2002a). Table 8-3 lists possible causes of anxiety in cancer patients, which serve as risk factors for increased anxiety.

Effective assessment for anxiety includes a thorough evaluation of the patient's experience. The familiar symptoms of anxiety are listed in Table 8-4.

Acute anxiety is an adjustment disorder. When patients develop behavior adjustment disorders, they experience maladaptive methods to offset their anxiety. These behaviors can include severe nervousness, worry, jitteriness, and impairment in normal functioning, such as the inability to work, attend school, or interact with others. In cancer patients, these periods of maladjustment can occur at critical times such as during the diagnostic workup, at diagnosis, or in relapse.

TABLE 8-3: POSSIBLE CAUSES OF ANXIETY

Medical Problem	Examples
Poorly controlled pain	Insufficient or as-needed pain medications.
Abnormal metabolic states	Hypoxia, pulmonary embolus, sepsis, delirium, hypoglycemia, bleeding coronary occlusion, or heart failure.
Hormone-secreting tumors	Pheochromocytoma, thyroid adenoma or carcinoma, parathyroid adenoma, adrenocorticotropic hormone-producing tumors, and insulinoma.
Anxiety-producing drugs	Corticosteroids, neuroleptics used as antiemetics, thyroxine, bronchodilators, beta-adrenergic stimulants, antihistamines, and benzodiazepines (paradoxical reactions often seen in elderly patients).
Anxiety-producing conditions	Substance withdrawal (from alcohol, narcotic analgesics, or sedative-hypnotics).

(NCI, 2003a; Massie, 1989)

TABLE 8-4: SYMPTOMS OF ANXIETY

- Intense fear
- Inability to absorb information
- Inability to cooperate with medical procedures
- Shortness of breath
- Sweating
- Lightheadedness
- Palpitations

TABLE 8-5: COMMONLY PRESCRIBED BENZODIAZEPINES (for cancer patients)

Short-acting	Alprazolam
	Oxazepam
	Lorazepam
	Temazepam
Intermediate-acting	Chlordiazepoxide
Long-acting	Diazepam
	Clorazepate
	Clonazepam

Anxiety-related conditions can include but are not limited to phobias, obsessive-compulsive disorders, and posttraumatic distress disorders. Further specialized interventions — medical and psychological — are appropriate to mobilize. In general, all patients, whether experiencing normal anxiety or adjustment disorders, respond to reassurance, relaxation techniques, low doses of short-acting benzodiazepines (see Table 8-5), and patient support and education programs (NCI, 2003a; Barsevick et al., 2000).

When dealing with patients displaying anxious behaviors, the nurse should keep in mind that acute onset of anxiety may be a precursor to a change in metabolic state or of another impending medical event. These can include myocardial infarction, infection, or pneumonia. Sepsis and electrolyte abnormalities can also cause anxiety symptoms. Sudden anxiety with chest pain or respiratory distress may suggest a pulmonary embolism. Patients who are hypoxic can experience anxiety; they may be fearful that they are suffocating. The patient may also experience a medication reaction that is manifested by motor restlessness, agitation and mania, as well as symptoms of severe depression (NCI, 2003a; Barsevick et al., 2000).

Assessment and Screening

To properly manage anxiety, the nurse begins with an assessment that leads to an accurate diagnosis. The normal fears and uncertainties associated with cancer are often intense. To assess the severity of the anxiety, it is important to understand to what extent the symptoms of anxiety are interfering with the patient's activities of daily living.

Toward establishing an anxiety assessment, Table 8-6 lists questions to help determine the type and severity of the patient's anxiety.

TABLE 8-6: QUESTIONS TO ASSESS ANXIETY

- Have you had any of the following symptoms since your cancer diagnosis or treatment? When do these symptoms occur (for example, how many days prior to treatment, at night, or at no specific time), and how long do they last?

- Do you feel shaky, jittery, or nervous?

- Have you felt tense, fearful, or apprehensive?

- Have you had to avoid certain places or activities because of fear?

- Have you felt your heart pounding or racing?

- Have you had trouble catching your breath when nervous?

- Have you had any unjustified sweating or trembling?

- Have you felt a knot in your stomach?

- Have you felt like you have a lump in your throat?

- Do you find yourself pacing?

- Are you afraid to close your eyes at night for fear that you may die in your sleep?

- Do you worry about the next diagnostic test, or the results of it, weeks in advance?

- Have you suddenly had a fear of losing control or going crazy?

- Have you suddenly had a fear of dying?

- Have you been confused or disoriented lately?

Note. From National Cancer Institute (NCI). (2003a). *Anxiety Disorder.* CancerNet (PDQ®) Web sites for health professionals. Retrieved April 1, 2003, from http://www.cancer.gov/cancerinfo/pdq/supportivecare/depression/healthprofessional/

DEPRESSION

Serious clinical depression has been estimated to be present in 15-25% of all cancer patients (NCI, 2003b; Barsevick, et al., 2000; DeLeeuw, DeGraeff, Ros, Winnubst, Blijham, & Hordijk, 2000). This level of depression should be treated with more than standard support and psychosocial interventions because the symptoms are more acute and last for a longer period of time (NCI, 2003b).

A cancer diagnosis undoubtedly brings fear of death, disbelief, denial, disruption of life plans, changes in body image and self-esteem, changes in social role and lifestyle, and financial and legal concerns. These feelings can last a few days to a few weeks. They may prompt changes in appetite and sleep disturbance, anxiety, and ruminative thoughts (Peterson & Quinlivan, 2002).

Myths concerning cancer exist, such as all people with cancer are depressed. It is worth emphasizing that some level of depression in a person with cancer is normal. Not all treatments are helpful and everyone with cancer does not necessarily face suffering and a painful death. In most cases the feeling of sadness, fear, and grief are normal reactions and transitions to other feelings and emotions over time (NCI, 2003b; Barsevick et al 2000).

Therefore, nurses need to know the difference between symptoms of normal, time-limited symptoms of "depression," and symptoms of "clinical depression." Once depression is diagnosed, treatment can begin — among the options are medication, support, psychotherapy, and counseling (NCI, 2003b; Shell & Karish, 2001). Table 8-7 provides a review of the indicators of depression.

Assessment and Screening

In addition to knowing and identifying patients at risk for depression, as well as knowing symptoms of depression, the nurse can use various assessment tools to determine the level of the patient's depression and possible interventions.

TABLE 8-7: INDICATORS OF DEPRESSION (requiring more focused or involved interventions)
• History of depression
• Weak social support system (not married, few friends, a solitary work environment); evidence of persistent irrational beliefs or negativistic thinking regarding the diagnosis
• More serious prognosis
• Greater dysfunction related to cancer
• A depressed mood for most of the day and on most days
In general, for more than 2 weeks:
• Diminished pleasure or interest in most activities
• Significant change in appetite and sleep patterns
• Psychomotor agitation or slowing
• Fatigue
• Feelings of worthlessness or excessive, inappropriate guilt
• Poor concentration
• Recurrent thoughts of death or suicide.
Note. From National Cancer Institute (NCI). (2003b). *Depression.* CancerNet (PDQ®) Web sites for health professionals. Retrieved April 1, 2003, from http://www.cancer.gov/cancerinfo/pdq/ supportivecare/depression/healthprofessional/

TABLE 8-8: EXAMPLES OF ASSESSMENT QUESTIONS FOR DEPRESSION AND SUICIDE
Depression
• How well are you coping with your cancer? Well? Poor?
• Do you cry sometimes? How often? Ever alone?
• What things do you still enjoy doing?
• Do you feel others would be better off without you?
• Is your pain under control?
• Do you feel you have any control over your care?
• Are you sleeping? Do you spend a lot of time in bed?
• What is your appetite like?
• Can you concentrate on things you want or need to do?
Suicide
• Have you ever had thoughts of not wanting to live or wishing you could hasten your death?
• Have you ever attempted suicide?
• Have you been treated for psychiatric problems before?
• Have you had a problem with alcohol or drugs?
Note. From National Cancer Institute (NCI). (2003b). *Depression.* CancerNet (PDQ®) Web sites for health professionals. Retrieved April 1, 2003, from http://www.cancer.gov/cancerinfo/pdq/ supportivecare/depression/healthprofessional/

Table 8-8 lists examples of questions to include when making a depression assessment.

Approaching the patient in a warm, supportive way is important in establishing a relationship of trust. Sometimes just asking these questions will express concern and increase the likelihood that the patient will be receptive to suggestions for further peer, spiritual, or professional counseling. An example of phrasing follows:

"Many people with cancer sometimes have these feelings. You are not alone. But talking to someone else about them can greatly help. I'd like to suggest that you consider doing that. Would you be willing to talk to someone who has a lot of experience helping people cope with the stress of having cancer?" (NCI, 2003b).

Any depression assessment needs to also include a suicide risk assessment. To determine if a patient is truly suicidal can be difficult. Table 8-9 lists cancer-related risk factors for depression and Table 8-10 reviews issues in suicide specific to cancer patients. One study has reported that more than 90% of patients said they preferred to discuss emotional issues with their physician, even though

TABLE 8-9: CANCER-RELATED RISK FACTORS FOR DEPRESSION

- Depression at time of cancer diagnosis
- Poorly controlled pain
- Advanced stage of cancer
- Additional concurrent life stressors
- Increased physical impairment or discomfort
- Pancreatic cancer
- Being unmarried and having head and neck cancer
- Treatment with certain medications. (See Table 8-11.)
- Metabolic changes
  - Hypercalcemia
  - Sodium/potassium imbalance
  - Anemia
  - Vitamin B_{12} or folate deficiency
  - Fever
- Endocrine abnormalities
  - Hyper- or hypothyroidism
  - Adrenal insufficiency

Note. From National Cancer Institute (NCI). (2003b). *Depression.* CancerNet (PDQ®) Web sites for health professionals. Retrieved April 1, 2003, from http://www.cancer.gov/cancerinfo/pdq/supportivecare/depression/healthprofessional/

TABLE 8-10: RISK FACTORS: SUICIDE IN CANCER PATIENTS

General Risk Factors

- History of psychiatric disorders, especially those associated with impulsive behavior (for example, borderline personality disorders)
- Family history of suicide
- History of previous/prior suicide attempts
- Depression
- Substance abuse
- Recent death of a friend or spouse
- Few social supports

Cancer-Specific Risk Factors

- Oral, pharyngeal, and lung cancers (often associated with heavy alcohol and tobacco use)
- Advanced stage of disease and poor prognosis
- Confusion/delirium
- Inadequately controlled pain
- Presence of deficit symptoms (for example, loss of mobility, loss of bowel and bladder control, amputation, sensory loss, paraplegia, inability to eat and to swallow, exhaustion, fatigue)

Note. From National Cancer Institute (NCI). (2003b). *Depression.* CancerNet (PDQ®) Web sites for health professionals. Retrieved April 1, 2003, from http://www.cancer.gov/cancerinfo/pdq/supportivecare/depression/healthprofessional/

one quarter of them wanted the physician to initiate the topic. The study further quantified that more than one quarter of the patients studied believed that the physician should initiate any discussion of suicide (Detmar, Aaronson, Wever, Muller, & Schornagel, 2000).

Any assessment of depression in cancer patients should also include evaluation of laboratory values, which may show the cause of depression as medical or organic. These values may show electrolyte or endocrine imbalances or nutritional deficits. Medication may also cause symptoms of depression. Examples include steroids and antibiotics. Table 8-11 reviews selected medications that can contribute to depression.

Interventions

Interventions for depression are based upon the severity of symptoms.

Psychiatric consultation, as an intervention, is appropriate when the patient presents with clinical features or behaviors that are beyond the scope of the standard oncology patient care team. An example of such a behavior is suicide ideation. Consider this type of consultation when

- The depressive symptoms are not responding to antidepressant medication after 2-4 weeks of treatment.

- The patient's depressive symptoms are worsening.

TABLE 8-11: POSSIBLE MEDICATION-BASED CAUSES OF DEPRESSION (with a cancer diagnosis) (also see Table 8-9)

Examples of treatment with certain medications.
- Corticosteroids
- Interferon alfa and aldesleukin (interleukin-2, IL-2)
- Methyldopa
- Reserpine
- Barbiturates
- Propranolol
- Some antibiotics (for example, amphotericin B)

Examples of treatment with certain chemotherapeutic agents.
- Procarbazine
- L-Asparaginase
- Interferon alfa
- Interleukin-2

Note. From National Cancer Institute (NCI). (2003b). *Depression.* CancerNet (PDQ®) Web sites for health professionals. Retrieved April 1, 2003, from http://www.cancer.gov/cancerinfo/pdq/supportivecare/depression/healthprofessional/

- The antidepressants are prompting adverse effects or dosing is not regulated.
- The patient's depression is making it difficult to treat the patient's cancer
(NCI, 2003b; Barsevick et al., 2000).

Pharmacologic Intervention

For some patients, antidepressant therapy is the appropriate intervention. Newer antidepressants, such as Zoloft,® Paxil,® Prozac,® or Celexa™, offer the patient quicker effectiveness and reduced adverse effects. Therefore, antidepressant therapy can be a simple, effective means to stop the spiral downward of depression in selected cancer patients. Still antidepressant use with cancer patients is underutilized. As a review, Table 8-12 lists common antidepressants that can be prescribed for cancer patients. Table 8-13 provides factors to take into account when choosing the appropriate antidepressant medication.

TABLE 8-12: COMMON ANTIDEPRESSANTS

Tricyclic antidepressants
- amitriptyline (Elavil®)
- clomipramine (Anafranil®)
- desipramine (Norpramin®)
- doxepin (Sinequan®)
- imipramine (Tofranil®)
- nortriptyline (Pamelor®)

Selective Serotonin Reuptake Inhibitors (SSRIs)
- citalopram (Celexa™)
- fluoxetine (Prozac®)
- fluvoxamine (Luvox®)
- paroxetine (Paxil®)
- sertraline (Zoloft®)

Monoamine Oxidase Inhibitors (MAOIs)
- tranylcypromine (Parnate®)
- phenelzine (Nardil®)

Atypical Antidepressants
- bupropion (Wellbutrin®)
- trazodone (Desyrel®)
- nefazodone (Serzone®)
- mirtazapine (Remeron®)
- maprotiline (Ludiomil®)
- venlafaxine (Effexor®)

Choosing the appropriate antidepressant depends on a patient's medical history and concomitant medical problems, the symptoms referable to depression, any prior responses to antidepressant medications, and the adverse effects associated with the agents available. Possible adverse effects from selected categories of antidepressants are listed in Table 8-14.

Typically antidepressant therapy is most effective when the patient continues treatment for 4-6 months. Tapering of doses is important — approximately 25% per week in most cases. Consult the drug's package information for more specific guidance (NCI, 2003b).

TABLE 8-13: FACTORS TO CONSIDER IN CHOOSING AN ANTIDEPRESSANT FOR ADULT CANCER PATIENTS

Comorbid Medical Conditions	SSRI	TCA	Analeptics	Other
Cardiac history	+	-		+ (a)
Hepatic dysfunction	+ (b)	+	- (e)	
Renal dysfunction (c)				
Glaucoma	+	- (d)		
Neuropathic pain	+	+		

Key:

(-) use of this medication may be a less appropriate choice

(+) use of this medication could relieve the symptom

Notes:

(a) In general, TCAs and analeptics can cause and exacerbate cardiac arrhythmia. SSRIs, bupropion, venlafaxine, and nefazodone are generally less likely to cause cardiac problems. ECGs should be obtained before starting TCA medication, and a cardiologist should be consulted if there is concern for cardiac compromise.

(b) The shorter-acting SSRIs (sertraline and paroxetine) are less problematic than fluoxetine in patients with hepatic dysfunction. There is less potential for adverse drug interactions and fewer problems related to drug accumulation due to a shorter half-life. Sertraline and nefazodone reportedly have less effect on hepatic P450 enzyme activity.

(c) Clinicians should consider whether antidepressant doses and administration schedules require modification for their patients with renal or hepatic insufficiency.

(d) The TCAs are contraindicated in closed-angle glaucoma.

(e) Pemoline should not be used in patients whose liver enzymes are elevated (2 times the upper limit of normal is often used clinically) before starting treatment.

Note. From National Cancer Institute (NCI). (2003b). *Depression.* CancerNet (PDQ®) Web sites for health professionals. Retrieved April 1, 2003, from http://www.cancer.gov/cancerinfo/pdq/supportivecare/depression/healthprofessional/

SOCIAL SUPPORT AND INTERVENTIONS

Many studies have shown that social support helps patients adapt to illness and treatment, particularly for women (Coward, 2003; Stacey et al., 2002; CancerSource, 2000; DeLeeuw et al., 2000). Support is multi-dimensional, translating into support that is psychosocial (providing affective support) or instrumental (programmatic, service-oriented).

Studies have shown that support for cancer patients can be categorized in three areas

1. Patient education (focusing on information control or case management).

2. Coping skills that lead to behavioral and cognitive management of emotions (primarily during treatment).

3. Support groups (focusing on diagnosis, treatment, rehabilitation, and continuing care; identifying, explaining, and expressing) (CancerSource, 2000).

In addition to support of the patient, support groups established for the women's family members (significant others, children) have also been shown to be effective in providing emotional and psychosocial support (Swenson et al., 2003; Petrie et al., 2001; Zahlis, 2001). For example, relaxation

TABLE 8-14: COMMON PHYSICAL ADVERSE EFFECTS FROM ANTIDEPRESSANTS				
Distressing Symptom	**SSRI**	**TCA**	**Analeptics**	**Other**
Fatigue	+ (a)		+	+ (a)
Insomnia (b)		+		+ (b)
Neuropathic pain (c)	+	+		
Opioid side effects	+		+	
Constipation	+		+	
Loss of appetite (weight loss)		+	+	
Akathisia	-	+ (d)	-	
Anxiety	+	+		+ (e)
Dry mouth/stomatitis	+	-	+	

Key:
(-) use of this medication could worsen the symptom
(+) use of this medication could relieve the symptom

Notes:
(a) Although all SSRIs have the potential paradoxical adverse effect of hypersomnia, fluoxetine is particularly activating. Bupropion is also somewhat activating.

(b) Sedating antidepressants are useful for insomnia, either alone or in addition to another antidepressant. Trazodone is often used as a sleep aid in combination with another antidepressant.

(c) Some antidepressants are useful in treating neuropathic pain. The most studied of these are the TCAs, particularly amitriptyline.

(d) The TCAs are the least likely to aggravate an existing condition of akathisia. SSRIs can cause akathisic reactions. Benzodiazepines and propranolol are first-line treatments for akathisia.

(e) Sedating antidepressants are most useful for anxious/agitated patients. These include the TCAs, trazodone, and nefazodone.

SSRI = Selective Serotonin-Reuptake Inhibitors

TCA = Tricyclic Antidepressants

In general, doses should start low and increase slowly. This list does not indicate absolute indications or contraindications for particular medications. A current *Physicians' Desk Reference* or another reliable drug information resource and experience should guide clinical decision-making.

Note. From National Cancer Institute (NCI). (2003b). *Depression.* CancerNet (PDQ®) Web sites for health professionals. Retrieved April 1, 2003, from http://www.cancer.gov/cancerinfo/pdq/supportivecare/depression/healthprofessional/

and counseling interventions have been shown to reduce psychological symptoms in women with a new diagnosis of gynecological cancer (Loerzel, 2004; Petersen & Quinlivan, 2002).

Support comes in many forms — informal, one-on-one among patients, professional (from a nurse or counselor), and group. The benefits of these forms of support are well documented in the literature, reporting that symptom distress,

increased self-concept, and returned sense of control are enhanced (Coward, 2003; Stacey et al., 2002). Education, problem-solving skills, decision-making skills, and clarification of emotions and feelings, are all part of supportive dynamics, no matter what the site of diagnosis or the individual involved (Barsevick et al., 2002).

In addition to face-to-face meetings, phone support and Internet support have gained in use and

TABLE 8-15: SELECTED ON-LINE SUPPORT GROUPS

(Listed on OncoLink, University of Pennsylvania Cancer Center Web site: www.oncolink.upenn.edu)

ACUP
A support list for anyone dealing with adenocarcinoma, identified in any location, for which the primary site cannot be determined.

ADEN-CYST
An unmoderated discussion list for parents, siblings, friends, researchers, and physicians, to discuss clinical and nonclinical issues and advances pertaining to Adenoid Cystic Carcinomas.

ALL-L
A list for Adult Acute Lymphocytic Leukemia.

AML
Acute Myeloid Leukemia Support Group.

BC-SUPPORTERS
Support list for husbands of breast cancer patients.

Bladder-Cancer-Cafe
Bladder cancer support and information group.

BMT-TALK
A moderated mailing list for the discussion of bone marrow transplants.

BRAINTMR List
A forum to discuss topics related to all types of brain tumors, whether benign or malignant.

BREAST-CANCER List
An open discussion list for any issue relating to breast cancer.

CAM-TRIALS
Complementary and Alternative Medicine trials.

CANCER
A general listserv maintained by ACOR (www.acor.org).

CANCER-DEPRESSION
This listserv is for the discussion of depression and cancer.

CANCER-ESP
Informacion para pacientes y sus familiares.

CANCER-FATIGUE
A list for the discussion of fatigue associated with cancer.

CANCER-FERTILITY
For discussion of fertility issues associated with cancer.

CANCER-FR
La liste francophone de support et d'information sur le cancer.

CANCER-HOSPICE
For the discussion of hospice as it relates to cancer patients.

CANCER-PAIN
For discussion of pain related to cancer.

CANCER-SEXUALITY
For discussion of sexual concerns related to cancer.

CA-PATIENTS
Forum for cancer patients.

CAREGIVERS
An unmoderated discussion list for parents, siblings or friends of cancer patients.

CaringKids - For Kids Who Know Someone Who is Ill
For kids who know someone who is ill, offers an open forum where kids may exchange information, share their feelings, and establish friendships with other kids dealing with similar issues.

CPCOS: Cancer Patients Christian Online Support Group

CLL - Chronic Lymphocytic Leukemia
An unmoderated discussion list for patients, family, friends, researchers, and physicians to disucss clinical and nonclinical issues, and advances pertinent to chronic lymphocytic leukemia.

CLL-CN: Canadian Chronic Lymphocytic Leukemia List
An adjunct to the original CLL list, this provides a forum to discuss treatment options for CLL using the Canadian Health system.

CML - Chronic Myelogenous Leukemia
An unmoderated discussion list for patients, family, friends, researchers, and physicians to disucss clinical and nonclinical issues, and advances pertinent to chronic myelogenous leukemia.

COLON CANCER
The stated purpose of the list is to encourage discussion amongst patients of colon cancer, their loved ones, and caregivers. Discussion will be of treatments and the effect of treatments as well as diseases related to colon cancer. The list is unmoderated.

CTCL-MF: Cutaneous T-Cell Lymphoma-Mycosis Fungoides Information/Support List
This list is for patients, family, friends, researchers, and physicians to discuss information pertaining to cutaneous T-cell lymphoma/mycosis fungoides. It includes patient experiences and support as well as information on new research, clinical trials, and discussions of current treatment practices.

EC-GROUP: Esophageal Cancer Discussion Group
A mailing list designed for physicians, patients, and their families to discuss problems, carry on dialogues about the good and bad aspects of any treatment, and offer individual support.

FACING-AHEAD: Helping to face the death of a loved one and its aftermath
Designed to provide support for those who are facing the death of a loved one as well as those who have experienced the death of a loved one. You will find support and help from others who are in the same situation.

GVHD: Graft Versus Host Disease Discussion Group
A moderated list for people who have had a bone marrow transplant and who suffer from graft-versus-host-disease. Anyone touched by GVHD is WELCOME!

GYN-ONC: Gynecologic Cancer Discussion Group
An unmoderated discussion list for patients, family, friends, researchers, and physicians, to discuss clinical and nonclinical issues and advances pertaining to gynecological cancers.

HAIRY-CELL
Hairy-cell leukemia support.

HEAD-NECK-ONC: Head and Neck Cancers On-line Support Group
An unmoderated discussion list for patients, family, friends, researchers, and physicians, to discuss clinical and nonclinical issues and advances pertaining to head and neck cancers.

HEM-ONC — Hematologic Diseases List
An unmoderated discussion list for patients, family, friends, researchers, and physicians to disucss clinical and nonclinical issues and advances pertinent to hematologic malignancies including leukemia, lymphoma, and multiple myeloma.

HODGKIN'S — Hodgkin's Disease List
The purpose of this unmoderated list is to exchange information, stories, hints, tidbits, and anything you can think of between fellow Hodgkin's disease patients.

HODGKINS
Hodgkin's Lymphoma Support Group (hosted by www.acor.org).

HOSPIC-L
The list is intended for all persons interested in discussing hospice care.

IBC — Inflammatory Breast Cancer List
This list is for friendly discussion about inflammatory breast cancer. Membership is primarily for people who have (or who are caring for people who have) IBC, although anyone with a genuine interest is welcome.

IROJC — Internet Radiation Oncology Journal Club
This list, designed for radiation oncologists, features an international board of well-known editors in the field who propose articles for discussion each month.

KIDNEY-ONC
An unmoderated discussion list for patients, family, friends, researchers, and physicians, to discuss clinical and nonclinical issues and advances pertaining to kidney cancer, including renal cell cancer, and transitional cell carcinoma of the renal pelvis.

LARYNX-C: Larynx Cancer On-line Support Group
An unmoderated discussion list for patients, parents, friends, researchers, and physicians, to discuss clinical and nonclinical issues and advances pertaining to cancer of the larynx.

LCL: Lesbian Cancer List
The list is for lesbian and bisexual women (regardless of birth gender) to discuss the impact of cancer in their lives. It is open to women who have or who have had cancer, and/or partners, family, and friends of people with cancer. Health care practioners working in this field are also welcomed.

L-SARCOMA
Liposarcoma support list.

L-M-SARCOMA: Leiomyosarcoma Online Support Group
An unmoderated discussion list for patients, family, friends, researchers, and physicians, to discuss clinical and nonclinical issues and advances pertaining to leiomyosarcoma, a rare form of cancer.

LI-FRAUMENI
This is a support group for people with Li-Fraumeni Syndrome.

LIVER-ONC: Liver Cancer Support Group
An unmoderated discussion list for parents, siblings, friends, researchers, and physicians, to discuss clinical and nonclinical issues and advances pertaining to liver cancers.

continued on next page

TABLE 8-15: SELECTED ON-LINE SUPPORT GROUPS (continued)

LT-SURVIVORS: Long-Term Survivors of Cancer
Long-term survivors of cancer face unique problems. Most will face social challenges (insurance and employment), some will have emotional challenges, and some will have ongoing health problems related to treatment. This discussion group addresses the unique needs of this group.

LUNG-ONC: The Lung Cancer Online Support Group
An unmoderated discussion list for patients, family, friends, researchers, and physicians, to discuss clinical and nonclinical issues and advances pertaining to lung cancers.

LUNG-BAC
A support group for patients with bronchioalveolar carcinoma and their loved ones.

LUNG-NSCLC
A support group for patients with non-small-cell lung cancer and their loved ones.

LUNG-SCLC
A support group for patients with bronchioalveolar carcinoma and their loved ones.

LYMPHEDEMA
An unmoderated discussion list for patients, parents, friends, researchers, and physicians, to discuss clinical and nonclinical issues and advances pertaining to lymphedema.

MaleBC: A Male Breast Cancer Discussion List
An unmoderated discussion list for patients, family, friends, physicians, researchers, and other interested persons to discuss clinical and nonclinical issues pertaining to male breast cancer.

Mantlecell: Mantle Cell Lymphoma Discussion List
Includes those diagnosed with mantle cell lymphoma or their relatives as well as interested health care professionals. Because this is an uncommon form of lymphoma whose treatment is in evolution, many oncologists are unfamiliar with it. The discussions aim to educate and empower all participants regarding all aspects of this disease.

MEDULLOBLASTOMA
List is for parents, patients, and professionals for discussion and support pertaining to Medulloblastoma and Primitive Neuroectodermal Tumor (PNET) brain tumors.

MEL-L: Melanoma Support Group
MEL-L is the melanoma mail list for melanoma patients, their loved ones, caregivers, physicians, and researchers to exchange information and offer support.

MESOTHELIOMA
Mesothelioma online support.

METASTATIC
General support for patients diagnosed with metastatic cancer.

MOL-CANCER — Consumer Discussion Group
Discussion group is open to anyone interested in cancer treatment discussion.

MYELOMA
An unmoderated discussion list for patients, family, friends, researchers, and physicians to discuss clinical and nonclinical issues and advances pertinent to multiple myeloma and other plasma cell neoplasms.

MYELOMA-DR
The purpose of this mailing list is to foster communication between health care professionals specializing in treatment of multiple myeloma.

N-BLASTOMA: Neuroblastoma Discussion Group
An unmoderated discussion list for patients, family, friends, researchers, and physicians, to discuss clinical and nonclinical issues and advances pertaining to neuroblastoma.

NHL-L: Non-Hodgkin's Lymphoma Discussion Group
For non-Hodgkin's lymphoma patients and care givers. Our purpose is to provide support, caring, information about lymphoma, and living with our disease.

O-SARCOMA
Osteosarcoma mailing list.

OVARIAN list
Unmoderated list is provided to support people who wish to discuss ovarian cancer and other ovarian disorders (such as ovarian cysts).

ORAL-ONC
An unmoderated discussion list for patients, family, friends, researchers, and physicians, to discuss clinical and nonclinical issues and advances pertaining to oral cancers.

PANCREAS-ONC: Pancreatic Cancer Support Group
An unmoderated discussion list for patients, friends, researchers, and physicians, to discuss clinical and nonclinical issues and advances pertaining to pancreatic cancer.

PARTB-L
Covers coding, billing, and reimbursement in Medicare, private insurance, and managed care plans. **Please note:** This list is designed to assist the needs of hospital administrators and is not intended for the use of patients.

RARE-CANCER
An unmoderated discussion list to discuss clinical and nonclinical issues and advances pertaining to rare cancers. This includes patient experiences, psychosocial issues, new research, clinical trials, and discussions of current treatment practices.

R-BLASTOMA: Retinoblastoma On-line Support Group
An unmoderated discussion list for patients, family, friends, researchers, and physicians, to discuss clinical and nonclinical issues and advances pertaining to retinoblastoma.

SARCOMA: Sarcoma On-line Support Group
An unmoderated discussion list for patients, parents, friends, researchers, and physicians, to discuss clinical and nonclinical issues and advances pertaining to all sarcomas.

SARCOMA-MED
Medical discussion of sarcoma.

SCAN-BC-LIST
Scandinavian language breast cancer list.

STOMACH-ONC: Stomach Cancer On-line Support Group
An unmoderated discussion list for patients, friends, researchers, and physicians, to discuss clinical and nonclinical issues and advances pertaining to stomach cancer.

THYROID-ONC: Thyroid Cancer On-line Support Group
An unmoderated discussion list for patients, family, friends, researchers, and physicians, to discuss clinical and nonclinical issues and advances pertaining to thyroid cancer.

effectiveness. Table 8-15 lists selected on-line support groups listed on the University of Pennsylvania Cancer care Web site, OncoLink. This list indicates how widespread on-line support avenues have become.

Worth noting, not all patients respond to social support. Studies focusing on multicultural aspects of care have shown that social support and programs for some demographic and racial groups may not be the most effective strategy to provide support (Katapodi, Facione, Miaskowski, Dodd, &

Water, 2002). Therefore, support needs to take into consideration multicultural and racial issues. Most of the research on support techniques and effectiveness have focused on Caucasian patients (Petrie et al., 2002). Because not all patients respond to support groups or counseling, more customized support strategies need to be considered (Dirkson & Erickson, 2002).

Other Support Interventions

Support can take many forms. One example of an ongoing, programmatic form of support is the "Reach to Recovery" program, an American Cancer Society (ACS)-sponsored group, which began in 1969. Anecdotal reports from participants in this program for women recovering from mastectomies indicate that the program continues to be helpful, although no data exists to verify improvement in the participating woman's emotional state.

Exercise intervention programs, such as walking and running, have also been reported to be helpful in rehabilitation by maintaining physical functioning and decreasing emotional distress. Studies on exercise for breast cancer patients have been shown to improve physical functioning and reduce symptom intensity, particularly in regard to fatigue, anxiety, and difficulty sleeping. Quality of life improvements from regular exercise have also been reported in the literature (Blanchard, Courneya, & Laing, 2001).

In addition to support through individual or group settings, individual counseling can offer cognitive and behavioral strategies to alleviate distress from mental, emotional and physical symptoms (Rawl et al., 2002; Stacey et al., 2002; Shell & Karish, 2001).

Complementary and alternative medicine (CAMs), brought to patients through counseling or support groups, have been shown to be effective, based on patients' anecdotal accounts. (See Chapter 10, CAM.) Many of the CAMs can be a form of support, based on cognitive and behavioral interventions. Examples of supportive CAMs include

- Relaxation training
- Biofeedback
- Contingency management
- Problem-solving
- Cognitive restructuring
- Distraction
- Thought stopping
- Coping self-statements
- Mental imagery exercises

(NCI, 2003c)

SUMMARY

Psychosocial issues are important elements of the cancer experience for women, affecting their outlook and ability to cope with their diagnosis and treatment.

Among psychosocial areas of focused study have been quality of life, hope, the search for meaning in the experience, relationship issues, and spirituality. As with other aspects of cancer care, careful assessment of the patient's psychosocial distress can help the nurse provide support for more effective adjustment and coping. Of special concern in oncology practice are the psychosocial disorders of anxiety and depression. Counseling and medication administration can profoundly help the cancer patient. For women, psychosocial support in the form of education, behavioral modification, and individual or group support are vital to a woman's navigation of her cancer experience.

EXAM QUESTIONS

CHAPTER 8

Questions 59-74

59. When responding to a stressor during an acute period, individuals may respond with

    a. higher blood pressures but lower respiratory rates.

    b. higher blood pressure and higher respiratory rates.

    c. lower epinephrine levels and higher blood pressure.

    d. higher epinephrine levels and lower respiratory rates.

60. An individual's ability to cope is affected by

    a. access to the Internet.

    b. computed tomography scan.

    c. hematacrit.

    d. diagnosis.

61. A marker of successful psychosocial adaptation is the

    a. complete blood count.

    b. opinion of the patient's family members.

    c. negative chest x-ray.

    d. maintaining active involvement in daily life.

62. An example of a maladjustment disorder, common in cancer patients, is

    a. obsessive-compulsive disorder.

    b. depression.

    c. addiction.

    d. claustrophobia.

63. According to the *DSM-IV-TR*, a chronic adjustment disorder should last more than

    a. 3 months.

    b. 6 months.

    c. 9 months.

    d. 1 year.

64. Two symptoms of anxiety are

    a. slow breathing, intense fear.

    b. lack of concentration, excessive sleeping.

    c. the inability to absorb information, palpitations.

    d. constipation, binge eating.

65. When assessing a cancer patient for anxiety, an appropriate question is

    a. Have you felt like you have a lump in your throat?

    b. Are you sleeping all the time?

    c. What did you have for lunch?

    d. Where is your leg pain?

66. A short-acting benzodiazepine is

    a. lorazepam.

    b. diazepam.

    c. clorazepate.

    d. chlordiazepoxide.

67. A risk factor for major depression, which suggests a need for further treatment in cancer patients is

    a. developmental stage.

    b. fever.

    c. abdominal pain.

    d. weak social support system.

68. In general, depressive symptoms that need to be assessed and treated last more than

    a. 2 days.

    b. 2 weeks.

    c. 2 months.

    d. 2 years.

69. A medication that can contribute to depression is

    a. Prozac.®

    b. corticosteroid.

    c. Xanax.®

    d. Zantac.®

70. A medical cause of depression can be

    a. hypercalcemia.

    b. hypocalcemia.

    c. hyperkalemia.

    d. hypokalemia.

71. Extra attention to the possibility of suicide in a cancer patient is heightened when during an assessment you hear the patient describe

    a. a family history of suicide.

    b. binge eating.

    c. regularly scheduled prayer.

    d. shortness of breath.

72. An effect of SSRI antidepressants is

    a. diarrhea.

    b. weight gain.

    c. insomnia.

    d. dry mouth.

73. Internet-based support groups are

    a. plentiful and can be specific to a diagnosis or problem.

    b. rare.

    c. mostly for those sophisticated in computer programming.

    d. not effective.

74. Based on many studies of psychosocial support, an effective support group for breast cancer survivors should include time for

    a. product endorsements.

    b. emotional connection.

    c. organization.

    d. complaining.

REFERENCES

American Psychiatric Association. (2000). *Diagnostic and Statistical Manual of Mental Disorders: (DSM-IV-TR), Test Revision,* 4th Edition. Washington, DC: American Psychiatric Association.

Barsevick, A.M., Sweeney, C., Haney, E., & Chung, E. (2002). A systematic qualitative analysis of psychoeducational interventions for depression in patients with cancer. *Oncology Nursing Forum, 29*(1):73-84.

Barsevick, A.M., Much, J., & Sweeney, C. (2000). Psychosocial responses to cancer. In C.H. Yarbro, M.H. Frogge, M. Goodman, & S.L. Groenwald (Eds.), *Cancer Nursing: Principles and Practice* (5th ed.), (pp. 1529-1549). Sudbury, MA: Jones & Bartlett Publishers.

Blanchard, C.M., Courneya, K.S., & Laing, D. (2001). Effects of acute exercise on state anxiety in breast cancer survivors. *Oncology Nursing Forum, 28*(10):1617-1621.

CancerSource. (2000). Breast Cancer: Social Support in Breast Cancer, A brief overview. *CancerSource.* Retrieved April 1, 2003, from http://www.cancersourcemd.com

Coward, D.D. (2003). Facilitation of self-transcendence in a breast cancer support group: II. *Oncology Nursing Forum, 30*(2):291-300.

DeLeeuw, J.R., DeGraeff, A., Ros, W.J., Winnubst, J.A., Blijham, G.H. & Hordijk, G.J. (2000). Negative and positive influences of social support on depression in patients with head and neck cancer: A prospective study. *Psycho-Oncology, 9*(1):20-28.

Detmar, S.B., Aaronson, N.K., & Wever, L.D., Muller, M., & Schornagel, J.H. (2000). How are you feeling? Who wants to know? Patients' and oncologists' preferences for discussing health-related quality-of-life issues. *Journal of Clinical Oncology, 18*(18): 3295-3301.

Dirkson, S. R. & Erickson, J.R. (2002). Well-being in Hispanic and non-Hispanic White survivors of breast cancer. *Oncology Nursing Forum, 29*(5):820-826.

Ebright, P.R., & Lyon, B. (2002). Understanding hope and factors that enhance hope in women with breast cancer. *Oncology Nursing Forum, 29*(3):561-568.

Ferrell, B.R., Smith, S.L., Juarez, G., & Melancon, C. (2003). Meaning of illness and spirituality in ovarian cancer survivors. *Oncology Nursing Forum, 30*(2):249-258.

Halstead, M.T., & Hull, M. (2001). Struggling with paradoxes: The process of spiritual development in women with cancer. *Oncology Nursing Forum, 28*(10):1534-1544.

Katapodi, M.C., Facione, N.C., Miaskowski, C., Dodd, M.J., & Water, C. (2002). The influence of social support on breast cancer screening in a multicultural community sample. *Oncology Nursing Forum, 29*(5):845-852.

Kessler, T.A. (2002). Contextual variables, emotional state and current and expected quality of life in breast cancer survivors. *Oncology Nursing Forum, 29*(7):1109-1116.

Lacey, M. (2002). The experience of using decisional support aids by patients with breast cancer. *Oncology Nursing Forum, 29*(10):1491-1497.

Loerzel, V.W. (2004). Support and survivorship issues. In K. Dow (Ed.), *Contemporary Issues in Breast Cancer* (2nd ed.), (pp. 313-322). Sudbury, MA: Jones & Bartlett Publishers.

Massie, M.J. (1989). Anxiety, panic and phobias. In J.C. Holland, & J.H. Rowland (Eds.), *Handbook of Psycho-oncology: Psychological Care of the Patient with Cancer* (pp. 300-309). New York: Oxford University Press.

National Cancer Institute (NCI). (2003a). Anxiety Disorder. CancerNet (PDQ®) Web sites for health professionals. Retrieved April 1, 2003, from http://www.cancer.gov/cancerinfo/pdq/supportivecare/depression/healthprofessional/

National Cancer Institute (NCI). (2003b). *Depression.* CancerNet (PDQ®) Web sites for health professionals. Retrieved April 1, 2003, from http://www.cancer.gov/cancerinfo/pdq/supportivecare/depression/healthprofessional/

National Cancer Institute (NCI). (2003c). *Normal Adjustment, Psychosocial Distress, and the Adjustment Disorders.* CancerNet (PDQ®) Web sites for health professionals. Retrieved May 1, 2003, from http://www.cancer.gov/cancerinfo/pdq/supportivecare/adjustment/healthprofessional

National Cancer Institute (NCI). (2002). Support groups may boost quality of life, not survival. Retrieved May 1, 2003, from http://www.cancer.gov/clinicaltrials/developments/support-groups0102

NCCN Practice Guidelines in Oncology: Distress Management. (2003). National Comprehensive Cancer Network. Retrieved July 3, 2003, from http://www.nccn.org/physician_gls/f_guidelines.html

Northouse, L.L., Mood, D., Kershaw, T., Schafenacker, A., Mellon, S., Galvin, E., et al. (2002). Quality of life of women with recurrent breast cancer and their family members. *Journal of Clinical Oncology, 20*(19):4050-4064.

Petrie, W., Logan, J., & Degrasse, C. (2001). Research review of the supportive care needs of spouses of women with breast cancer. *Oncology Nursing Forum, 28*(10):1601-1607.

Petersen, R.W., & Quinlivan, J.A. (2002). Preventing anxiety and depression in gynecological cancer: A randomised controlled trial. *British Journal of Obstetrics & Gynecology, 109*(4):386-94.

Rawl, S.M., Given, B.A., Given, C., Champion, V.L., Kozachik, S.L., Barton, D., Emsley, C.L. & Williams, S.D. (2002). Intervention to improve psychological functioning for newly diagnosed patients with cancer. *Oncology Nursing Forum, 29*(6):967-975.

Shell, J.A., & Karish, S. (2001). Psychosocial Care. In S. Otto (Ed.), *Oncology Nursing* (4th ed.), (pp. 948-972). St. Louis, MO: Mosby, Inc.

Spencer, S.M., Carver, C.S., & Price, A.A. (1998). Psychological and social factors in adaptation. In J.C. Holland, W. Breitbart, & P.B. Jacobsen, (Eds.), *Psycho-Oncology,* (pp. 211-222). New York: Oxford University Press.

Stacey, D., DeGrasse, C., & Johnston, L. (2002). Addressing the support needs of women at high risk for breast cancer: Evidence-based care by advanced practice nurses. *Oncology Nursing Forum, 29*(6). Retrieved May 1, 2003, from www.ons.org/forum/

Swenson, M.M., MacLeod, J.S., Williams, S.D., Miller, A.M., & Champion, V.C. (2003). Quality of living among ovarian germ cell cancer survivors: A narrative analysis. *Oncology Nursing Forum, 30*(3):380. Retrieved May 1, 2003, from http://ons.org/xp6/ONS/Library.xml/ONS_Publications.xml/ONF.xml

Winningham, M. (2000). *Fatigue in Cancer.* CancerSource. Retrieved March 1, 2003, from http://www.cancersourcemd.com

Zahlis, E.H. (2001). The child's worries about the mother's breast cancer: Sources of distress in school-age children. *Oncology Nursing Forum, 28*(6):1019-1025.

CHAPTER 9

SEXUALITY: WOMEN WITH CANCER

CHAPTER OBJECTIVE

After completing this chapter on sexuality issues, the reader will be able to discuss psychologic, functioning, and fertility associated with sexuality in women with cancer and identify interventions to address these issues.

LEARNING OBJECTIVES

After studying this chapter, the reader will be able to

1. recognize two stresses that affect a woman's sexuality when diagnosed with cancer.

2. cite two psychological factors that affect a woman's ability to cope, thus affecting her sexuality.

3. identify two treatments that can affect the woman's sexual functioning.

4. recognize two chemotherapy agents that can adversely affect the woman's fertility.

5. list three medications that can affect a woman's sexuality.

6. identify two questions to ask during a sexual assessment.

7. describe two interventions to support women with cancer.

INTRODUCTION

Sexuality is defined by each patient and his/her partner within a context of gender, age, personal attitudes, and religious and cultural values (NCI, 2003). We know that sexuality is an important component to quality of life no matter what the age, experience, or status in life (NCI, 2003; Bedell, 2000). When a woman faces a serious illness such as cancer, her sexuality is affected in many ways.

This chapter reviews issues related to women with cancer and their sexuality. Those issues are framed as psychological and affect the ability of the woman to cope with changes to her sexuality, sexual functioning and, for those women still in the reproductive phase, her fertility.

As with any issue that patients face, nurses can support them by approaching their sexual assessment in a competent, open, and caring manner. This chapter will review strategies of assessment and briefly review interventions that can help patients face sexuality issues.

PSYCHOLOGICAL ASPECTS

A person's sexuality is part of being normal (Buckman, 2001; Griffo, Branas, Cheville, & Packel, 2000). Sexuality is an integral part of our personalities and life roles. With cancer patients, it can be a powerful distraction to pain and misery, offering a means of human contact, intimacy, or escape (NCI, 2003; CancerSource, 2001a).

Because the diagnosis of cancer inevitably increases stress for the woman, her sexuality is a major target of that stress. Relationships can be strained — both for the patient and her partner. The patient can be experiencing pain, hair loss, nausea, or profound fatigue. Fear, uncertainty, grief, and depression can contribute to or accompany a person's normal sexual feelings, libido, or coping response (NCI, 2003; Buckman, 2001; Stead et al., 2001; Bedell, 2000).

Cancer and its treatments affect a woman's emotional equilibrium, her body image, and sense of attractiveness (Krebs, 2000). Study data suggests that younger women are generally more distressed psychologically by changes in sexuality than are older women (CancerSource, 2001b).

One of the most important factors in adjustment after being diagnosed with cancer is the person's feelings about his or her sexuality prior to cancer (CancerSource, 2001a; Krebs, 2000). Whatever the past experience, exploring sexuality issues during diagnosis and treatment is a prime opportunity to help women deal with their sexuality here and now (NCI, 2003; Stead et al., 2001).

A cancer diagnosis and treatment can affect sexual desire, and cause vaginal dryness or weight gain or loss (NCI, 2003; Krebs, 2000; Bruner & Iwamoto, 2000). Especially with surgeries, such as mastectomies or colonoscopies, the woman may think of herself as mutilated, inadequate, and unappealing (Buckman, 2001, CancerSource, 2001a; Krebs, 2000).

In addition, the woman's partner brings his or her own issues of concern — fear of losing the partner to cancer, coping with physical changes, concern about getting the cancer from the woman during intercourse, and general attitudes toward the changes that a cancer diagnosis brings to the situa-

tion (changing roles, income, attitudes). Strained relations before the woman is diagnosed with cancer can only be exacerbated with a cancer diagnosis, affecting the patient's sexual health (NCI, 2003; Buckman, 2001; CancerSource, 2001b; Bedell, 2000).

In addition to a partner losing interest in sex, both the woman and her partner may believe, although incorrectly, that past sexual activity, an extramarital affair, a sexually transmitted disease, or an abortion has caused their cancer. And some believe, again incorrectly, that sexual activity may promote a recurrence of their cancer (CancerSource, 2001a; Bedell, 2000).

This misconception is especially common in individuals with a malignancy of the pelvic or genital area. For example, women with squamous cell carcinoma of the cervix have read or been told that this cancer is associated with the sexually transmitted human papilloma virus (HPV). (See Chapter 5, Cervical Cancer.) Information is the best antidote to this guilt — in this case, the emphasis on accuracy is important — the virus is transmittable through sexual contact, not the cancer (CancerSource, 2001a).

As reviewed in Chapter 8, Psychosocial Issues, depression can be prevalent in cancer patients (estimated that 15-25% of cancer patients suffer from depression). With depression, a common presenting symptom is loss of sexual desire (NCI, 2003). In some cases, patients will identify sexual dysfunction as the problem, when it is a secondary effect of depression. Thus appropriate assessment and treatment of the patient's condition should follow — if it is depression, treat it. If the loss of desire is an adverse effect of antidepressant therapy, also treat this symptom (NCI, 2003; Krebs, 2000; Griffo et al., 2000). Always, offer support — it is key to the patient's ability to cope. (Table 9-1 lists coping with changes that affect sexuality. Also see Chapter 8.)

TABLE 9-1: COPING WITH CHANGES THAT AFFECT SEXUALITY

- Focus on physical recovery, including diet and physical activities.
- Ask your physician or nurse about maintaining or resuming sexual activity.
- Include your partner in discussions.
- Discuss fertility and birth control with your physician.
- Report vaginal discharge or bleeding, fever, or pain to your physician or nurse.
- Choose a time for intimacy when you and your partner are rested and free from distractions.
- Create a romantic mood.
- Try different positions until you find one that is more comfortable and less tiring for you.
- Use a water-soluble lubricant (Astroglide, K-Y jelly, Lubrin), if needed.
- Use pain medications, if needed.
- Remember that cancer is not contagious.
- Remember that being intimate will not make the cancer come back or grow.
- Remember that your partner is also affected by your cancer, so talk about both of your feelings and fears.
- Explore different ways of showing love (hugging and holding, stroking and caressing, talking).
- If needed, find humor where you can.

Note. From CancerSource. Ovarian Cancer: Sexuality and the Woman with Cancer. Retrieved May 1, 2003, from http://www.cancersource md.com

ISSUES OF FUNCTIONING AND TREATMENT

Sexual functioning can be at the core of problems related to sexuality related to cancer treatment. Table 9-2 reviews some of these changes, based on the diagnosis or treatment that can affect sexual functioning.

TABLE 9-2: SELECTED CAUSES OR SOURCES OF SEXUAL DYSFUNCTION RELATED TO CANCER TREATMENT

Chemotherapy
Loss of desire and decreased frequency of intercourse
Nausea, vomiting
Diarrhea, constipation
Mucositis
Weight changes (gain or loss)
Altered sense of taste and smell
Alopecia
Vaginal dryness
Dyspareunia
Reduced ability to reach orgasm

Estrogen deprivation
Vaginal atrophy
Thinning of the vulvar tissues and vagina
Loss of tissue elasticity
Decreased vaginal lubrication
Hot flashes
Increased frequency of urinary tract infections
Mood swings
Fatigue
Irritability

Surgery
Sexual and urinary dysfunctions (after resection for rectal cancer)

Pain from pelvic surgeries including hysterectomy/oophorectomy, cystectomy, vulvectomy, and abdominoperineal resection

Radiation
Fatigue
Nausea and vomiting
Diarrhea
Vaginal stenosis and vascular fibrosis

Other issues
Catheter placement and interference

One researcher estimated that more than 90% of women with cancer may experience sexual dysfunction, especially related to the body site of diagnosis (CancerSource, 2001a). Sexual dysfunction is associated with many types of cancer and cancer therapies. Moreover, researchers have estimated that sexual dysfunction from various treatments affect 40-100% of patients not only during their treatments but after as well (NCI, 2003; CancerSource, 2001b).

Even if sexual functioning is disrupted, the majority of patients can be treated effectively (CancerSource, 2001b; Krebs, 2000; Bedell, 2000). Several predictors of postoperative sexual functioning include the patient's age, premorbid sexual and bladder functioning, tumor location, tumor size, and the extent of surgical resection (NCI, 2003).

These changes in functioning may not resolve quickly and can linger for years, well after the woman is considered a survivor of her cancer (NCI, 2003; CancerSource, 2001; Bedell, 2000). In studying women with cancer, researchers have most frequently looked at the experience of breast and gynecological cancer patients (NCI, 2003; CancerSource, 2001; Krebs, 2000; Bedell, 2000).

TREATMENTS AND THEIR EFFECTS

Women with cancer face various issues related to their sexuality. Each treatment modality has the potential to cause changes in sexual functioning.

Fertility Issues

Sterility can be related to a number of factors including the individual's gender, age at the time of treatment, type of therapeutic agent, total dose, single versus multiple agents, and length of time since treatment. Not all women are profoundly affected by fertility challenges, but many women — despite not wanting to bear children — can find these changes emotionally distressful. Thus, the woman may be anxious, depressed, and grieving with the changes to her fertility. Treatment-generated changes stem from chemotherapy administration and radiation therapy.

Chemotherapy

Studies have found that patients who are age 35-40 are most susceptible to changes in their ovarian function due to chemotherapy. The ovaries of younger women can tolerate greater doses, although clear predictors of outcomes and failure are not well defined (CancerSource, 2001a; Bedell, 2000).

Alkylating agents have been shown to be particularly damaging to fertility. They include busulfan, melphalan, cyclophosphamide, nitrosureas, cisplatin, chlorambucil, mustine, carmustine, lomustine, cytarabine, and procarbazine (NCI, 2003).

For women treated for breast cancer, studies indicate that chemotherapy-induced premature ovarian failure occurs in approximately 63-85% of women (NCI, 2003). The alkylating chemotherapeutic agents — cyclophosphamide (cumulative dose 5.2 grams) — is the primary cause of ovarian failure (NCI, 2003). Table 9-3 provides a list of chemotherapy agents that can affect sexuality related to ovarian function.

Radiation Therapy

For women, no matter what age, a dose of 5-20 Gy administered to the ovary can completely impair gonadal function. In 60% of women younger than age 26, a dose of 30 Gy can provoke premature menopause (NCI, 2003).

The factors that determine ovarian failure include menstrual and reproductive history, measurements of serum hormone levels, and clinical evidence of ovarian function.

To protect the ovaries during high-dose radiation therapy, shielding the ovaries by moving them

TABLE 9-3: SELECTED CHEMOTHERAPY AGENTS THAT AFFECT SEXUALITY

Agent	Effect
Busulfan Cyclophosphamide Melphalan 5FU Methotrexate Doxorubicin Vincristine Vinblastine Procarbazine Estrogens Progestins	Amenorrhea, decreased libido, ovarian dysfunction
Corticosteroids	Irregular menses, acne

out of the field of radiation (ovariopexy) — either laterally, toward the iliac crest, or behind the uterus — may help preserve fertility. Despite shielding, 5-10% of the ovary can be irradiated (NCI, 2003).

Pregnancy

For women diagnosed and treated for their cancer who carry pregnancies to term, the outcomes have not shown any increase in genetically mediated birth defects, birth weight effects, and sex ratios (CancerSource, 2001a). Thus it has been shown that some individuals treated with cytotoxic chemotherapy can remain fertile and are not at an increased risk of having children with genetic abnormalities.

Based on several studies over the past 10 years, data has shown that some women having children after breast cancer treatment can survive equally as well as women who do not have a subsequent pregnancy (NCI, 2003). So pregnancy does not necessarily have an adverse impact on the clinical course of disease (CancerSource, 2001a).

Many of these studies looked at the experience of pregnancy as well as parenthood. Major concerns of study subjects during pregnancy were (a) living long enough to see their child grow up, (b) receiving proper treatment for their breast cancer,

(c) their breast cancer worsening with pregnancy, (d) the potential future effects of chemotherapy on their child, and (e) the possibility of having to terminate their pregnancy. Subjects were least concerned about what other people would say about their breast cancer diagnosis and decision to become pregnant (CancerSource, 2001a).

Preserving the Ability to Reproduce

Because cancer and its treatment can permanently affect the woman's ability to reproduce, some patients of reproductive age may want to preserve their reproductive options. These options may not be appropriate for all patients. Counseling is an important part of the decision-making process for patients. The struggle to take on their cancer and the following treatment period can be enough stress for many women. To keep reproductive options open, patients need to consider costs, stress, time, emotions, and potential inclusion of another individual in the pregnancy process (in other words, a surrogate) (NCI, 2003; Bedell, 2000; Gossfeld, 2000).

Cryopreservation is an option that can preserve ovarian tissue (follicles and embryos). As part of exploring options of maintaining reproduction for patients, oncology professionals may want to discuss reproductive cell and tissue banking with their cancer patients. To offer the best preparation and strategies, the patient may be referred to a reproductive endocrinologist before chemotherapy and/or radiation (NCI, 2003; Gossfeld, 2000).

Keep in mind that these processes can be expensive and further in vitro fertilization procedures do not guarantee a child (NIC, 2003). One study with a limited sample size, reported that the oocytes from patients with malignant disorders were of a poorer quality and exhibited a significantly impaired fertilization rate compared to age-matched controls (NCI, 2003).

MEDICATION FACTORS

Various common medications can affect sexual function that may be prescribed for women undergoing treatment or during the follow-up period for their malignancies. Medications may adversely affect one or more of the physiologic mechanisms (vascular, hormonal, neurologic) that underlie normal sexual function, as well as affect mental alertness, mood state, and/or social interactions (NCI, 2003). Table 9-4 lists medications that can affect sexuality or sexual function.

Patients may be on multiple medications that can cause diminished desire or other difficulties in sexual functioning, which can add to the impact of surgery, radiation, and chemotherapy on sexuality (NCI, 2003).

ASSESSMENT

Too often, health care professionals ignore the issues of sexuality when caring for patients (Reuters, 2001). To offset these practices, a standard, thorough approach to assessment when dealing with patients is important.

Any assessment should take into account the patient's demographic and diagnostic information that may influence sexuality. This information can include gender, age, socioeconomic status, education level, cultural and ethnic background, diagnosis and treatment, concomitant medical and psychiatric problems, and medications (NCI, 2003; Krebs, 2000; Bedell, 2000).

One of the acronyms used to organize a sexual assessment and plan for intervention is the P-LI-SS-IT model, which represents the levels of Permission, Limited Information, Specific Suggestion, and Intensive Therapy (NCI, 2003). The tone and setting of assessment can be as important as the questions asked. The goal is to build trust in the patient and protect confidentiality. The nurse should also be aware of verbal and non-

TABLE 9-4: MEDICATIONS THAT AFFECT SEXUAL RESPONSE

- Endocrine medications (hormones)
- Antihypertensive drugs
- Diuretics
- Antipsychotics
- Anti-anxiety drugs
- Narcotics
- Cocaine
- Hallucinogens
- Antidepressants
- Sedatives and hypnotics
- Beta blockers

verbal communication that can influence data gathered on sexual health such as self-esteem and body image (NCI, 2003; Krebs, 2000; Bedell, 2000).

Another acronym for organizing an assessment is B-E-T-T-E-R. This stands for *B*ring up topics so the patient knows sexuality can be discussed; *E*xplain concern about all aspects of the patient's life; *T*ell the patient that sexual dysfunction can occur and that resources are available; *T*iming of sexual issue discussions during a visit or over many visits; *E*ducate patients about adverse effects of treatment; *R*ecord assessments and interventions (Mick, Cohen, & Hughes, 2003).

A common strategy of assessment is to move from less sensitive to more sensitive issues. One line of questioning is as follows:

1. Has your role as a parent, spouse, or intimate friend changed since you were diagnosed with or treated for cancer?

2. Do you feel different about yourself or your body since you were diagnosed with or treated for cancer?

3. Has your sexual functioning changed (or do you think it will change) due to your diagnosis

or cancer treatment? [If yes] How has it/will it change?

Many tools are available to establish or guide a sexual health history and assessment. For women with cancer, these tools review the impact of the cancer diagnosis on the patient as well as issues of functioning, relationships, arousal and activity level. Tools should take into account the partner's sexuality issues, also (Bruner & Iwamoto, 2000; Krebs, 2000; Bedell, 2000).

INTERVENTIONS

Many guidelines can address sexuality during the stages of disease and its treatment. When therapeutic decisions are being made, health care providers should always offer education and information to their patients (NCI, 2003; Bruner & Iwamoto, 2000, Krebs, 2000).

Health care providers can help educate couples by offering practical suggestions to overcome changes in responsiveness to sexual stimulation. Couples should allow plenty of time for sexual expression with sufficient foreplay to develop the fullest possible sexual arousal.

Health care providers need to reassure patients and their significant others that even when intercourse is difficult or impossible, their sex lives are not over. Couples can give and receive pleasure and satisfaction by expressing their love and intimacy with their hands, mouths, tongues, and lips. Health care providers should encourage couples to express affection in alternative ways (hugging, kissing, nongenital touching) until they feel ready to resume sexual activity. Couples should be encouraged to communicate honest feelings, concerns, and preferences (NCI, 2003).

For some couples, early morning may be a good restful time for sexual expression. Conditions that facilitate sexual pleasure should be explored and may include relaxation, dreams, fantasy, deep breathing, and recalling positive experiences with the partner (NCI, 2003; CancerSource, 2001a; Griffo et al., 2000; Bruner & Iwamoto, 2000; Krebs, 2000).

More specific information for the evaluation and treatment of female sexual dysfunction including painful intercourse (dyspareunia), vaginismus, inhibited orgasm, sexual arousal, and desire disorders is available in other resources (NCI, 2003; Bruner & Iwamoto, 2000).

Specific suggestions are included as nursing interventions for phase-specific problems. However, whenever an identified problem is beyond the realm of expertise for the nurse, a referral should be made to an appropriate therapist (NCI, 2003; CancerSource, 2000; Krebs, 2000; Bedell, 2000). Lubricants, appliances, and medications are available to help women with functioning

---

TABLE 9-5: STRATEGIES FOR HELPING WOMEN WITH SEXUAL FUNCTION

Lubricants (vaginal dryness and irritation)

- Vaginal moisturizers (for example, Replens)
- Water-based lubricants (for example, Astroglide and K-Y Liquid)
- Estradiol-releasing vaginal ring (Estring)*, containing a slow-release preparation, 2 mg micronized 17beta-estradiol, may also provide a less risky alternative to systemic estrogen replacement
- 25-mcg 17beta-estradiol vaginal tablet (Vagifem)*
- Conjugated equine estrogen vaginal cream (Premarin)* (relieving symptoms of atrophic vaginitis)

Exercises

- Kegel exercises

Appliances

- Vaginal dilators

* Check with physician, based on controversies with hormone replacement therapies

issues related to their sexuality. Some of these strategies are listed in Table 9-5.

NOTE: Some interventions suggest hormone replacement therapy (HRT) to offset sexually-related adverse effects from the disease or treatment. HRT can mitigate the effects of osteoporosis and cardiovascular disease, but its use in women with a history of breast cancer is considered controversial. In addition, women taking HRT have a slightly elevated risk of endometrial cancer. (See Chapter 3, Endometrial Cancer.)

SUMMARY

Sexuality in a woman's life is important no matter what her age, experience, or status in life. Women with a cancer diagnosis need information about how their cancer and its treatment phases will affect sexuality. Any effort to support the woman with information or tools to optimize functioning should be preceded by a thorough, sensitive assessment. Above all, support about these issues helps her and her partner cope with changes in her sexuality, sexual functioning, and the impact of cancer on her fertility.

EXAM QUESTIONS

CHAPTER 9

Questions 75-84

75. When a woman is diagnosed with cancer, examples of stresses that can affect her sexuality are

    a. fear, uncertainty, grief, depression.

    b. changes in relationships and changes in roles.

    c. support and education.

    d. time and distance.

76. A major psychological factor, affecting her ability to cope as well as her sexuality, is

    a. body image.

    b. insurance coverage.

    c. time management.

    d. children.

77. A woman's sexual function can be affected by

    a. her reading level.

    b. her participation in support groups.

    c. dryness during intercourse.

    d. her vision.

78. Studies indicate that chemotherapy-induced premature ovarian failure can occur in as many as

    a. 20-33% of women.

    b. 35-42% of women.

    c. 43-60% of women.

    d. 63-85% of women.

79. A woman receiving chemotherapy as treatment for breast cancer

    a. can never have a healthy child.

    b. can never get pregnant.

    c. may be able to get pregnant.

    d. should avoid getting pregnant during treatment.

80. A chemotherapy agent that can affect a woman's sexuality is

    a. cyclophosphamide.

    b. cisplatin.

    c. epoeitin.

    d. leukovorin.

81. A medication class, which can affect a woman's sexuality is

    a. antihypertensives.

    b. multivitamins.

    c. antihistamines.

    d. aspirin.

82. During a sexual assessment, a first step, initial question to ask would be

    a. What are you expecting from treatment, which may affect your sexuality or sexual function?

    b. How often do you engage in sexual activity?

    c. When can I talk with your partner about your sexual relations?

    d. What medications do you now take, that affect your sexual functioning?

157

83. To best support a woman with cancer, the nurse can offer

    a. analgesics.

    b. materials about religion.

    c. education about her diagnosis, treatment, and adverse effects.

    d. a second opinion.

84. To help a woman with vaginal dryness, recommend

    a. oil-based lubrication.

    b. water-based lubrication.

    c. rest.

    d. heat.

REFERENCES

Bedell, C. (2000). Sexuality, body image and cancer. In B. Nevidjon, & B.K. Sowers (Eds.), *A Nurse's Guide to Cancer Care* (pp. 272-283). Philadelphia: Lippincott.

Bruner, D.W., & Iwamoto, R.R. (2000). Altered sexual health. In S.L. Groenwald, M.H. Frogge, M. Goodman, & C. Yarbro. *Cancer Symptom Management,* (2nd ed.), Sudbury, MA: Jones & Bartlett Publishers.

Buckman, R. (2001). Coming to Terms With Sexual Relationship Problems. CancerSource. Retrieved May 1, 2003, from http://www.cancer sourcemd.com

CancerSource. (2000). Nursing Assessment of Sexual Dysfunction. CancerSource. Retrieved May 1, 2003, from http://www.cancer sourcemd.com.

CancerSource. (2001a). Ovarian cancer: Sexuality and the woman with cancer. CancerSource. Retrieved May 1, 2003, from http://www.cancer sourcemd.com

CancerSource. (2001b). Uterine Cancer: Sexuality and the woman with cancer. CancerSource. Retrieved May 1, 2003, from http://www.cancer sourcemd.com.

Gossfeld, L. (2000). Cervical cancer: Introduction to sexuality and fertility issues. CancerSource. Retrieved May 1, 2003, from http://www.cancer sourcemd.com

Griffo, C.L., Branas, A., Cheville, A., & Packel, L. (2000). About gynecologic cancer and sexuality. OncoLink, University of Pennsylvania Cancer Center. Retrieved May 1, 2003, from http://www.oncolink.com.

Krebs, L. (2000). Sexual and reproductive dysfunction. In C.H. Yarbro, M.H. Frogge, M. Goodman, & S.L. Groenwald (Eds.), *Cancer Nursing: Principles and Practice* (5th ed.), (pp. 831-854). Boston: Jones & Bartlett Publishers.

Mick, J., Cohen, M.A., & Hughes, M. (2003). Sexuality and cancer: How oncology nurses can address BETTER [Abstract #180]. ONS 28th Annual Congress. *Oncology Nursing Forum, 30*(2):70.

National Cancer Institute (NCI). (2003). Sexuality and reproductive issues. CancerNet (PDQ®) Web sites for health professionals. Retrieved March 1, 2003, from http://www.cancer.gov/cancerinfo/pdq/supportivecare/sexuality/Health Professional#Section_1

Reuters Health Information (2001). *Physicians urged to address sexual problems of ovarian cancer patients* (published 10/12/2001). Retrieved March 1, 2003 from http:/www.reuters.com

Stead, M.L., Fallowfield, L., Brown, J.M., & Selby, P. (2001). Communication about sexual problems and sexual concerns in ovarian cancer: qualitative study. *British Medical Journal, 323*(7317) 836-837.

CHAPTER 10

COMPLEMENTARY AND ALTERNATIVE MEDICINE

CHAPTER OBJECTIVE

After completing this chapter on complementary and alternative medicine (CAM), the reader will be able to discuss why cancer patients seek out CAM options, list some common CAMs, and identify ways to evaluate their merit and usefulness.

LEARNING OBJECTIVES

After studying this chapter, the reader will be able to

1. recognize motivations for cancer patients to try CAMs.

2. identify established CAMs.

3. list CAMs that are being studied through research coordinated by the National Center for Complementary and Alternative Medicine (NCCAM) or other clinical trial sites.

4. list criteria that the research community uses to evaluate CAMs.

5. list questions that patients can ask when evaluating CAM effectiveness.

6. list criteria to evaluate CAM-related Web sites.

INTRODUCTION

No discussion of cancer in women is complete without addressing the attraction and use of CAMs for treatment of adverse effects.

Complementary, as the word implies, refers to methods used with conventional treatment to augment treatment or lessen a treatment's adverse effects (for example, aromatherapy used after surgery to reduce discomfort) (NIH, 2003; NCI, 2002). The term alternative medicine is used in place of conventional medical treatments. For example, patients may use a special diet as a component of their treatment for cancer instead of undergoing conventional surgery, radiation, or chemotherapy (NCI, 2003; NCCAM, 2001).

To date, no CAM has been proven universally effective to treat cancer, based on scientific method and criteria such as double-blind placebo-controlled studies (NCI, 2003; NCCAM. 2001). But for many patients, they offer profound benefits, especially when integrated with a total approach to patient treatment and care (Creagan, 2003; Harpham, 2001; Ades & Yarbro, 2000).

Claims and testimonials abound about the merits and effectiveness of CAMs (Lengacher et al., 2002; Jordan & Delunas, 2001; NCCAM, 2001; Rosenthal & Ades, 2001). The advantages and issues that are relevant when considering CAMs are reliability, their ability to integrate with standard treatment protocols, and the benefits they offer in better quality of life for the patient (NCI, 2003; Harpham, 2001; Lerner, 2002). Based on many surveys of CAM use, few cancer patients confront their disease — especially women — without hearing about and trying many of the variations of

TABLE 10-1: SELECTED COMPLEMENTARY AND ALTERNATIVE MEDICINES (CAMs)

Mind-Body Interventions
Relaxation Techniques
Creative Arts Therapies
Prayer
Music

Bioelectromagnetic Therapies
Electromagnetic Field Therapy
Cymatics/Aquasonics
Magnet Therapy
Pulsed Electromagnetic Energy
Transcutaneous Electrical Nerve Stimulation
Acupuncture
Hyperthermia
Phototherapy/Light Therapy
Color Therapy
Polarity Therapy

Alternative Systems of Medical Practice
Folk Medicine
Homeopathic Medicine
Latin American Rural Practices
Native American Practices
Naturopathic Medicine
Past Life Therapy
Tibetan Medicine

Manual Healing Methods
Acupressure
Alexander Technique
Applied Kinesiology
Biodynamic Therapy
Chiropractic
Feldenkrais Method
Massage Therapy
Osteopathy
Reflexology and Zone Therapy
Rolfing (Structural Integration)
Trager Method (Psychophysical Integration)
Therapeutic Touch
Reiki

Pharmacologic and Biologic Therapies
Oxidation
Chelation Therapy
Antineoplastons
Shark Cartilage
Bovine Cartilage
Mistletoe (Iscador)
Herbal Medicine
Aloe
Astragalus
Bilberry
Burdock
Capsicum
Chamomile
Comfrey
Cranberry
Echinacea
Ephedra
Evening Primrose
Garlic
Ginger
Ginkgo
Ginseng
Kava Kava
Licorice
Myrtle
Psyllium
Saw Palmetto
St. John's Wort
Valerian

Diets, Nutrition
Vegetarian Diets
Macrobiotic Diets
Gerson Therapy
Nutritional Supplements
Water-Soluble Vitamins
Fat-Soluble Vitamins
Supplemental Minerals

CAMs. (Lengacher et al., 2002; NCCAM. 2001). Table 10-1 provides a listing of selected CAMs.

CAMs AS OPTIONS

CAMs are attractive to patients — and can be personally effective — because they include such a wide range of physical, emotional, and spiritual strategies (diet, mind-body connection, rest, exercise, support, homeopathy). Moreover, they have been shown to improve the feeling and reality of well-being for many patients. (Creagan, 2003; Harpham, 2001; Lengacher et al., 2002; NCCAM, 2001, Ades & Yarbro, 2000).

The National Institutes of Health (NIH) categorizes CAMs in five areas: alternative medical systems; mind-body interventions, biologically-based treatments; manipulative and body-based methods; and energy therapies (NCI, 2003). Table 10-2 lists those categories and offers specific examples of therapies.

Some consider CAMs to be more natural and gentle in approach than conventional treatment or therapies. Others rely on the non-Western medicine foundation of many CAMs as proof of effective-

---

TABLE 10-2: FIVE DOMAINS OF CAMs

Alternative medical systems
Ayurvedic medicine (India's traditional medical system, based on health achieved by restoring innate harmony of the individual)

Mind-body interventions
Meditation, hypnosis, prayer; forms of art, music, and dance therapy

Biologically-based therapies
Herbal remedies, special diets, and food products

Manipulative and body-based methods
Chiropractic manipulation

Energy therapies
Qi gong, Reiki, and Therapeutic Touch

Note. From "Cancer facts: Complementary and alternative medicines in Cancer treatment: Questions and answers, 2003". Retrieved April 1, 2003, from http://cis.nci.nih.gov/fact/9_14.htm

---

ness. Because CAMs can be self-chosen — or at the least — socially encouraged, they offer a means for the patient to gain control and empowerment (Harpham, 2001; Lengacher, et al., 2002; NCCAM, 2001; Ades & Yarbro, 2000). For patients who are weary and discouraged when initially diagnosed or when their cancer progresses with conventional treatments, CAMs offer them a personal and real perception of healing (Lengacher, et al., 2002; Ades & Yarbro, 2000).

Thus the challenge of nurses and other health care providers is to be supportive of patients who use CAMs, while also being appropriate advocates. CAMs can be promoted by charlatans who seek out the vulnerable (NCI, 2003). The obligation of health care providers is to help patients sort through information, focus on those promising and effective options and support studies that generate documented effectiveness data (Harpham, 2001; NCCAM, 2001).

PREVALENCE

Studies show that CAM use is widespread and increasing (NCI, 2003; NCCAM, 2001). Between 1990 and 1997, the number of Americans using CAM increased by 38% from 60 million to 83 million. (NCI, 2003; NCCAM, 2001). Since then, CAM interest and use has risen (Ades & Yarbro, 2000).

An M.D. Anderson survey of cancer patients reports that 70% of patients had tried CAMs (Perez, 2003). In 2000, a study of CAM use by patients with different types of cancer reported that 83% of 453 cancer patients had used at least one CAM therapy as part of their cancer treatment (including special diets, psychotherapy, spiritual practices, and vitamin supplements) (Ades & Yarbro, 2000). Omitting psychotherapy and spiritual practices, 69% of patients had used at least one CAM therapy in their cancer treatment.

In 1997, conservative estimates put expenditures for alternative medicine professional services at $21.2 billion, with at least $12.2 billion paid out-of-pocket. At that time, Americans spent more out-of-pocket for CAMs than they paid out-of-pocket for all hospitalizations — an amount comparable to the projected 1997 out-of-pocket expenditures for all U.S. physician services (NCI, 2003; NCCAM, 2001).

With women, the interest and use of CAMs is high. For example, a 2002 study of women diagnosed with breast cancer (Lengacher et al., 2002), reported that 64% of all participants reported regular use of vitamins and minerals and 33% regularly used antioxidants, herbs, and health foods. Among stress-reducing techniques, 49% of all participants regularly used prayer and spiritual healing, followed by support groups (37%), and humor or laughter therapy (21%).

In the 2002 study, women rarely used traditional and ethnic medicine therapies with the exception of massage, which 27% of all participants used at least once after diagnosis. The study indicated that CAM use was more frequent with those who had undergone previous courses of chemotherapy and had an education beyond high school.

Yet another study (Jordan & Delunas, 2001) reported that more than one-third of cancer patients studied had initiated some CAMs after receiving their diagnosis and that the majority of those patients were female and more highly educated.

SOUND FOUNDATION FOR STUDY

In 1998, the NIH established the NCCAM. The NCCAM was established to conduct basic and clinical research, train researchers, and educate and communicate findings concerning therapeutic and preventive CAMs. Table 10-3 lists cancer-related CAM studies currently coordinated out of the NCCAM.

TABLE 10-3: SELECTED CAM-RELATED STUDIES

Cancer or cancer treatment conditions

Acupuncture to Reduce Symptoms of Advanced Colorectal Cancer

Effects of Ginseng and Ginkgo on Drug Disposition in Man

Massage Therapy for Cancer-Related Fatigue (Breast, Ovarian, Prostate, Colorectal)

Macrobiotic Diet and Flax Seed: Effects on Estrogens, Phytoestrogens, and Fibrinolytic Factors (Breast, Endometrial Cancer)

Mindfulness-Based Art Therapy for Cancer Patients

Shark Cartilage in Treating Patients with Advanced Colorectal or Breast Cancer

Mistletoe Extract and Gemcitabine for the Treatment of Solid Tumor Cancers

Note. From National Center for Complementary and Alternative Medicine (NCCAM), (NCI, 2003).

Based on its charter, the NCCAM strives to use evidence-based standards in its research and studies to prove CAM effectiveness. The strategic plan for the NCCAM, published in 2001, intends to make CAMs more integrative therapies, based on scientifically driven studies (NCCAM, 2001). Toward making CAMs acceptable to a wider health care community, those research studies and targets are in the midst of early phases of evaluation and analytical rigor. Table 10-4 lists the criteria NCCAM used to evaluate CAM studies.

TABLE 10-4: CRITERIA TO EVALUATE CAM STUDIES

• Strength of Study Design (randomized, double-blinded)

• Strength of Endpoints Measured (total mortality, disease-free survival, progression-free survival, quality of life, tumor response rate)

(NCCAM, 2001)

Evaluation of Studies

To provide a sound foundation to determine the effectiveness of CAMs, several evaluation strategies are in place.

In 1991, NCI began its Best Case Series Program out of the Office of Cancer Complementary and Alternative Medicine (OCCAM). Health care providers who offer CAM services submit their patients' medical records and related materials to OCCAM. Then OCCAM provides a critical review of the materials and develops follow-up research strategies for approaches that have therapeutic potential.

In addition to OCCAM as a source of government-sponsored information evaluation, many other government agencies have Web sites. Among them are

- NCI's PDQ® Clinical Trials Database — The search form at [http://cancer.gov/search/clinical_trials/] on the Cancer.gov Web site

- NCCAM Clinical Trials Web page — [http://nccam.nih.gov/clinicaltrials/]

- OCCAM Clinical Trials Web page — [http://cancer.gov/occam/trials.html]

HELPFUL CAMS IN CANCER PATIENT CARE

CAM use is subjective and so their benefits are of unique benefit to the individual. Although the positive track record of many CAMs is reported, few reports document the benefits of certain CAMs related to cancer and cancer treatment.

The following list is not exhaustive and only highlights some common CAMs, which cancer patients and clinicians report to be safe and helpful. Few studies have actually evaluated safety, dosing, scheduling, technique, or outcomes (Ades & Yarbro, 2000). Accepted therapies, based on anecdotal reports so far, are

Aromatherapy
Art Therapy
Biofeedback
Herbals
    Ginger Tea for nausea or heartburn
    Camomile Tea for indigestion
    Valerian Tea for Sleep
Massage Therapy
Meditation
Music Therapy
Physical Activity
Prayer, spiritual practices
Support Groups
Tai chi
Yoga
Well-balanced Diet.

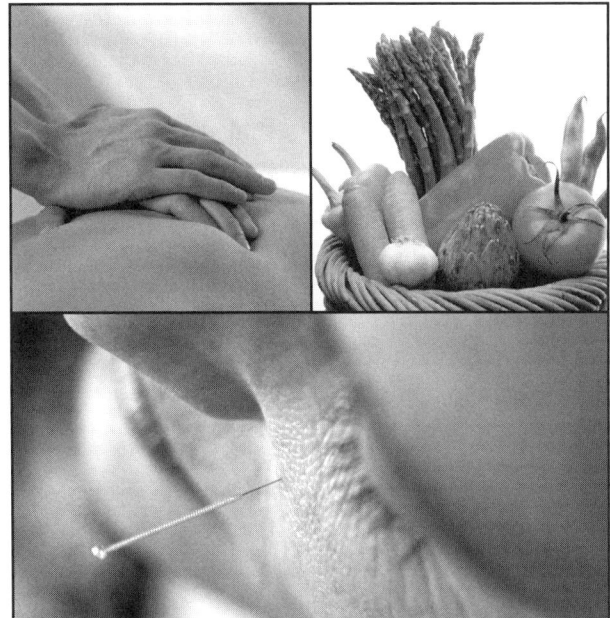

CAMs in Practice, Two Abstracts

Two abstracts presented at the Oncology Nursing Society Congress in 2003 represent the state of practice with CAMs. One abstract reviewed components of an educational project that is based on practice guidelines for providing aromatherapy (Perez, 2003). The second abstract described the tasks and timeline necessary to launch a modest CAM program at three locations in community cancer facilities (Kostka, Coughlin, & Jackson, 2003).

Aromatherapy Program Curriculum

The aromatherapy program emphasized the need for accredited education that practitioners need before offering aromatherapy in a practice setting. Among components of the curriculum include

- knowing the safety and toxicity profile of essential oils used in aromatherapy

- understanding the way that essential oils are processed and absorbed by the patient (using the Limbic System and dermal absorption)

- obtaining reliable information and products from credible vendors

- knowing credible sources of information — from books, experts, Web sites

- understanding the therapeutic nature of individual essential oils (Table 10-5)

- understanding factors that can decrease the quality and purity of essential oils

- using precautions with essential oils (Table 10-6)

- targeting symptom management areas studied, to date: pain (postoperative, arthritis, cancer related), dermatology, anxiety, depression, nausea, and vomiting, wound care

(Perez, 2003).

TABLE 10-5: THERAPEUTIC NATURE OF SELECTED ESSENTIAL OILS

Essential Oil	Therapeutic Nature
Terpenes	Antiviral, antiseptic, bactericidal, and anti-inflammatory
Esters	Fungicidal, sedative
Aldehydes	Sedative, antiseptic
Ketones	Can be toxic, but can ease congestion
Alcohols	Nontoxic (generally), antiseptic, antiviral, and uplifting qualities
Phenols	Irritate, but can stimulate
Oxides	Expectorant

TABLE 10-6: PRECAUTIONS WHEN USING ESSENTIAL OILS

- Skin irritation, rash (allspice, aniseed, sweet basil, borneol, cajeput, careway, thyme, cinnamon, leaf, black pepper, clove, cornmint, eucalyptus, garlic, ginger, lemon, parsley, peppermint, pine needle, tumeric)

- Photosensitivity (bergamot, lemon, lime, ginger, angelica, cumin, lovage, mandarin, orange, and verbena)

- Diabetes (angelica may interfere with insulin)

- Nervous system stimulant (fennel, hyssop, rosemary, and sage)

- Uterine stimulants* (angelic, star anise, basil, bay laurel, celery seed, cedarwood, cinnamon left, clary sage, citronella, clove, cumin, fennel, hyssop, juniper, labdanum, lovage, marjoram, myrrh, nutmeg, parsley, snakeroot, Spanish sage, tarragon, and white thyme)

- Circulatory stimulant (rosemary, sage, thyme, and hyssop)

* Do not use during pregnancy. (During last weeks of pregnancy, can use rosemary, sage and thyme)

Note. From "Aromatherapy: Guidelines for safe incorporation into nursing practice," by C. Perez, 2003, [Abstract #125]. ONS 28th Annual Congress, *Oncology Nursing Forum, 30*(2):140.

CAMs in Community Practice

CAM practice in the community cancer center setting began with two pilot studies — one offering massage to patients and caregivers for 20 hours/week at one infusion center site over a 3-month period. Later the program branched to a medical oncology practice and radiation oncology offices.

The program began with massage only, then expanded its offerings to aromatherapy, reflexology, and Therapeutic Touch. Program planning began 4 years before any pilot studies were launched.

Patient satisfaction data from program surveys is listed in Table 10-7. Among comments cited from the survey

"Healing touch/massage is a crucial component in the process of getting well — it's been the

TABLE 10-7: PATIENT SATISFACTION AND EFFECTIVENESS DATA

Pilot CAM Program in Oncology, 2003

	Massage	Reflexology	Aromatherapy	Therapeutic Touch
# of patients	50	34	6	35
Reported Benefit				
Decreased Pain	15	20	3	18
Decreased Nausea	5	10	5	11
Decreased Anxiety	17	34	6	33
Decreased Fatigue	12	20	6	18
Increased Comfort	8	28	6	25

Note. From "Launching a complementary therapy program in oncology: A nursing initiative in holistic care," by J. Koska, B. Coughlin, J. Jackson (2003), *Oncology Nursing Forum, 30*(2):140.

single oasis in the ordeal of my treatment. More, more, more."

"It was a pleasant experience, helping to accept the chemo treatment with lower stress."

"Need more therapists each day. My one session this morning dropped my blood pressure 20 points."

The experience described in this abstract indicated that worthwhile and well-run CAM programs need time to become established. With little documentation available about CAM effectiveness, proactive surveys of patients and clinicians are key to any program's success (Koska et al., 2003).

PATIENT EVALUATION OF CAMs

With CAM availability and use so sweeping, patients appear to be left to navigate the territory alone. Thus, advocacy for the patient — in the form of helping her evaluate CAMs — becomes the appropriate focus of nurses and other health care providers.

Table 10-8 provides a list of questions that patients can ask when considering CAMs. The NIH also publishes guidelines when selecting a CAM practitioner, listed on Table 10-9. With the amount of CAM information and publicity on the Internet, no coaching of patients about CAMs is complete without guidance in reviewing Web sites (NCCAM, 2002). Table 10-10 provides questions for the patient to keep in mind when visiting CAM-related Web sites. (See Chapter 11, Health Care and the Internet, for more on accessing the Web for CAM-related information.)

TABLE 10-8: QUESTIONS TO ASK WHEN CONSIDERING CAMs

• What benefits can be expected from this therapy?

• What are the risks associated with this therapy?

• Do the known benefits outweigh the risks?

• What adverse effects can be expected?

• Will the therapy interfere with conventional treatment?

• Is this therapy part of a clinical trial? If so, who is sponsoring the trial?

• Will the therapy be covered by health insurance?

Note. From "Cancer facts: Complementary and alternative medicines in Cancer treatment: Questions and answers, 2003." Retrieved April 1, 2003, from http://cis.nci.nih.gov/fact/9_14.htm

TABLE 10-9: SELECTING A CAM PRACTITIONER

Issues to consider when selecting a Complementary and Alternative Medicine (CAM) Practitioner

• If you are seeking a CAM practitioner, speak with your primary health care provider(s) or someone you believe to be knowledgeable about CAM regarding the therapy in which you are interested. Ask if they have a recommendation for the type of CAM practitioner you are seeking.

• Make a list of CAM practitioners and gather information about each before making your first visit. Ask basic questions about their credentials and practice. Where did they receive their training? What licenses or certifications do they have? How much will the treatment cost?

• Check with your insurer to see if the cost of therapy will be covered.

• After you select a practitioner, make a list of questions to ask at your first visit. You may want to bring a friend or family member who can help you ask questions and note answers.

• Come to the first visit prepared to answer questions about your health history, including injuries, surgeries, and major illnesses, as well as prescription medicines, vitamins, and other supplements you may take.

• Assess your first visit and decide if the practitioner is right for you. Did you feel comfortable with the practitioner? Could the practitioner answer your questions? Did he respond to you in a way that satisfied you? Does the treatment plan seem reasonable and acceptable to you?

Note. From National Center for Complementary and Alternative Medicine (NCCAM). (2002). Are you considering using complementary and alternative medicine (CAM)? Retrieved April 1, 2003, from http://nccam.nih.gov/about/plans/fiveyear/fiveyear.pdf

TABLE 10-10: EVALUATING MEDICAL RESOURCES ON THE WEB

1. Who runs this site?
2. Who pays for the site?
3. What is the purpose of the site?
4. Where does the information come from?
5. What is the basis of the information?
6. How is the information selected?
7. How current is the information?
8. How does the site choose links to other sites?
9. What information about you does the site collect, and why?
10. How does the site manage interactions with visitors?

Note. From National Center for Complementary and Alternative Medicine (NCCAM). (2002). Are you considering using complementary and alternative medicine (CAM)? Retrieved April 1, 2003, from http://nccam.nih.gov/about/plans/fiveyear/fiveyear.pdf

SUMMARY

The use of CAMs is widespread, especially with women. Although no CAM has been shown to be effective in replacing conventional cancer treatment, CAMs have been shown to boost the perceived effectiveness of treatment and help patients better deal with treatment adverse effects. CAMs provide physical, emotional, and spiritual methods — mind-body interventions, biologically-based treatments, manipulative and body-based methods, and energy therapies. CAM programs in practice are in their infancy. Clinicians are still educating themselves about what is needed to provide CAM options to patients. When integrating CAMs in practice, clinicians should help patients assess their reliability, their ability to blend with standard treatment protocols, and their real and perceived benefits to quality of life.

EXAM QUESTIONS

CHAPTER 10
Questions 85-92

85. Women diagnosed with cancer choose to use CAM cancer treatments because they

    a. offer a sense of control.

    b. are inexpensive.

    c. are harmless.

    d. are pure.

86. An established form of complementary therapy is

    a. group intervention.

    b. relaxation through massage.

    c. counseling.

    d. narcotics.

87. Examples of CAM include the

    a. paxitaxel.

    b. gamma knife radiation.

    c. sentinel node biopsy.

    d. homeopathic diets.

88. CAMS being studied by the NCCAM for their efficacy for cancer patients include

    a. shark cartilage in breast cancer patients.

    b. shark cartilage for lung cancer patients.

    c. acupuncture for ovarian cancer patients.

    d. macrobiotic diet for pancreatic cancer patients.

89. The NCCAM is studying massage in ovarian and breast cancer patients to see if it helps reduce

    a. pain.

    b. fatigue.

    c. blood clots.

    d. bed sores.

90. An NCCAM-established criteria for CAM studies, which gives a study more strength is

    a. several variables.

    b. to use a study design.

    c. targeting multiple populations in the study.

    d. to make sure investigators are vested.

91. When evaluating a CAM practitioner about clinical benefits of the therapy, include questions about

    a. the cost of the therapy.

    b. adverse effects from therapy.

    c. his/her address and phone number.

    d. opinions on the Internet.

92. When evaluating CAM-related Web sites, look for

    a. size of font, ease of use, timeliness of information.

    b. source and timeliness of information, and who pays for the site.

    c. links to government sources.

    d. ways the site asks you questions.

REFERENCES

Ades, T.B., & Yarbro, C.H. (2000). Alterations and complementary therapies in cancer management. In C.H. Yarbro, M.H. Frogge, M. Goodman, & S.L. Groenwald (Eds.), *Cancer Nursing: Principles and Practice* (5th ed.), (pp. 616-630, 1116). Sudbury, MA: Jones & Bartlett Publishers.

Creagan, E.T. (2003). Complementary and alternative care for cancer. MayoClinic.com. Retrieved April 15, 2003, from http://www.mayoclinic.com

Harpham, W.S. (2001). Alternative therapies for curing cancer: What do patients want? What do patients need? *CA Cancer Journal for Clinicians, 51*:131-136.

Jordan, M.L., & Delunas, L.R. (2001). Quality of life and patterns of nontraditional therapy use by patients with cancer. *Oncology Nursing Forum, 28*(7):1107-1113.

Koska, J., Coughlin, B., & Jackson, J. (2003). Launching a complementary therapy program in oncology: A nursing initiative in holistic care [Abstract #127] ONS 28th Annual Congress. *Oncology Nursing Forum, 30*(2):140.

Lengacher, C.A., Bennett, M.P., Kip, K.E., Keller, R., LaVance, M.S., Smith, L., & Cox, C.E. (2002). Frequency of use of complementary and alternative medicine in women with breast cancer. *Oncology Nursing Forum, 29*:10:1445-1452.

Lerner, M. (2002). Complementary and conventional medicine go hand-in-hand. CancerSource. Retrieved April 15, 2003, from http://www.cancersourcemd.com

National Cancer Institute (NCI). (2003). Cancer Facts: Complementary and alternative medicine in cancer treatment: Questions and answers. Retrieved April 1, 2003, from http://cis.nci.nih.gov/fact/9_14.htm

National Center for Complementary and Alternative Medicine (NCCAM). (2001). Expanding horizons of healthcare, five-year strategic plan, 2001-2005. Retrieved April 1, 2003, from http://nccam.nih.gov/about/plans/fiveyear/fiveyear.pdf

National Center for Complementary and Alternative Medicine (NCCAM). (2002). Are you considering using complementary and alternative medicine (CAM)? Retrieved April 1, 2003, from http://nccam.nih.gov/health/decisions/

Perez, C. (2003). Aromatherapy: Guidelines for safe incorporation into nursing practice [Abstract #125] ONS 28th Annual Congress. *Oncology Nursing Forum, 30*(2):140.

Rosenthal, D., & Ades, T. (2001). Complementary & alternative methods. *CA Cancer Journal for Clinicians, 51*:316-320.

CHAPTER 11

HEALTH CARE AND THE INTERNET

CHAPTER OBJECTIVE

After completing this chapter, the reader can discuss ways for the clinician and patient to evaluate and access content available on the Internet, which best mobilizes appropriate and effective care for cancer patients.

LEARNING OBJECTIVES

After studying this chapter, the reader will be able to

1. identify a section of the population that most frequently seeks health-related information on-line.

2. list criteria to evaluate Web sites that present health care and patient information.

3. specify one site, which provides accurate and timely cancer-related information.

4. indicate one way to coach patients, who also seek cancer-related information on the Internet.

5. discuss methods to optimize e-mail communication between the health care provider and patient.

6. identify two ways that patients can use the Web for support.

INTERNET — A COMMUNICATION TOOL

The World Wide Web has become an integral part of the way our world communicates. For health care providers and their patients, the World Wide Web offers an unprecedented tool of contact, convenience, and personal control. Information is abundant, available anytime, providing disease reviews, treatments, clinical trials, latest research news, decision-making tools, discussion groups, coping strategies, and a means to directly communicate with a health care provider (Sharp, 2001). (Table 11-1 provides a listing of trends related to seeking health care information on the Web.)

In this, the second consumer-related decade of life with the Internet, we face complexities that rise from that ready access — privacy issues, accuracy of information, timeliness of information, and sheer volume of data that can be overwhelming, especially to patients diagnosed with cancer.

In the past 10 years there has been a revolution of information spurred by the increase in home computers and access to the Internet. In 2002, worldwide Internet users were estimated at 407.1 million and climbing (Dickerson & Brennan, 2002). Of those, 167.12 million users live in the United States and Canada; 113.14 million live in Europe (Dickerson & Brennan, 2002).

In 2001, about 47.5% adults in the United States had access to the Internet. Data from another

TABLE 11-1: TRENDS — INTEGRATION OF TECH HEALTH CARE BEHAVIORS

	2002	2001	1999
Seek out information on medical professionals sites	77%, (n=1206)	77% (n=1594)	
Discussed their Internet finding with their physician	62% (n=1216)	64% (n=1635)	69% (n=2137)
Search drug information	81% (n=1249)	82% (n=1574)	79% (n=3195)
Buy drugs on-line	13% (n=1244)	14% (n=1613)	15% (n=3115)
Use the Internet for 2nd opinion	49% (n=1252)	43% (n=1649)	41% (n=2010)
E-mail their own physician	23% (n=1253)	14% (n=1509)	21% (n=2103)

Note. From "Highlights of the 8th HON Survey of Health and Medical Internet Users." Health On the Net Foundation, (2002) by C. Boyer, M. Provost, & V. Baujard (2002). Retrieved from http://www.hon.ch/Survey/8th_HON_results.html

2001 survey estimated that as many as 75% of patients had direct access to the Internet — or access through a friend or family member (Cumbo et al., 2001; Brooks, 2001).

By 2005, 88.5 million adults are expected to communicate about health care using the Internet (HON, 2002a; Sharp, 2001; Brooks, 2001). On any given day, 59 million Americans are on-line with an estimated 7% seeking some type of health care information (Dickerson & Brennan, 2002). The majority of those seeking health information online are aging baby boomers who are either experiencing health problems or searching for answers for family and friends (Sharp, 2001; Clarke & Gomez, 2001). The fastest growing age group of Internet users is age 55 and older, estimated to be 20% of all new Internet users by 2004 (Martin & Youngren, 2002). This age group, as health care statistics attest, is the age group of the majority of patients diagnosed with cancer.

Additionally in 2002, we know more about who has been left behind as Internet use expands. Nearly one fourth of Americans have Internet direct access at home with White Americans more likely to have access than African Americans or Hispanics. Users have been surveyed, showing that those with less education (< 12 years school) are less likely to use the Internet (HON, 2002a; Cumbo et al., 2001). Efforts to bring the world on-line continue with Internet access available in libraries, shopping malls, and other public places. Still, the ready access to the Internet remains yet another benefit for patients who are white, not poor, and have some education (Boyer, Provost, & Baujard, 2002; Brooks, 2001).

Health care professionals have now become their own sophisticated data librarians, able to search the Web for the latest in research findings, new treatments and information to better understand their patients' diseases. One study estimates that the Internet posts more than 70,000 health care related Web sites (Martin & Youngren, 2002). Where do they go for that information? A recent survey indicated that 67% of the health care providers asked seek information from Web sites sponsored by nonprofit organizations (e.g., ONS Online, Cancer Care, Oncolink) and 38% used hospital Web sites (Clark & Gomez, 2001).

For those with Web access in their home, on-line health care information has its advantages. Accessing it can be convenient and can be done in private. In an at-home venue accessing the Web, the patient benefits from a sense of control (Clark & Gomez, 2001).

The sense of control goes hand in hand with patients wanting more control of their health care choices and dollars. Yet, it's worth emphasizing, there is no substitute for the relationship that develops face to face, clinician to patient. So Internet based information should always — and only — augment that information that comes from sound, evidence-based clinical care.

A 2002 survey showed that those who seek health care information online search for disease-related information (HON, 2002b). Cancer tops this list of information topics; about one third of disease information seekers are looking for cancer-related content (HON, 2002b). In 2001, Sharp proposed two main challenges in searching the Internet for cancer information: 1) How does one find relevant information specific to one's diagnosis, stage of disease, treatment options, and where to obtain quality treatment? and 2) How does one determine the reliability of the information found and present it to the oncology team?

FINDING INFORMATION

Search engines and directories on the Web provide easy portals for Internet users. Yet only 50% of available Web information is accessed this way, thus limiting how adequate any search can be (Sharp, 2001). Methods to focus a search help increase the effectiveness of a search (making the words in a search line as precise as possible — depending on the search engine, for example, instead of leukemia, type "chemotherapy for leukemia"). Still, a search may be deficient. Figure 11-1 illustrates the difference in search engine choices for professionals and patients.

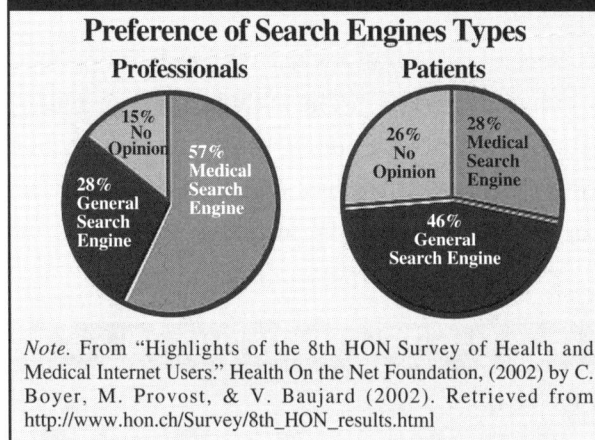

FIGURE 11-1: SEARCH ENGINE PREFERENCES

Note. From "Highlights of the 8th HON Survey of Health and Medical Internet Users." Health On the Net Foundation, (2002) by C. Boyer, M. Provost, & V. Baujard (2002). Retrieved from http://www.hon.ch/Survey/8th_HON_results.html

Therefore, visiting reliable cancer Web sites, available to update news and to package contents well, is a worthy strategy. Examples of these sites include the American Cancer Society (www.cancer.org) or the National Cancer Institute (www.nci.nih.gov). Yet another way to access reliable sites is through sites that link or filter their information from reliable sites. Examples of these include Oncolink, the University of Pennsylvania Cancer Center site (www.oncolink.com), which also passes on news from the Reuters health news service.

More advanced users — or professionals seeking a more clinical level of information — can find information posted on professional journal sites or through MEDLINE sites available at most medical center libraries. PubMed (National Library of Medicine site) and Medscape are examples of sites that provide a thorough gateway for updated clinical information.

Evaluating Internet-Based Information

As of 2003, Internet-based information remains unregulated with no oversight body guaranteeing the veracity of information. The nature of the Internet will not change this. Therefore, those using the Internet for health care information need to continue to be vigilant with themselves and their patients. The quest is always to find information using sound criteria to identify reliable information and health care advice (Stapleton, 2001; Martin et al., 2002).

Several organizations have offered criteria lists to guide Internet searches. Table 11-2 provides Health on the Net Foundation Code of Conduct Principles. Table 11-3 lists organizations that have proposed guidelines and principles.

In a question-based approach, Sharp (2001) suggests asking the following to help evaluate a Web site's veracity:

- Who is the author?
- When was the information updated?
- Does the site have a medical advisory board?

TABLE 11-2: HEALTH ON THE NET FOUNDATION (HON) CODE OF CONDUCT

PRINCIPLES

1. Authority
Any medical or health advice provided and hosted on this site will only be given by medically trained and qualified professionals unless a clear statement is made that a piece of advice offered is from a nonmedically qualified individual or organization.

2. Complementarity
The information provided on this site is designed to support, not replace, the relationship that exists between a patient/site visitor and his/her existing physician.

3. Confidentiality
Confidentiality of data relating to individual patients and visitors to a medical/health Web site, including their identity, is respected by this Web site. The Web site owners undertake to honour or exceed the legal requirements of medical/health information privacy that apply in the country and state where the Web site and mirror sites are located.

4. Attribution
Where appropriate, information contained on this site will be supported by clear references to source data and, where possible, have specific HTML links to that data. The date when a clinical page was last modified will be clearly displayed (for example, at the bottom of the page).

5. Justifiability
Any claims relating to the benefits/performance of a specific treatment, commercial product, or service will be supported by appropriate, balanced evidence in the manner outlined above in Principle 4.

6. Transparency of authorship
The designers of this Web site will seek to provide information in the clearest possible manner and provide contact addresses for visitors that seek further information or support. The Webmaster will display his/her E-mail address clearly throughout the Web site.

7. Transparency of sponsorship
Support for this Web site will be clearly identified, including the identities of commercial and noncommercial organisations that have contributed funding, services or material for the site.

8. Honesty in advertising & editorial policy
If advertising is a source of funding it will be clearly stated. A brief description of the advertising policy adopted by the Web site owners will be displayed on the site. Advertising and other promotional material will be presented to viewers in a manner and context that facilitates differentiation between it and the original material created by the institution operating the site.

Note. From Health on the Net Foundation. (2002). Principles, version 1.6. Retrieved from http://www.hon.ch/HONcode/Conduct.html

- Does the site generate its own material or does it have a partnership with another organization or Web site?

- Is the author someone with current knowledge of this particular field of oncology?

- Does the site accept sponsorship from pharmaceutical or medical companies and does this influence their content?

- For news items, what is the source of the research findings?

For reports on new treatments, additional questions can include:

- Does the summary information about the treatment match how the information was reported in a peer review journal?

- How many patients were treated? Is the treatment in its initial trials, thus the report addresses preliminary results?

- Was a major cancer center involved in the clinical trial?

- Are both sides of the study presented? (promising results, as well as adverse effects)

- An additional tip sheet, developed by the Internet Coalition, is listed in Table 11-4.

QUERIES FROM CANCER PATIENTS

Cancer patients (and survivors) typically search the net for two types of information — new treatments and CAM therapies (Sharp, 2001; Stapleton, 2001). (Chapter 10, Complementary and Alternative Medicine, provides an overview of these therapies.) The most complete information is available on the Web sites of hospitals, cancer centers, pharmaceutical companies, or cancer or profession-

---

TABLE 11-3: HEALTH ORGANIZATIONS DEVELOPING GUIDELINES FOR HEALTH CARE CONSUMERS TO EVALUATE ON-LINE SOURCES OF HEALTH INFORMATION

1. The Science Panel on Interactive Communication and Health (SciPICH) was convened by the Office of Disease Prevention and Health Promotion of the U.S. Department of Health and Human Services (DHHS). This panel has created a checklist of questions to help consumers judge whether health information offered by an interactive health communication (IHC) application is useful and reliable. The checklist can be found at http://www.scipich.org/IHC/checklist.htm

2. The mission of the Internet Healthcare Coalition is quality health care resources on the Internet. Their tips for health care consumers can be found at http://www.ihealthcoalition.org/content/tips.html

3. Health On the Net Foundation's mission is to guide the growing community of health care consumers and providers on the World Wide Web to sound, reliable medical information and expertise. This Swiss-based, not-for-profit organization has developed principles for ethical conduct on the Internet located at http://www.hon.ch/HONcode/Conduct.html

4. These guidelines are the American Medical Association's policy for its Web sites but also are intended to provide guidance for creators of Web sites that provide medical and health information for professionals and consumers. http://jama.amaassn.org/issues/v283n12/ffull/jsc00054.htm

5. Healthfinder® is a Web site from the U.S. Department of Health and Human Services. It helps consumers find reliable health information that can help them stay healthy, understand diagnoses, explore treatment options, find support, and generally become more informed about health and medical topics. http://www.healthfinder.gov/smartchoices/onlineinfo/checklist.htm

6. Hi-Ethics, or Health Internet Ethics, has a goal to establish and comply with the highest standards for privacy, security, credibility, and reliability so that consumers can realize the fullest benefits of the Internet. Hi-Ethics Principles for Health Web sites are located at http://www.hiethics.org/Principles/index.asp

TABLE 11-4: TIPS FOR HEALTH SURFING ON-LINE

Finding Quality Health Information on the Internet

• Choosing an on-line health information resource is like choosing your physician. You wouldn't go to just any physician and you may get opinions from several physicians. Therefore you shouldn't rely on just any one Internet site for all of your health needs. A good rule of thumb is to find a Web site that has a person, institution, or organization in which you already have confidence. If possible, you should seek information from several sources and not rely on a single source of information.

• Trust what you see or read on the Internet only if you can validate the source of the information. Authors and contributors should always be identified, along with their affiliations and financial interests, if any, in the content. Phone numbers, e-mail addresses, or other contact information should also be provided.

• Question Web sites that credit themselves as the sole source of information on a topic as well as sites that disrespect other sources of knowledge.

• Don't be fooled by a comprehensive list of links. Any Web site can link to another and this in no way implies endorsement from either site.

• Find out if the site is professionally managed and reviewed by an editorial board of experts to ensure that the material is both credible and reliable. Sources used to create the content should be clearly referenced and acknowledged.

• Medical knowledge is continually evolving. Make sure that all clinical content includes the date of publication or modification.

• Any and all sponsorship, advertising, underwriting, commercial funding arrangements, or potential conflicts should be clearly stated and separated from the editorial content. A good question to ask is: Does the author or authors have anything to gain from proposing one particular point of view over another?

• Avoid any on-line physician who proposes to diagnose or treat you without a proper physical examination and consultation regarding your medical history.

• Read the Web site's privacy statement and make certain that any personal medical or other information you supply will be kept absolutely confidential.

• Most importantly, use your common sense. Shop around, always get more than one opinion, be suspicious of miracle cures, and always read the fine print.

Note. From Internet Healthcare Coalition. (2002). Retrieved from http://www.ihealthcoalition.org/content/tips.html

FIGURE 11-5: TYPES OF WEB SITES

Coupled with a sound criteria for evaluating Web sites, reliable sources of cancer information on the Web include:

• Familiar resources
  National Cancer Institute (www.nci.nih.gov)
• Activist organizations
  American Cancer Society (www.cancer.org)
• Health portals
  CancerSource RN (www.Cancersourcern.com)
• Pharmaceutical/biotechnology companies
  Amgen, Bristol Myers Squibb, Novartis
  (www.amgen.com; www.bms.com;
  www.novartis.com)
• Professional organizations
  ONS Online www.ons.org; American Society of
  Clinical Oncology (http://www.asco.org)

al organizations associated with the treatment or presentation. Table 11-5 lists examples of the type of cancer-related Web sites, which clinicians and patients use. (Appendix I provides a list of several reputable cancer-related Web sites.)

When seeking valid information about complementary and alternative therapies, the challenge is daunting. Many reports are based on personal testimonies rather than scientific inquiry and testing. Sites that proclaim effectiveness need to be corroborated by other sites, or by sources that can give equal weight to the therapy's limitations. (NOTE: Some promising treatments undergo testing abroad; but have not gone through rigorous testing to establish effectiveness in the United States.)

Two sources to check about complementary therapies are the National Center for Complementary and Alternative Medicine (http://www.nccam.nih.gov) and Quack Watch (http://www.quackwatch.com). They provide reviews of such therapies. Clinicians need to be vigilant in helping patients gather information about alternative therapies that can boost the effectiveness of proven therapies, or, at the very least, do no harm.

E-MAIL TO COMMUNICATE

E-mail, as a method to communicate, is one of the primary reasons Internet use grows. Today, communication is still its main purpose through e-mail, which accounts for about 75% of all traffic on the Internet (Jenkins, 2001).

E-mail provides an immediate way for clinicians to support patients, offering them ready feedback and reliable patient information. It also provides a built-in form of documentation for exchanges with patients. That said, Internet users have become more aware about the need to protect patient confidentiality. Clark & Gomez (2001) offers technical ground rules for using e-mail as a method of clinician-patient communication:

- Turn-around time — Both parties should agree on an acceptable turn-around time for e-mail and conditions under which a telephone call or a page should be used instead of e-mail.

- Privacy — Patients should be notified if office staff triages e-mail and be given the opportunity to "opt-out" of e-mail communication for this reason.

- Content — HIV testing, workers' compensation, mental illness, and other sensitive issues are best discussed in person or at least over the telephone.

- Archiving messages — Patients should know what happens to their e-mail messages after

they are received, whether they are placed in the medical record or archived in some other way (Clark & Gomez, 2001).

OPEN FORUMS

The Internet also provides a wealth of support groups, which take many forms such as news groups, discussion groups (listservs), and chat rooms. These forums provide the opportunity for patients to share advice and so-called facts on the health care experience. But these forums have no quality control that guarantees accuracy or offers perspective. Patients desperate to sort out their situations constantly need to be reminded about the open forum limitations. Table 11-6 lists advantages and disadvantages of Internet-based support groups.

Proposed criterion when searching for an Internet-based support group may include:

- Demonstrated sustainability (online history more than 1 year),

- Sponsor is a not-for-profit organization or an individual rather than a commercial operation, and

- No prominent advertising to sell products (Martin et al., 2002).

Another avenue to connect to reputable Internet-based cancer support groups is the Association for Cancer Online Resources (http://www.acor.org). This organization sponsors 79 such groups and has developed a specialty in rare cancers (Sharp, 2000).

Patients familiar with navigating the Internet and open-forum sites will present clinicians with all sorts of information. Clinicians cannot dissuade patients from visiting these forums, but coaching them on evaluating what they read is important. To better guide patients as they visit these sites, share the criteria approaches which Internet experts have developed (Clark & Gomez, 2001).

FIGURE 11-6: ADVANTAGES AND DISADVANTAGES OF INTERNET-BASED SUPPORT GROUPS

Advantages
• Eliminate prejudices that sometimes rise from face-to-face support groups (such as age, gender, dress, or social status)
• Around-the-clock availability
• Reasonable cost
• Ability to read others' comments without responding until the user is comfortable with the group
• Ability to avoid being seen while affected by chemotherapy or the disease
• A reduction in the hesitancy male patients have about participating in support groups
• Geography is not a limitation

Disadvantage
• Typically no professional facilitator
• Inability to include (assess) nonverbal behavior
• Potential for nonpatients or non-cancer-related patients to present themselves falsely
• Language may be offensive
• Lag time between comments (postings)
• For some, delay in developing relationship, trust because of online communication only

SUMMARY

The Internet is an integral way in which our modern day world communicates. For health care professionals and their patients, the World Wide Web offers accessible, abundant information, a means for discussion and the ability to directly communicate using e-mail. Such an unregulated medium of communication and data begs for health care professionals to rise up to practice as knowledgeable educators and vigilant advocates, so that patients can distinguish sound information from hype and rumor. The nurse can serve as a credible guide and coach for the patient, as more patients navigate through their health care experience using the Web.

EXAM QUESTIONS

CHAPTER 11

Questions 93-100

93. The majority of those seeking health information online are

   a. women.

   b. aging baby boomers.

   c. kids.

   d. elderly patients.

94. A Web site that provides accurate health-related information is

   a. www.fccc.edu (Fox Chase Cancer Center).

   b. www.Laetrile.org (Laitrile interest group).

   c. www.foxnews.com (Fox News Service).

   d. www.docinabox.com (Private MD).

95. When accessing Internet health care Web sites, be leery if

   a. respected physicians and nurses are on its editorial review board.

   b. the Web site credits itself as the sole source of information on a topic.

   c. it was updated in the past 3 days.

   d. the affiliations of the editorial review board are posted.

96. A Web site that provides accurate cancer information is

   a. www.curestoday.com

   b. www.cancer.org

   c. www.osteoporosis.org

   d. www.historychannel.com

97. When seeking cancer-related information on the Internet, patients should be coached to

   a. visit reliable sites, that are well-known and respected by clinicians and researchers.

   b. visit sites only accessed through Google.

   c. visit sites that are financed by pharmaceutical companies.

   d. visit every 3rd site they surf to.

98. The Health on the Net Foundation Code of Conduct Principles include principles about

   a. Transparency of Citizenship.

   b. Transparency of Personality.

   c. Transparency of Purpose.

   d. Transparency of Sponsorship.

99. To optimize e-mail communication between health care professional and patients,

   a. clarify turnaround time between e-mail communications.

   b. use only at night.

   c. use only for sensitive information.

   d. use for all patients.

100. The World Wide Web can provide the cancer patient with

   a. a physical assessment.

   b. remission of her disease.

   c. always accurate information.

   d. access to national and worldwide support groups.

REFERENCES

Boyer, C., Provost, M., & Baujard, V. (2002). Highlights of the 8th HON Survey of Health and Medical Internet Users. *Health On the Net Foundation.* Retrieved March 1, 2003, from http://www.hon.ch/Survey/8th_HON_results.html

Brooks, B.A. (2001). Using the Internet for patient education. *Orthopedic Nursing,* Sep-Oct; 20(5):69-77.

Clark, P.M., & Gomez, E.G. (2001). Details on demand: consumers, cancer information, and the Internet. *Clinical Journal of Oncology Nursing,* 5(1):19-24.

Clinical Journal of Oncology Nursing. (2000). Updated Internet site provides information to patients with small-cell lung and ovarian cancers, 4(5):199.

Cumbo, A., Agre, P., Dougherty, J., Callery, M., Tetzlaff, L., Pirone, J., & Tallia, R. (2002). Online cancer patient education: Evaluating usability and content. *Cancer Practice, 10*(3):155-61.

Cyberdialogue. (2000). *Health Data at a Glance.* Retrieved March 1, 2003, from http://www.cyberdialogue.com/resource/data/cch/data.html/

Dickerson, S.S., & Brennan, P.F., (2002). The internet as a catalyst for shifting power in provider-patient relationships. *Nursing Outlook, 50*(5):195-203.

Health On the Net Foundation. (2002a). *HON Code of Conduct: Principles. ver. 1.6.* Retrieved March 1, 2003, from http://www.hon.ch/HONcode/Conduct.html

Health On the Net Foundation. (2002b). *Policing the HON Code.* Retrieved March 1, 2003, from http://www.hon.ch/HONcode/policy.html/

Jenkins, D. (2001). Finding your way on the Internet. *Clinical Nurse Specialist, 15*(5):215-216.

Martin, S.D., & Youngren, K.B. (2002) Help on the net: Internet support groups for people dealing with cancer. *Home Healthcare Nurse, 20*(12):771-777.

Sharp, J.W. (2001) Locating and evaluating cancer information on the Internet. *Cancer Practice, 9*(3):151-154.

Sharp, J.W. (2000). The Internet. Changing the way cancer survivors receive support. *Cancer Practice, 8*(3):145-147.

Stapleton, J.L. (2001) A comprehensive review of selected cancer websites. *Canadian Oncology Nursing Journal, 11*(3):146-148.

Tips for healthy surfing online: Finding quality health information on the Internet (2002). *Internet Healthcare Coalition.* Retrieved March 1, 2003, from http://www.ihealthcoalition.org/content/tips.html

APPENDIX I

CANCER RESOURCES FOR PATIENTS AND THEIR FAMILIES

Alliance for Lung Cancer Advocacy, Support, and Education (ALCASE)
Post Office Box 849
Vancouver, WA 98666
Telephone: 360-696-2436
        1-800-298-2436
E-mail: info@alcase.org
Web site: http://www.alcase.org

American Cancer Society (ACS)
1599 Clifton Road, NE.
Atlanta, GA 30329-4251
Telephone: 404-320-3333
        1-800-227-2345 (1-800-ACS-2345)
Web site: http://www.cancer.org

American Cancer Society (ACS) Supported Programs:
Cancer Survivors Network
(http://www.acscsn.org)
I Can Cope
Look Good. . .Feel Better (http://www.lookgood-feelbetter.org)
Reach to Recovery

Cancer Care, Inc.
275 Seventh Avenue
New York, NY 10001
Telephone: 212-712-8080
        1-800-813-4673 (1-800-813-HOPE)
        212-712-8400 (Administration)
info@cancercare.org
Web site: http://www.cancercare.org

Cancer Hope Network
Two North Road
Chester, NJ 07930
Telephone: 1-877-467-3638 (1-877-HOPENET)
E-mail: info@cancerhopenetwork.org
Web site: http://www.cancerhopenetwork.org

Cancer Research Foundation of America
Suite 110
1600 Duke Street
Alexandria, VA 22314
Telephone: 703-836-4412
        1-800-227-2732 (1-800-227-CRFA)
E-mail: info@crfa.org
Web site: http://www.preventcancer.org

Colon Cancer Alliance (CCA)
175 Ninth Avenue
New York, NY 10011
Telephone: 212-627-7451 (Main office)
        1-877-422-2030 (Helpline)
E-mail: info@ccalliance.org
Web site: http://www.ccalliance.org

Colorectal Cancer Network
Post Office Box 182
Kensington, MD 20895-0182
Telephone: 301-879-1500
E-mail: ccnetwork@colorectal-cancer.net
Web site: http://www.colorectal-cancer.net

Gilda's Club® Worldwide
Suite 1402
322 Eighth Avenue
New York, NY 10001
Telephone: 1-888-445-3248 (1-888-GILDA-4-U)
E-mail: info@gildasclub.org
Web site: http://www.gildasclub.org

Gynecologic Cancer Foundation
Telephone: 1-800-444-4441
Web site: http://www.sgo.org/gcf

Living Beyond Breast Cancer (LBBC)
Suite 204
10 East Athens Avenue
Ardmore, PA 19003
Telephone: 610-645-4567
          1-888-753-5222 (1-888-753-LBBC)
          (Survivors' Helpline)
E-mail: mail@lbbc.org
Web site: http://www.lbbc.org

**National Alliance of Breast Cancer
Organizations (NABCO)**
10th Floor
Nine East 37th Street
New York, NY 10016
Telephone: 212-889-0606
          1-888-806-2226 (1-888-80-NABCO)
E-mail: NABCOinfo@aol.com
Web site: http://www.nabco.org

**National Asian Women's Health Organization
(NAWHO)**
Suite 900
250 Montgomery Street
San Francisco, CA 94104
Telephone: 415-989-9747
E-mail: nawho@nawho.org

National Cervical Cancer Coalition
1-800-685-5531
Web site: http://www.nccc-online.org/

**National Coalition for Cancer Survivorship
(NCCS)**
Suite 770
1010 Wayne Avenue
Silver Springs, MD 20910-5600
Telephone: 301-650-9127
          1-877-622-7937 (1-877-NCCS-YES)
E-mail: info@canceradvocacy.org
Web site: http://www.canceradvocacy.org

National Lymphedema Network (NLN)
Suite 1111
1611 Telegraph Avenue
Oakland, CA 94612-2138
Telephone: 510-208-3200
          1-800-541-3259
E-mail: nln@lymphnet.org
Web site: http://www.lymphnet.org

National Ovarian Cancer Coalition (NOCC)
Suite 14
500 Northeast Spanish River Boulevard
Boca Raton, FL 33431
Telephone: 561-393-0005
          1-888-682-7426 (1-888-OVARIAN)
E-mail: NOCC@ovarian.org
Web site: http://www.ovarian.org

Ovarian Cancer National Alliance (OCNA)
Suite 413
910 17th Street, NW.
Washington, DC 20006
Telephone: 202-331-1332
E-mail: ocna@ovariancancer.org
Web site: http://www.ovariancancer.org

Pancreatic Cancer Action Network (PanCAN)
Suite 131
2221 Rosecrans Avenue
El Segundo, CA 90245
Telephone: 301-725-0025
          1-877-272-6226 (1-877-2-PANCAN)
E-mail: information@pancan.org
Web site: http://www.pancan.org

R. A. Bloch Cancer Foundation, Inc.
4400 Main Street
Kansas City, MO 64111
Telephone: 816-932-8453 (816-WE-BUILD)
        1-800-433-0464
E-mail: hotline@hrblock.com
Web site: http://www.blochcancer.org

Sisters Network®, Inc.
Suite 4206
8787 Woodway Drive
Houston, TX 77063
Telephone: 713-781-0255
E-mail: sisnet4@aol.com
Web site: http://www.sistersnetworkinc.org

The Susan G. Komen Breast Cancer Foundation
Suite 250
5005 LBJ Freeway
Dallas, TX 75244
Telephone: 972-855-1600
        1-800-462-9273 (1-800-IM AWARE®)
E-mail: helpline@komen.org
Web site: http://www.breastcancerinfo.com

United Ostomy Association, Inc.
Suite 200
19772 MacArthur Boulevard
Irvine, CA 92612-2405
Telephone: 949-660-8624
        1-800-826-0826 (6:30 a.m.- 4:30 p.m.,
        Pacific time)
E-mail: uoa@deltanet.com

The Wellness Community
Suite 412
35 East Seventh Street
Cincinnati, OH 45202
Telephone: 513-421-7111
        1-888-793-9355 (1-888-793-WELL)
E-mail: help@thewellnesscommunity.org
Web site: http://www.thewellnesscommunity.org

Y-ME National Breast Cancer Organization, Inc.
Suite 500
212 West Van Buren Street
Chicago, IL 60607
312-986-8338
Telephone: 1-800-221-2141 (English)
        1-800-986-9505 (Spanish)
E-mail: askme@y-me.org (English);
        latino@y-me.org (Spanish)
Web site: http://www.y-me.org

APPENDIX II

SELECTED INTERNET RESOURCES

GENERAL

American Cancer Society
http://www.cancer.org

Fox Chase Cancer Center
http://www.fccc.edu

Harvard Medical School Consumer Health Information (Intelihealth Partnership)
http://www.intelihealth.com

MayoClinic
http://www.mayoclinic.com

National Cancer Institute of the National Institutes of Health
http://www.cancer.gov

National Institutes of Health
http://www.nci.nih.gov

National Coalition for Cancer Survivorship
http://www.canceradvocacy.org

OncoLink
http://www.oncolink.upenn.edu/

WOMEN'S CANCERS

Women's Cancer Network
http://www.wcn.org

COMPLEMENTARY THERAPIES

National Center for Complementary and Alternative Medicine (NCCAM)
http://nccam.nih.gov

BREAST HEALTH

Breast Cancer Education Network
http://www.healthtalk.com/bcen/index.html

Breast Cancer.Net
http://www.breastcancer.net

Y-Me
http://www.y-me.org

APPENDIX III

SELECTED NURSING DIAGNOSES

SELECTED NURSING DIAGNOSES FOR SURGERY*

*Focus: After abdominal surgeries (Endometrial, Ovarian, and Cervical Cancer)

Nursing Diagnoses	Possible Nursing Interventions
Impaired skin integrity	1. Assess skin reactions. 2. Instruct patient and family to keep skin clean. 3. Instruct patient to avoid shaving within area of treatment. 4. Apply moisturizing lotion as directed for skin dryness. 5. If pruritus occurs, apply a thin layer of hydrocortisone cream. 6. If moist desquamation occurs, use Burrow compresses 3-4 times a day.
Activity intolerance	1. Assess level of fatigue. 2. Advise patient to plan rest periods throughout the day. 3. Maintain nutritional intake. 4. Utilize resources to conserve energy. 5. Obtain assistance for chores and transportation as needed.
Altered nutrition, less than body requirements related to anorexia	1. Assess appetite. 2. Monitor weight. 3. Recommend frequent, small meals. 4. Advise on use of nutrient-dense foods such as nutritional supplements.
Pain	Pain typically is located in lower pelvis, radiating down the back of the leg (sciatic nerve or pain occurs because of metastasis to bone or other organs). 1. Assess level of pain using appropriate tools. 2. Assess level of insomnia using appropriate tools. 3. Assess level of anxiety using appropriate tools. 4. Teach patient and family about principles of pain management) — addiction versus tolerance, medication (dose, route, steady state of medication), synergy of adjunct medications, cognitive/behavioral techniques to decrease pain, tolerance and addiction, adverse effects (constipation). 5. Administer narcotics to cover pain, including breakthrough pain.
Preoperative: Bowel	For women preparing for hysterectomy, the nurse can review the following: 1. Bowel rest before surgery; enemas and NPO, as ordered.
Postoperative: Bowel	Postoperative 1. Stimulate bowel function, walking heating pads, bowel stimulants. 2. Monitor bowel sounds every 8 hours. 3. Until bowel sounds return, limit food and fluid intake. 4. After bowel sounds, promote fluid intake.
Complication: Ascites and pleural effusions	(Typical of ovarian cancer or its treatment, when ovarian tumor seeds in the serous peritoneal membrane and diaphragm.) 1. Assess for signs and symptoms — weight gain, trouble breathing, SOB, nausea/vomiting, increased pain over 2-4 days. 2. Encourage proper diet, pain control, and activity. 3. Report symptoms to physician. 4. Support postoperative para or pleurocentesis. 5. Administer oral diuretics, as prescribed. 6. Support the patient pre- and post-sclerosing procedures.
Complication: Pericardial effusion	1. Assess for signs and symptoms — cough, weakness, weight gain, trouble breathing, SOB, nausea/vomiting, chest pain, dizziness, swollen hands/feet, feeling restless, change in memory or being confused. 2. Report symptoms to physician.

SELECTED NURSING DIAGNOSES FOR SURGERY (CONTINUED)

Nursing Diagnoses	Possible Nursing Interventions
Complication: Pulmonary Embolism and Deep Vein Thrombosis (DVT)	(Bedrest and immobility after pelvic surgery increases the risk) 1. Assess for pulmonary embolism and DVT. 2. Administer anticoagulation therapy. 3. Administer pneumatic calf compression. 4. Support non-weight bearing leg movement.
Complication: Wound Breakdown	1. Assess wound areas for infection — genitourinary and GI tracts near surgical incisions. 2. Prevent infection and contamination with monitoring, hygiene, and frequent dressing changes and as needed debridement.
Complication: Bleeding	(Bleeding may be associated with all post-surgical courses and also with cramping, which may be a sign of bowel obstruction — especially in ovarian cancer.) 1. Monitor sites of bleeding for signs and symptoms — mouth, skin, urine, vomit, and vaginal bleeding. 2. Support prevention through skin care (avoiding falls, protecting skin from cuts and scrapes), mouth care, digestive support (stool softeners, diet, exercise). 3. Manage bleeding: Apply pressure to bleeding areas, ice. 4. Note color, amount of bleeding. 5. Report bleeding occurrences, as needed, to physician.

SELECTED NURSING DIAGNOSES FOR RADIATION THERAPY

Nursing Diagnoses	Possible Nursing Interventions
Impaired skin integrity	1. Assess skin reactions. 2. Instruct patient and family to keep skin clean. 3. Instruct patient to avoid shaving within area of treatment. 4. Apply moisturizing lotion as directed for skin dryness. 5. If pruritus occurs, apply a thin layer of hydrocortisone cream. 6. If moist desquamation occurs, use Burrow compresses three to four times a day.
Complication (Intestinal): Enteritis and Proctitis, changed innervation to bladder and bowel	(Bladder and bowel hypercontractility can occur 2-3 weeks postradiation) 1. Educate patient before surgery (changes in sense to urge, incontinence — may need catheter, appliances). 2. Monitor for signs and symptoms. *Voiding:* 3. Restrict fluid intake to 2L/daily. 4. Promote regular scheduled for voiding. 5. Provide analgesics and antispasmotics. *Bowel:* 6. Manage with antidiarrheals, as needed. 7. Support low residue diets; avoid fruits and vegetables that promote diarrhea.
Complication (Bladder): Chronic Cystitis	1. Monitor and assess for signs and symptoms — pain, infection, urgency, frequency, and inability to empty bladder. 2. Promote fluid intake. 3. Use good hygiene. 4. Instruct patient to avoid caffeine. 5. Support warm baths. 6. Administer medication, as ordered.
Complication: Constipation, Small Bowel Obstruction	1. Monitor for signs and symptoms — pain, consistency of stools, and bloody stools. 2. Administer nasogastric (NG) suction and IV fluids, as needed. 3. Support patient while NPO while NG tube in place; manage nausea and vomiting. 4. Promote fluid intake, as appropriate. 5. Perform mouth care. 6. Report symptoms to physician, as needed.
Complication: Diarrhea	1. Monitor for signs and symptoms — pain, infection, and reduced bowel pattern. 2. Promote fluid intake, as appropriate. 3. Promote low-residue diet. 4. Monitor for signs of infection. 5. Administer antidiarrheal medication, as ordered. 6. Avoid fatty foods, rich desserts. 7. Administer medication, as ordered. 8. Report symptoms to physician, as needed.
Complication: Vaginitis	1. Monitor for signs and symptoms — pain, drainage, and infection. 2. Promote fluid intake. 3. Use good hygiene. 4. Instruct patient to avoid caffeine.
Complication: Leg Edema, Thrombophlebitis	1. Monitor for signs and symptoms — pain, redness, inflammation, and swelling.
Complication: Fistula Formation	(Vaginal or cervical radiation can form vaginal fistulas — both resigovaginal (bladder) and rectovaginal (bowel) — because radiation thins the vaginal wall). 1. Monitor signs of fistula. 2. Advocate for surgical closure. 3. Manage temporary urinary or fecal diversions. 4. Promote wound healing of fistula, manage necrosis of tissue. 5. Support cleanliness with sitz baths, pad changes, protecting skin, and dryness. 6. Administer antibiotics, as prescribed.

SELECTED NURSING DIAGNOSES FOR RADIATION THERAPY (CONTINUED)

Nursing Diagnoses	Possible Nursing Interventions
Activity intolerance, fatigue	1. Assess level of fatigue. 2. Advise patient to plan rest periods throughout the day. 3. Maintain nutritional intake. 4. Utilize resources to conserve energy. 5. Obtain assistance for chores and transportation, as needed.
Altered nutrition, less than body requirements related to anorexia	(Maybe especially pronounced in ovarian cancer, due to ascites, early satiation (from increased girth and protein loss) 1. Assess appetite. 2. Monitor weight. 3. Recommend frequent, small meals, and cold foods. 4. Advise on use of nutrient-dense foods such as nutritional supplements. 5. Administer appetite stimulants, as prescribed (Megace, corticosteroids and metoclopramide).

SELECTED NURSING DIAGNOSES FOR CHEMOTHERAPY

Nursing Diagnoses	Possible Nursing Interventions
Risk for fluid volume deficit related to nausea and vomiting	1. Assess for nausea and vomiting. 2. Instruct patient to use antiemetics before chemotherapy and as needed. 3. Monitor hydration status. 4. Encourage fluids. 5. Utilize nonpharmacologic measures to manage nausea and vomiting: relaxation exercises, or distraction. 6. Encourage small frequent meals. 7. Provide diet that is low in fat and nonsweet; encourage fluids. 8. Provide mouth care frequently during the day.
Risk for injury related to nephrotoxicity of cisplatin	(Many gynecologic malignancies include cisplatin-based chemotherapy protocols) 1. Monitor laboratory values, electrolytes, especially creatinine and blood urea nitrogen levels. 2. Provide hydrating intravenous fluids and medications, as ordered. 3. Monitor intake and output. 4. Encourage fluids. 5. Control nausea and vomiting. 6. Observe and monitor "glove and stocking" anesthesia after chemotherapy treatments end, also gait changes — encourage patient to prevent falls and promote safety.

Altered oral mucous membrane	1. Assess oral cavity: tenderness, ulceration, bleeding, and infections.
	2. Instruct patient about mouth care:
	    Brush teeth after each meal.
	    Floss teeth at bedtime, if patient normally practices flossing.
	    Perform frequent oral rinses with warm normal saline.
	3. Advise on diet consisting of nonspicy, non acidic, room-temperature, or cool foods.
	4. Maintain hydration.

Risk for infection related to neutropenia	1. Monitor blood counts: white blood count, neutrophils; assess for neutropenia.
	2. Institute neutropenia precautions when white blood cell count is decreased.
	3. Instruct patient about risk for infection:
	    Monitor temperature: be alert for fever, chills, sweats, myalgias; report these occurrences.
	    Avoid crowds.
	    Avoid persons with colds or other respiratory infections.
	    Avoid sharing eating utensils, beverage containers.
	    Avoid handling animal excreta (for example, cat litter box, bird cage).
	    Preserve and protect skin integrity.

Risk for injury related to thrombocytopenia	1. Monitor platelet count. 2. Institute bleeding precautions when platelet count is decreased. 3. Assess skin, mucous membranes, bowel movements, urine, emesis, and secretions for signs of bleeding. 4. Assess signs of hemorrhage: hypotension, changes in consciousness, headache, vomiting, and tachycardia. 5. Protect skin integrity: avoid venipuncture, intramuscular injections. 6. Perform mouth care, avoid traumatizing oral mucosa. 7. Institute bowel program to prevent constipation. 8. Avoid trauma to rectal tissues: avoid rectal medication, rectal thermometer, enemas. 9. Use electric razor. 10. Provide safe environment that eliminates hazards for injury.

Risk for activity intolerance related to anemia	1. Assess for fatigue.
	2. Monitor blood counts: red blood cells, hematocrit.
	3. Recommend measures to minimize fatigue:
	    Pace activities.
	    Plan rest periods during the day.
	4. Administer blood products, as ordered.
	5. Ensure adequate nutritional intake.

Knowledge deficit related to chemotherapy and self-care measures	1. Assess level of understanding about chemotherapy. 2. Provide information about chemotherapy: effects, adverse effects, and self-care measures, as well as symptoms to report. 3. Provide educational booklets, videotapes, and audiotapes as they are available. 4. Evaluate comprehension of patient education.

MISCELLANEOUS NURSING DIAGNOSES

Nursing Diagnoses	Possible Nursing Interventions
Sleep Disturbances, Insomnia	1. Assess sleep patterns through sleep log. 2. Instruct patient and family about optimal sleep preparation — relaxation, no alcohol, avoid heavy or spicy foods, avoid nicotine, exercise. 3. Medicate, as directed, by physician. 4. Develop a routine for sleep — schedule and place. 5. Avoid day-time napping.
Lymphedema	1. Focus on prevention — exercise, skin care, and prevent injury. 2. Report signs of infection (redness, warmth, red streaks, inflamed areas). 3. Reports signs of swelling — tightness of clothing, rings; numbness, pain. 4. Support massage and stretching, as appropriate. 5. Elevate extremity, as needed. 6. Use compression sleeve or stocking to limit swelling, promote drainage.

NURSING DIAGNOSES: PSYCHOSOCIAL ISSUES

Nursing Diagnoses	Possible Nursing Interventions
Anxiety	1. Assess level of anxiety. 2. Allow patient and family to verbalize issues and concerns. 3. Provide education about illness and treatment.
Body image disturbance	1. Assess patient understanding about body image changes. 2. Provide education about changes and rehabilitative measures available. 3. Allow patient and family to discuss issues and concerns about body image changes.
Knowledge deficit related to surgery and self-care measures	1. Assess patient's and family's understanding about surgery and self-care measures. 2. Provide education about surgery and self-care measures; utilize available multimedia patient . education tools: booklets, videos, and audiotapes. 3. Evaluate patient's comprehension of education materials.
Depression	1. Monitor signs and symptoms (see Chapter 8). 2. Administer medications, as prescribed. 3. Provide support for improved sleep, diet, and exercise. 4. Provide support for patient and family to move through short-and long-term grieving process.

GLOSSARY

acupressure: The application of pressure or localized massage to specific sites on the body to control symptoms such as pain or nausea. Also used to stop bleeding.

acupuncture: The technique of inserting thin needles through the skin at specific points on the body to control pain and other symptoms.

acustimulation: Mild electrical stimulation of acupuncture points to control symptoms, such as nausea and vomiting.

adenocarcinoma: Cancer that begins in cells that line certain internal organs and that have glandular (secretory) properties.

adenoma: A noncancerous tumor.

adjuvant therapy: Treatment given after the primary treatment to increase the chances of a cure. Adjuvant therapy may include chemotherapy, radiation therapy, hormone therapy, or biological therapy.

AJCC staging system: A system developed by the American Joint Committee on Cancer for describing the extent of cancer in a patient's body. The descriptions include TNM: T describes the size of the tumor and if it has invaded nearby tissue, N describes any lymph nodes that are involved, and M describes metastasis (spread of cancer from one body part to another).

alkylating agents: A family of anticancer drugs that interferes with the cell's deoxyribonucleic acid and inhibits cancer cell growth.

alopecia: The lack or loss of hair from areas of the body where hair is usually found. Alopecia can be an adverse effect of some cancer treatments.

alternative medicine: Practices not generally recognized by the medical community as standard or conventional medical approaches and used instead of standard treatments. Alternative medicine includes the taking of dietary supplements, megadose vitamins, and herbal preparations; the drinking of special teas; and practices such as massage therapy, magnet therapy, spiritual healing, and meditation.

antidepressant: A drug used to treat depression.

antiestrogen: A substance that blocks the activity of estrogens, the family of hormones that promote the development and maintenance of female sex characteristics.

aromatase inhibition: Prevention of the formation of estradiol, a female hormone, by interfering with an aromatase enzyme. Aromatase inhibition is a type of hormone therapy used in postmenopausal women who have hormone-dependent breast cancer.

axillary dissection: Surgery to remove lymph nodes found in the armpit region. Also called axillary lymph node dissection.

axillary lymph node dissection: Surgery to remove lymph nodes found in the armpit region. Also called axillary dissection.

axillary lymph nodes: Lymph nodes found in the armpit that drain the lymph channels from the breast.

benign proliferative breast disease: A group of noncancerous conditions that may increase the risk of developing breast cancer. Examples include ductal hyperplasia, lobular hyperplasia, and papillomas.

biofeedback: A method of learning to voluntarily control certain body functions such as heartbeat, blood pressure, and muscle tension with the help of a special machine. This method can help control pain.

biopsy: The removal of cells or tissues for examination under a microscope. When only a sample of tissue is removed, the procedure is called an incisional biopsy or core biopsy. When an entire lump or suspicious area is removed, the procedure is called an excisional biopsy. When a sample of tissue or fluid is removed with a needle, the procedure is called a needle biopsy or fine needle aspiration.

brachytherapy: A treatment which allows radioactive material — sealed in needles, seeds, wires or cathetors — to be placed in or near a tumor. The treatment is also called internal radiation, implant radiation or interstitial radiation.

BRCA1: A gene on chromosome 17 that normally helps to suppress cell growth. A person who inherits an altered version of the BRCA1 gene has a higher risk of getting breast, ovarian, or prostate cancer.

BRCA2: A gene on chromosome 13 that normally helps to suppress cell growth. A person who inherits an altered version of the BRCA2 gene has a higher risk of getting breast, ovarian, or prostate cancer.

breast cancer in situ: Abnormal cells that are confined to the ducts or lobules in the breast. There are two forms, called ductal carcinoma in situ (DCIS) and lobular carcinoma in situ (LCIS).

breast implant: A silicone gel-filled or saline-filled sac placed under the chest muscle to restore breast shape.

breast reconstruction: Surgery to rebuild a breast's shape after a mastectomy.

breast-conserving surgery: An operation to remove the breast cancer but not the breast itself. Types of breast-conserving surgery include lumpectomy (removal of the lump), quadrantectomy (removal of one quarter of the breast), and segmental mastectomy (removal of the cancer as well as some of the breast tissue around the tumor and the lining over the chest muscles below the tumor).

c-erbB-2: The gene that controls cell growth by making the human epidermal growth factor receptor 2; also called HER-2/neu.

cervical intraepithelial neoplasia (CIN): A general term for the growth of abnormal cells on the surface of the cervix. Numbers from 1-3 may be used to describe how much of the cervix contains abnormal cells.

cervix: The lower, narrow end of the uterus that forms a canal between the uterus and vagina.

colon: The long, tube-like organ that is connected to the small intestine and rectum. The colon removes water and some nutrients and electrolytes from digested food. The remaining material, solid waste called stool, moves through the colon to the rectum and leaves the body through the anus. Also called the large intestine.

colon cancer: A disease in which malignant (cancer) cells are found in the tissues of the colon.

colon polyps: Abnormal growths of tissue in the lining of the bowel. Polyps are a risk factor for colon cancer.

colonoscope: A thin, lighted tube used to examine the inside of the colon.

colonoscopy: An examination of the inside of the colon using a thin, lighted tube (called a colonoscope) inserted into the rectum. If abnormal areas are seen, tissue can be removed and examined under a microscope to determine whether disease is present.

colostomy: An opening into the colon from the outside of the body. A colostomy provides a new path for waste material to leave the body after part of the colon has been removed.

complementary and alternative medicine (CAM): Forms of treatment that are used in addition to (complementary) or instead of (alternative) standard treatments. These practices are not considered standard medical approaches. CAM includes dietary supplements, megadose vitamins, herbal preparations, special teas, acupuncture, massage therapy, magnet therapy, spiritual healing, and meditation.

complementary medicine: Practices not generally recognized by the medical community as standard or conventional medical approaches and used to enhance or complement standard treatments. Complementary medicine includes dietary supplements, megadose vitamins, herbal preparations, special teas, acupuncture, massage therapy, magnet therapy, spiritual healing, and meditation.

complete hysterectomy: Surgery to remove the entire uterus, including the cervix. Sometimes, not all of the cervix is removed. Also called total hysterectomy.

computed tomography (CT scan): A series of detailed pictures of areas inside the body taken from different angles; the pictures are created by a computer linked to an x-ray machine. Also called computerized tomography and computerized axial tomography (CAT) scan.

cone biopsy: Surgery to remove a cone-shaped piece of tissue from the cervix and cervical canal. Cone biopsy may be used to diagnose or treat a cervical condition. Also called conization.

corpus: The body of the uterus.

curettage: Removal of tissue with a curette, a spoon-shaped instrument with a sharp edge.

cutaneous breast cancer: Cancer that has spread from the breast to the skin.

cyst: A sac or capsule filled with fluid.

DCIS: Ductal carcinoma in situ. Abnormal cells that involve only the lining of a duct. The cells have not spread outside the duct to other tissues in the breast. Also called intraductal carcinoma.

Diethylstilbestrol (DES): A synthetic hormone that was prescribed from the early 1940s until 1971 to help women with complications of pregnancy. DES has been linked to an increased risk of clear cell carcinoma of the vagina in daughters of women who used DES. DES may also increase the risk of breast cancer in women who used DES.

digital rectal examination (DRE): An examination in which a doctor inserts a lubricated, gloved finger into the rectum to feel for abnormalities.

dilation and curettage (D&C): A minor operation in which the cervix is expanded enough (dilation) to permit the cervical canal and uterine lining to be scraped with a spoon-shaped instrument called a curette (curettage).

distal pancreatectomy: Removal of the body and tail of the pancreas.

ductal carcinoma: The most common type of breast cancer. It begins in the cells that line the milk ducts in the breast.

ductal carcinoma in situ (DCIS): Abnormal cells that involve only the lining of a duct. The cells have not spread outside the duct to other tissues in the breast. Also called intraductal carcinoma.

ductal lavage: A method used to collect cells from milk ducts in the breast. The cells are looked at under a microscope to check for cancer. A hair-size catheter (tube) is inserted into the nipple. A small amount of salt water flows into the duct and is then removed with the cells in it. Ductal lavage may be used in addition to physical breast examination and mammography to detect breast cancer.

Dukes' classification: A staging system used to describe the extent of colorectal cancer. Stages range from A (early stage) to D (advanced stage).

endocervical curettage: The scraping of the mucous membrane of the cervical canal using a spoon-shaped instrument called a curette.

endometrial: Having to do with the endometrium (the layer of tissue that lines the uterus).

endometrial disorder: Abnormal cell growth in the endometrium (the lining of the uterus).

endometriosis: A benign condition in which tissue that looks like endometrial tissue grows in abnormal places in the abdomen.

endometrium: The layer of tissue that lines the uterus.

endoscope: A thin, lighted tube used to look at tissues inside the body.

endoscopic retrograde cholangiopancreatography (ERCP): A procedure to x-ray the pancreatic duct, hepatic duct, common bile duct, duodenal papilla, and gallbladder. In this procedure, a thin, lighted tube (endoscope) is passed through the mouth and down into the first part of the small intestine (duodenum). A smaller tube (catheter) is then inserted through the endoscope into the bile and pancreatic ducts. A dye is injected through the catheter into the ducts, and an x-ray is taken.

epithelial ovarian cancer: Cancer that occurs in the cells lining the ovaries.

epithelium: A thin layer of tissue that covers organs, glands, and other structures within the body.

estrogen receptor (ER): Protein found on some cancer cells to which estrogen will attach.

estrogen receptor positive (ER+): Breast cancer cells that have a protein (receptor molecule) to which estrogen will attach. Breast cancer cells that are ER+ need the hormone estrogen to grow and will usually respond to hormone (antiestrogen) therapy that blocks these receptor sites.

estrogen receptor negative (ER-): Breast cancer cells that do not have a protein (receptor molecule) to which estrogen will attach. Breast cancer cells that are ER- do not need the hormone estrogen to grow and usually do not respond to hormone (antiestrogen) therapy that blocks these receptor sites.

estrogens: A family of hormones that promote the development and maintenance of female sex characteristics.

estrogen replacement therapy (ERT): Hormones (estrogen, progesterone, or both) given to postmenopausal women or to women who have had their ovaries surgically removed. Hormones are given to replace the estrogen no longer produced by the ovaries.

external-beam radiation: Radiation therapy that uses a machine to aim high-energy rays at the cancer. Also called external radiation.

fallopian tubes: Part of the female reproductive tract. The long slender tubes through which eggs pass from the ovaries to the uterus.

familial adenomatous polyposis (FAP): An inherited condition in which numerous polyps (growths that protrude from mucous membranes) form on the inside walls of the colon and rectum. It increases the risk for colon cancer. Also called familial polyposis.

familial polyposis: An inherited condition in which numerous polyps (growths that protrude from mucous membranes) form on the inside walls of the colon and rectum. It increases the risk for colon cancer. Also called familial adenomatous polyposis or FAP.

fibroid: A benign smooth-muscle tumor, usually in the uterus or gastrointestinal tract. Also called leiomyoma.

genetic counseling: A communication process between a specially trained health professional and a person concerned about the genetic risk of disease. The person's family and personal medical history may be discussed, and counseling may lead to genetic testing.

genetic testing: Analyzing DNA to look for a genetic alteration that may indicate an increased risk for developing a specific disease or disorder.

gonads: The part of the reproductive system that produces and releases eggs (ovaries) or sperm (testicles/testes).

gynecologic: Having to do with the female reproductive tract (including the cervix, endometrium, fallopian tubes, ovaries, uterus, and vagina).

gynecologic cancer: Cancer of the female reproductive tract, including the cervix, endometrium, fallopian tubes, ovaries, uterus, and vagina.

gynecologic oncologist: A physician who specializes in treating cancers of the female reproductive organs.

gynecologist: A physician who specializes in treating diseases of the female reproductive organs.

Halsted radical mastectomy: Surgery for breast cancer in which the breast, chest muscles, and all of the lymph nodes under the arm are removed. For many years, this was the operation most used, but it is used now only when the tumor has spread to the chest muscles. Also called radical mastectomy.

HER-2/neu: Human epidermal growth factor receptor 2. The HER-2/neu protein is involved in growth of some cancer cells. Also called c-erbB-2.

hereditary nonpolyposis colon cancer (HNPCC): An inherited disorder in which affected individuals have a higher-than-normal chance of developing colon cancer and certain other types of cancer, usually before age 60. Also called Lynch syndrome.

high-grade squamous intraepithelial lesion (HSIL): A precancerous condition in which the cells of the uterine cervix are moderately or severely abnormal.

hormone receptor: A protein on the surface of a cell that binds to a specific hormone. The hormone causes many changes to take place in the cell.

hormone receptor test: A test to measure the amount of certain proteins, called hormone receptors, in cancer tissue. Hormones can attach to these proteins. A high level of hormone receptors may mean that hormones help the cancer grow.

hormone replacement therapy (HRT): Hormones (estrogen, progesterone, or both) given to postmenopausal women or women who have had their ovaries surgically removed, to replace the estrogen no longer produced by the ovaries.

hormone responsive: In oncology, describes cancer that responds to hormone treatment.

hormone therapy: Treatment that adds, blocks, or removes hormones. For certain conditions (such as diabetes or menopause), hormones are given to adjust low hormone levels. To slow or stop the growth of certain cancers (such as prostate and breast cancer), hormones may be given to block the body's natural hormones. Sometimes surgery is needed to remove the source of hormones. Also called hormonal therapy, hormone treatment, or endocrine therapy.

hormones: Chemicals produced by glands in the body and circulated in the bloodstream. Hormones control the actions of certain cells or organs.

hysterectomy: An operation in which the uterus is removed.

in situ cancer: Early cancer that has not spread to neighboring tissue.

in vitro: In the laboratory (outside the body). The opposite of in vivo (in the body).

in vivo: In the body. The opposite of in vitro (outside the body or in the laboratory).

incidence: The number of new cases of a disease diagnosed each year.

incision: A cut made in the body to perform surgery.

incisional biopsy: A surgical procedure in which a portion of a lump or suspicious area is removed for diagnosis. The tissue is then examined under a microscope.

infiltrating ductal carcinoma: The most common type of invasive breast cancer. It starts in the cells that line the milk ducts in the breast, grows outside the ducts, and often spreads to the lymph nodes.

inflammatory breast cancer: A type of breast cancer in which the breast looks red and swollen and feels warm. The skin of the breast may also show the pitted appearance called peau d'orange (like the skin of an orange). The redness and warmth occur because the cancer cells block the lymph vessels in the skin.

internal radiation: A procedure in which radioactive material sealed in needles, seeds, wires, or catheters is placed directly into or near a tumor. Also called brachytherapy, implant radiation, or interstitial radiation therapy.

interstitial radiation therapy: A procedure in which radioactive material sealed in needles, seeds, wires, or catheters is placed directly into or near a tumor. Also called brachytherapy, internal radiation, or implant radiation.

intraductal carcinoma: Abnormal cells that involve only the lining of a duct. The cells have not spread outside the duct to other tissues in the breast. Also called ductal carcinoma in situ.

invasive cervical cancer: Cancer that has spread from the surface of the cervix to tissue deeper in the cervix or to other parts of the body.

jaundice: A condition in which the skin and the whites of the eyes become yellow, urine darkens, and the color of stool becomes lighter than normal. Jaundice occurs when the liver is not working properly or when a bile duct is blocked.

laparoscopy: The insertion of a thin, lighted tube (called a laparoscope) through the abdominal wall to inspect the inside of the abdomen and remove tissue.

lobular carcinoma in situ (LCIS): Abnormal cells found in the lobules of the breast. This condition seldom becomes invasive cancer; however, having lobular carcinoma in situ increases one's risk of developing breast cancer in either breast.

lumpectomy: Surgery to remove the tumor and a small amount of normal tissue around it.

magnetic resonance imaging (MRI): A procedure in which a magnet linked to a computer is used to create detailed pictures of areas inside the body. Also called nuclear magnetic resonance imaging.

mammogram: An x-ray of the breast.

mammography: The use of x-rays to create a picture of the breast

medullary breast carcinoma: A rare type of breast cancer that often can be treated successfully. It is marked by lymphocytes (a type of white blood cell) in and around the tumor that can be seen when viewed under a microscope

microcalcifications: Tiny deposits of calcium in the breast that cannot be felt but can be detected on a mammogram. A cluster of these very small specks of calcium may indicate that cancer is present.

modified radical mastectomy: Surgery for breast cancer in which the breast, some of the lymph nodes under the arm, the lining over the chest muscles, and sometimes part of the chest wall muscles are removed.

needle biopsy: The removal of tissue or fluid with a needle for examination under a microscope. Also called fine needle aspiration.

negative axillary lymph nodes: Lymph nodes in the armpit that are free of cancer.

neoadjuvant therapy: Treatment given before the primary treatment. Examples of neoadjuvant therapy include chemotherapy, radiation therapy, and hormone therapy.

node-negative: Cancer that has not spread to the lymph nodes.

node-positive: Cancer that has spread to the lymph nodes.

nodule: A growth or lump that may be cancerous or noncancerous.

oophorectomy: Surgery to remove one or both ovaries.

ovarian: Having to do with the ovaries, the female reproductive glands in which the ova (eggs) are formed. The ovaries are located in the pelvis, one on each side of the uterus.

ovarian ablation: Surgery, radiation therapy, or a drug treatment to stop the functioning of the ovaries. Also called ovarian suppression.

ovarian epithelial cancer: Cancer that occurs in the cells lining the ovaries.

ovarian suppression: Surgery, radiation therapy, or a drug treatment to stop the functioning of the ovaries. Also called ovarian ablation.

ovaries: The pair of female reproductive glands in which the ova, or eggs, are formed. The ovaries are located in the pelvis, one on each side of the uterus.

Paget's disease of the nipple: A form of breast cancer in which the tumor grows from ducts beneath the nipple onto the surface of the nipple. Symptoms commonly include itching and burning and an eczema-like condition around the nipple, sometimes accompanied by oozing or bleeding.

Papanicolaou (Pap) test: The collection of cells from the cervix for examination under a microscope. It is used to detect changes that may be cancer or may lead to cancer, and can show noncancerous conditions, such as infection or inflammation. Also called a Pap smear.

partial mastectomy: The removal of a cancer as well as some of the breast tissue around the tumor and the lining over the chest muscles below the tumor. Usually some of the lymph nodes under the arm are also taken out. Also called segmental mastectomy.

peau d'orange: A dimpled condition of the skin of the breast, resembling the skin of an orange, sometimes found in inflammatory breast cancer.

positive axillary lymph nodes: Lymph nodes in the area of the armpit (axilla) to which cancer has spread. This spread is determined by surgically removing some of the lymph nodes and examining them under a microscope to see whether cancer cells are present.

progesterone: a female sex hormone released by the ovaries during every menstrual cycle to prepare the uterus for pregnancy and the breasts for milk production (lactation). In breast cancer, tumor growth may depened on progesterone. If the woman's tumor does rely on progesterone for growth, she is progesterone receptor positive (PR+). If it does not, she is progesterone receptor negative (PR-).

progesterone receptor positive (PR+): In breast cancer, if the woman's tumor growth is affected by progesterone.

progesterone receptor positive (PR-): In breast cancer, if the woman's tumor growth is not affected by progesterone.

preventive mastectomy: Surgery to remove one or both breasts in order to decrease the risk of developing breast cancer. Also called prophylactic mastectomy.

prophylactic mastectomy: Surgery to remove one or both breasts in order to decrease the risk of developing breast cancer. Also called preventive mastectomy.

prophylactic oophorectomy: Surgery intended to reduce the risk of ovarian cancer by removing the ovaries before disease develops.

quadrantectomy: Surgical removal of the region of the breast (approximately one quarter) containing cancer.

radiation therapy: The use of high-energy radiation from x-rays, gamma rays, neutrons, and other sources to kill cancer cells and shrink tumors. Radiation may come from a machine outside the body (external-beam radiation therapy), or from materials called radioisotopes. Radioisotopes produce radiation and can be placed in or near the tumor or in the area near cancer cells. This type of radiation treatment is called internal radiation therapy, implant radiation, interstitial radiation, or brachytherapy. Systemic radiation therapy uses a radioactive substance, such as a radiolabeled monoclonal antibody, that circulates throughout the body. Also called radiotherapy, irradiation, and x-ray therapy.

radical lymph node dissection: A surgical procedure to remove most or all of the lymph nodes that drain lymph from the area around a tumor. The lymph nodes are then examined under a microscope to see if cancer cells have spread to them.

radical mastectomy: Surgery for breast cancer in which the breast, chest muscles, and all of the lymph nodes under the arm are removed. For many years, this was the operation most used, but it is used now only when the tumor has spread to the chest muscles. Also called the Halsted radical mastectomy.

raloxifene: A drug that belongs to the family of drugs called selective estrogen receptor modulators (SERMs) and is used in the prevention of osteoporosis in postmenopausal women. Raloxifene is also being studied as a cancer prevention drug.

reconstructive surgery: Surgery that is done to reshape or rebuild (reconstruct) a part of the body changed by previous surgery.

regional lymph node dissection: A surgical procedure to remove some of the lymph nodes that drain lymph from the area around a tumor. The lymph nodes are then examined under a microscope to see if cancer cells have spread to them.

resection: Removal of tissue or part or all of an organ by surgery.

salpingo-oophorectomy: Surgical removal of the fallopian tubes and ovaries.

Schiller test: A test in which iodine is applied to the cervix. The iodine colors healthy cells brown; abnormal cells remain unstained, usually appearing white or yellow.

segmental mastectomy: The removal of a cancer as well as some of the breast tissue around the tumor and the lining over the chest muscles below the tumor. Usually some of the lymph nodes under the arm are also taken out. Also called partial mastectomy.

selective estrogen receptor modulator (SERM): A drug that acts like estrogen on some tissues but blocks the effect of estrogen on other tissues. Tamoxifen and raloxifene are SERMs.

sentinel lymph node: The first lymph node to which cancer is likely to spread from the primary tumor. Cancer cells may appear first in the sentinel node before spreading to other lymph nodes.

sentinel lymph node biopsy: Removal and examination of the sentinel node(s) (the first lymph node(s) to which cancer cells are likely to spread from a primary tumor). To identify the sentinel lymph node(s), the surgeon injects a radioactive substance, blue dye, or both near the tumor. The surgeon then uses a scanner to find the sentinel lymph node(s) containing the radioactive substance or looks for the lymph node(s) stained with dye. The surgeon then removes the sentinel node(s) to check for the presence of cancer cells.

sentinel lymph node mapping: The use of dyes and radioactive substances to identify the first lymph node to which cancer is likely to spread from the primary tumor. Cancer cells may appear first in the sentinel node before spreading to other lymph nodes and other places in the body.

staging: Performing examinations and tests to learn the extent of the cancer within the body, especially whether the disease has spread from the original site to other parts of the body. It is important to know the stage of the disease in order to plan the best treatment.

tamoxifen: An anticancer drug that belongs to the family of drugs called antiestrogens. Tamoxifen blocks the effects of the hormone estrogen in the body. It is used to prevent or delay the return of breast cancer or to control its spread.

total estrogen blockade: Therapy used to eliminate estrogen in the body. This may be done with surgery, radiation therapy, chemotherapy, or a combination of these procedures.

total hysterectomy: Surgery to remove the entire uterus, including the cervix. Sometimes, not all of the cervix is removed. Also called complete hysterectomy.

total mastectomy: Removal of the breast. Also called simple mastectomy.

transvaginal ultrasound: A procedure used to examine the vagina, uterus, fallopian tubes, and bladder. An instrument is inserted into the vagina, and sound waves bounce off organs inside the pelvic area. These sound waves create echoes, which a computer uses to create a picture called a sonogram. Also called TVS.

ultrasound: A procedure in which high-energy sound waves (ultrasound) are bounced off internal tissues or organs and make echoes. The echoes form a picture of body tissues called a sonogram. Also called ultrasonography.

vulva: The external female genital organs, including the clitoris, vaginal lips, and the opening to the vagina.

vulvar cancer: Cancer of the vulva (the external female genital organs, including the clitoris, vaginal lips, and the opening to the vagina).

Whipple procedure: A type of surgery used to treat pancreatic cancer. The head of the pancreas, the duodenum, a portion of the stomach, and other nearby tissues are removed.

INDEX

A

ACS (American Cancer Society), 72, 114, 115*t*
ACS (American Cancer Society) website, 175
acute anxiety, 131
adjustment disorders
    acute anxiety as, 131
    described, 131
    diagnosis of, 128*t*
    prevalence of, 131
AJCC (American Joint Committee on Cancer), 39
alternative medical systems, 163*t*
Amsterdam Criteria-II, 111*t*
antidepressants
    common physical adverse effects from, 138*t*
    common types of, 136*t*
    factors to consider in choosing, 137*t*
anxiety
    assessment and screening of, 133*t*
    commonly prescribed benzodiazepines for, 132*t*
    overview of cancer and, 131-132
    possible causes of, 132*t*
    symptoms of, 132*t*
APC (adenomatous polyposis coli), 110
Aredia, 25
aromatherapy program, 166*t*
ASCUS/LSIL Triage Study (ALTS), 70
Association for Cancer Online Resources website, 179

B

BCPT (Breast Cancer Prevention Trial), 13
Bethesda Criteria, 111*t*
Bethesda system, 74, 75*t*
B-E-T-T-E-R assessment, 154
biologically-based therapies (CAMs), 163*t*
biological therapy (breast cancer), 23
brachytherapy (intracavitary irradiation), 77-78
BRCA1 mutation
    breast cancer associated with, 16, 18, 19*t*
    ovarian cancer associated with, 53*t*, 54
BRCA2 mutation
    breast cancer associated with, 16, 18, 19*t*
    ovarian cancer associated with, 53*t*, 54
breast anatomy, 10, 11*fig*

breast cancer
    CAMs used by patients with, 164
    case study of, 26-27
    diagnosing, 19-20
    epidemiology of, 9-10
    genetic risk for, 17-19*t*
    lifetime probability of being diagnosed with, 10*t*
    morality risk according to age, 10*t*
    noninvasive, 10-11
    pregnancy and, 153
    rehabilitation process, 25-26
    risk categories with node-negative, 23*t*
    risk factors for, 11-13
    staging of, 20*t*, 23*t*-25
    statistical trends of, 3
    treatment of, 20-25*t*
    trends regarding, 2-3
breast cancer genetic risks
    assessing, 17
    counseling and risk models, 18-19*t*
    overview of, 17
    risk assessment of BRCA1/BRCA2 mutation, 16, 18, 19*t*
breast cancer screening
    BSE (breast self-examination), 14*fig*-15
    CBE (clinical breast examination), 15
    impact on incidence and mortality, 16-17
    mammography, 15-16
    recommended guidelines for, 15*t*
breast cancer stages
    listed, 20*t*
    treatment during early, 23
    treatment during III, 23-24
    treatment during recurrent breast cancer and advanced, 24-25
breast cancer treatments
    for axillary node-negative breast cancer, 24*t*
    biological therapy, 23
    chemotherapy, 22*t*-23
    hormone therapy, 22*t*
    radiation therapy, 21-22
    SLNB (sentinel lymph node biopsy), 20-21
    during specific stages of cancer, 23*t*-25
    surgery, 20, 21*fig*

breastfeeding, 12
breast prosthesis, 26
breast reconstruction, 25-26
BSE (breast self-examination), 14*fig*

C

CA-125 levels, 59
CA-125 testing, 55, 56
CAM practitioners, 168*t*
CAMs (complementary and alternative medicine)
  anecdotal accounts of, 141, 161, 163
  evaluating website resources on, 168*t*
  five domains of, 163*t*
  helpful in care of cancer patients, 165-167*t*
  increasing interest in, 161, 163
  NCCAM studies on, 164*t*-165
  patient evaluation of, 167*t*
  prevalence of, 163-164
  reliable website sources on, 179
  selected therapies listed, 162*t*
  selecting a practitioner of, 168*t*
cancer
  psychosocial issues of, 125-141
  research contributions to prevention of, 3
  resources for patients and their families, 185-187
  selected Internet resources on, 189
  trends regarding women and, 1-3
Cancer Genetics Studies Consortium Task Force (NIH), 16
cancer incidence rates
  age-related breast cancer, 9-10
  breast cancer screening and, 16-17
  estimated for colorectal cancer, 108*fig*, 109t
  estimated for endometrial cancer, 34*fig*
  estimated for lung cancer, 88*fig*
  estimated for ovarian cancer, 49-50*fig*
  listed by sex and age, 2*fig*
cancer mortality rates
  age-related breast cancer, 10*t*
  breast cancer screening and, 16-17
  estimated for cervical cancer, 67
  estimated for colorectal cancer, 108*fig*, 109*t*
  estimated for endometrial cancer, 34*fig*
  estimated for females (2003), 3*fig*
  estimated for lung cancer, 88*fig*
  estimated for ovarian cancer, 49-50*fig*
CBE (clinical breast examination), 15

cervical cancer
  case study on, 80-81
  chemotherapy for, 79
  CIN (cervical intraepithelial neoplasia) and, 70-71
  described, 71-72
  epidemiology of, 67-68
  preinvasive cervical conditions of, 70-71
  radiotherapy for, 77, 79
  recurrent, 79
  risk factors for, 68*t*-69
  screening for, 72*t*-74, 76-77
  signs and symptoms of, 70*t*
  staging of, 77, 78*t*-79*t*
  surgical treatment for, 77
  treatments for benign tumors, 69-70
cervical cancer screening
  nursing role in, 72-73
  Pap test used in, 73*t*-74, 76*t*
  recommendations/guidelines for, 72*t*
cervix anatomy, 68*fig*
chemotherapy
  affecting sexuality, 152, 153*t*
  breast cancer, 22*t*-23
  cervical cancer, 79
  colorectal cancer, 117, 118*t*
  endometrial cancer, 42
  lung cancer, 99*t*, 100
  ovarian cancer, 58-59
CIN (cervical intraepithelial neoplasia), 70-71
Claus model, 18, 19*t*
colon anatomy, 110*fig*
colon cancer, 37-38
colonoscopy, 114
colorectal cancer
  case study for, 119-120
  described, 109-110
  epidemiology of, 107-109*t*, 108*fig*
  follow-up care after treatment, 119
  genetic origins of, 110, 111*t*-112
  hepatic involvement of, 118
  HNPCC (hereditary nonpolyposis colorectal cancer), 38, 53, 110, 112
  protective strategies in case of, 115, 116*t*
  risk factors for, 110-113, 111*t*
  screening and detection of, 113-115*t*, 114*t*
  staging and diagnosis of, 115, 116*t*
  symptoms of, 113
  treatments for, 116-118*t*
  women and, 109*fig*
colposcopy, 76
community cancer center CAM pilot studies, 166-167

coping
  with changes affecting sexuality, 151*t*
  cognitive model of coping theory on, 127
  factors affecting, 127-129
  selected studies of cancer patients and their, 129-130
  See also psychosocial issues; stress
Cowden syndrome, 53
cryopreservation, 153

D

D&C (dilation & curettage), 76-77
DCBE (Double Contrast Barium Enema), 117
DCC gene, 110
DCIS (ductal carcinoma in situ), 10-11
depression
  assessment and screening of, 133-135, 134*t*
  indicators of, 134*t*
  interventions in case of, 135-136
  medication-based causes of, 136*t*
  overview of, 133
  pharmacologic treatment of, 136*t*-137*t*, 138*t*
  understanding clinical depression vs., 133
DRE (Digital Rectal Examination), 113

E

ECC (endocervical curettage), 76
e-mail communication, 179
endometrial cancer
  case study on, 43
  cell types, 36*t*
  colon cancer relationship to, 37-38
  detection of, 38-39
  diagnosis of, 39
  epidemiology of, 33-34
  hormone metabolism and, 37
  prevention of, 36
  risk factors for, 36-37*t*
  staging of, 39, 40*t*
  symptoms of, 35-36
  tamoxifen linked to, 37, 38
  treatments for, 39-42
  tumor development, 35
  uterus anatomy and, 35*fig*
endometrial cancer treatments
  chemotherapy, 42
  hormone therapy, 42
  hysterectomy, 36, 39-41
  radiation therapy, 41-42
endometrial hyperplasia, 35, 38
endometrioid adenocarcinoma, 35
endometriosis, 35
endoscopic visualization methods, 113-114
energy therapies, 163*t*

essential oils, 166*t*
estrogen
  breast cancer and long-term exposure to, 12
  cervical cancer and, 69
  endometrial cancer and, 37
  See also HRT (hormone replacement therapy)
estrogen receptor test, 19
ethnic differences
  in cancer rates, 3
  colorectal cancer and, 109*t*
  endometrial cancer and, 33-34
  ovarian cancer and, 54
  See also racial differences
exercise rehabilitation, 25
external radiation therapy, 42, 77

F

family history
  breast cancer and, 12
  colorectal cancer and, 110, 111*t*-112
  endometrial and colon cancers and, 38
  lung cancer and, 95
  ovarian cancer and, 52, 53-54
  See also genetic carcinogenesis
female patients
  cancer incidence rates of, 2*fig*
  leading cancer cases estimated for, 2*fig*
  leading cancer deaths estimated for, 3*fig*
  psychosocial framework supporting, 1
  unique characteristics of, 1
fertility issues
  preserving ability to reproduce, 153
  sterility resulting from treatment, 152
fibroids, 35
FIGO (International Federation of Gynecology and Obstetrics), 39
FOBT (Fecal Occult Blood Test), 113, 114*t*

G

Gail model, 18, 19*t*
gender differences
  in breast cancer, 11
  cancer statistical trends and, 3-4
  colorectal cancer and, 108, 109*fig*
  lung cancer and, 87-88
gene therapy, 59
genetic carcinogenesis, 95
  See also family history

H

HDR (high dose brachytherapy), 77, 79
HER-2 gene, 20, 23
HER-2/neu, 23

Herceptin, 23
HIV (human immunodeficiency virus), 69, 73
HNPCC (hereditary nonpolyposis colorectal cancer), 38, 53, 110, 112
hormone metabolism, 37
hormone therapy
    breast cancer, 22*t*
    endometrial cancer, 42
    as ovarian cancer treatment, 59
hot flashes, 40
HPVs (human papillomaviruses), 68-69, 150
HRT (hormone replacement therapy)
    cervical cancer and, 69
    colorectal cancer reduced by, 115
    conflicting data regarding, 13*b*
    endometrial cancer prevention using, 37
    as endometriosis treatment, 35
    to mitigate sexually-related adverse effects, 156
    raloxifene, 14
    tamoxifen (Nolvodex), 13-14, 37, 38
    See also estrogen; medication
HSV-2 (herpes simplex virus type 2), 68, 69
hyperplasia, 8
hysterectomy
    as endometrial cancer treatment, 36, 39-41
    as endometriosis treatment, 35
    impact on sexuality by, 40-41

I
internal radiation therapy, 42, 77
Internet
    evaluating information found on the, 175-177*t*
    finding information on the, 175
    HON (Health on the Net Foundation) principles for using the, 176*t*
    integration of tech health care behaviors using the, 174*t*
    on-line support groups found on, 139*t*-140*t*, 179-180*fig*
    search engine preferences, 175*fig*
    selected resources on cancer listed, 189
    tips for health surfing on the, 178*t*
    as valuable communication tool, 173-175
    See also websites
isthmus, 35

L
LCIS (lobular carcinoma in situ), 11, 12, 13
LEEP (loop electrosurgical excision procedure), 70, 76
lifestyle
    as breast cancer risk, 12
    cancer statistical trends and, 3
    colorectal cancer and, 112-113

lobectomy, 98
LPA (lysophosphatidic acid), 56
Lung anatomy, 94*fig*
lung cancer
    case study for, 100-101
    complications of, 100
    diagnosis and staging of, 96*t*-97*t*
    epidemiology of, 87-88
    genetic carciogenesis and, 95
    growth in epidemic of, 88*fig*
    histopathologic cell types, bronchogenic, and lung carcinomas, 94*t*
    myths regarding, 88-89
    NSCLC (non-small cell lung cancer), 94, 95, 98, 99
    prevention/detection strategies, 95-96
    prognosis of, 98*t*
    risk factors for, 92*t*, 94-95
    SCLC (small cell lung cancer), 94, 95, 98, 99, 100
    signs and symptoms of, 96
    statistical trends of, 3-4
    treatments for, 98-100
    women, tobacco and, 89*fig*, 90
Lung Cancer Profile, 93*t*
lung cancer treatments
    chemotherapy, 99*t*, 100
    radiation therapy, 99
    during Stage III and Stage IV disease, 99
    surgery, 98-99
lymphedema, 25

M
mammography, 15-16
manipulative and body-based methods, 163*t*
medication
    affecting sexual response, 154*t*-155
    antidepressants, 136*t*, 137*t*, 138*t*
    anxiety, 132*t*
    selected CAMs types of, 162*t*
    See also HRT (hormone replacement therapy)
MEDLINE, 175
Medscape, 175
menopause (hysterectomy-induced), 39-41
mind-body interventions, 163*t*

N
National Center for Complementary and Alternative Medicine website, 179
NCCAM studies, 164*t*-165
NCCN (National Comprehensive Cancer Network), 126
NCI Best Case Series Program, 165
NCI (National Cancer Institute), 16, 114
NCI (National Cancer Institute) website, 175
Nolvodex, 13-14, 37, 38

nonepithelial ovarian cancer, 51
noninvasive breast cancers
 ductal carcinoma in situ (DCIS), 10-11
 lobular carcinoma in situ (LCIS), 11, 12, 13
NSABP (National Surgical Adjuvant Breast and Bowel
 Project) B-14 study, 13
NSCLC (non-small cell lung cancer)
 described, 94, 95
 treatments for, 98, 99
nurses
 role in cervical cancer screening, 72-73
 selected nursing diagnoses listed, 191-192
 suicide assessment by, 134*t*

O

obesity risk factor, 36, 37
OCCAM (Office of Cancer Complementary and
 Alternative Medicine), 165
Oncology Nursing Society Congress (2003), 165
on-line support groups
 advantages/disadvantages of, 180*fig*
 listed of selected, 139*t*-140*t*
 open forums/information available through, 179
oral contraceptives, 36
ovarian cancer
 case study on, 59-61
 complications from, 59
 diagnosis, treatment, prognosis of, 56*t*-59
 epidemiology of, 49-51
 overview of, 51-52
 prevention of, 52
 risk factors for, 52-54, 53*t*
 screening for, 54-56
 signs and symptoms of, 52
 staging criteria for, 57*t*
ovarian cancer survivorship, 130*t*
ovarian cysts, 51
ovary anatomy, 51*fig*

P

p53 molecular marker, 55
pamidronate (Aredia), 25
Pap test
 Bethesda system of interpreting, 74, 75*t*
 causes of inflamed cervical tissue affecting, 76*t*
 cervical cancer screening using, 73-74, 76
 classifications of abnormalities in, 75*t*
 technique used in, 74
 terms, follow-up, and strategies of, 73*t*
P-LI-SS-IT model, 154
pneumonectomy, 98
polyps, 111
pregnancy issues, 153

preinvasive cervical conditions, 70-71
progesterone, 37
progesterone receptor test, 19, 39
prophylactic mastectomy, 12
prophylactic oophorectomy, 56
psychosocial issues
 adjustment disorders as, 128*t*, 131
 anxiety as, 131-133*t*, 132*t*
 assessing and screening patients for, 126-127
 depression as, 133-137*t*
 importance of understanding, 125-126
 meaning in ovarian cancer survivorship, 130*t*
 selected studies of cancer patients and, 129-130
 social support/interventions for, 137-141
 stress as, 126
 surviving cancer and, 126-127
 See also coping
PubMED (National Library of Medicine site), 175

Q

Quack Watch website, 179

R

racial differences
 breast cancer risk and, 11
 cancer incidence rates and, 3
 cervical cancer and, 68
 colorectal cancer and, 108, 109*t*
 endometrial cancer and, 33-34
 See also ethnic differences
radiation therapy
 breast cancer, 21-22
 cervical cancer, 77, 79
 colorectal cancer, 117
 endometrial cancer, 41-42
 as ovarian cancer treatment, 59
 sexuality and, 152-153
raloxifene, 14

S

SCLC (small cell lung cancer)
 chemotherapy and, 100
 described, 94, 95
 treatments for, 98, 99
segmentectomy, 98
SERM (selective estrogen receptor modulator), 38
sexual dysfunction
 interventions for, 155*t*-156
 issues of, 151-152
 medication factors causing, 154*t*-155
 selected causes related to cancer treatment, 151*t*

sexuality
    coping with changes affecting, 151*t*
    impact of hysterectomy on, 40-41
    importance to quality of life, 149
    issues of functioning and treatment, 151*t*-152
    postmastectomy, 26
    psychological aspects of, 149-150
sexuality/treatment effects
    chemotherapy and, 152, 153*t*
    fertility issues, 152, 153
    pregnancy, 153
    radiation therapy, 152-153
SILs (squamous intraepithelial lesions), 69-70
sleeve resection, 98
smoking
    additional health risks of, 90
    cancer statistical trends and, 3
    colorectal cancer and, 113
    endometrial cancer linked to, 36
    global spread of, 92*fig*
    lung cancer and, 89-90
    teenagers and, 90
    ways to quit, 91*t*
    women and, 89*fig*, 90
social support/interventions
    benefits of different types of, 137-138, 140
    exercise, counseling, CAMs used in, 141
    on-line support groups, 139*t*-140*t*, 179-180*fig*
    studies on categories of, 137
staging
    breast cancer, 20t, 23*t*-25
    cervical cancer, 77, 78*t*-79*t*
    colorectal cancer, 115, 116*t*
    endometrial cancer, 39, 40*t*
    lung cancer, 96*t*-97*t*
    ovarian cancer, 57*t*
STAR trial, 14
stress, 126
    See also coping
suicide assessment, 134*t*
surgery
    breast cancer, 20, 21*fig*
    cervical cancer, 77
    colorectal cancer, 116-117*t*
    hysterectomy, 35, 36, 39-41
    lung cancer, 98-99
    as ovarian cancer treatment, 57-58
    prophylactic mastectomy, 12
    prophylactic oophorectomy, 56
    selected nursing diagnoses on, 191-192

T
tamoxifen (Nolvodex), 13-14, 37, 38
teenage smokers, 90
Therapeutic Touch, 166
tobacco. *See* smoking
trastuzumab (Herceptin), 23
tumors
    development in the uterus, 35
    endometrial cancer, 35-36
    treatment for benign cervical, 69-70

U
uterine cancer. *See* endometrial cancer
uterus
    anatomy of, 35
    tumor development in, 35

W
websites
    American Cancer Society, 175
    Association for Cancer Online Resources, 179
    evaluating CAM resource, 168*t*
    evaluating health information found on, 175-177*t*
    HON (Health on the Net Foundation) principles for health, 176*t*
    Medscape, 175
    National Cancer Institute, 175
    National Center for Complementary and Alternative Medicine, 179
    on OCCAM studies, 165
    PubMED (National Library of Medicine site), 175
    Quack Watch, 179
    queries from cancer patients to, 177-179
    reliable sources on CAMs, 179
    tips on finding quality health information, 178*t*
    types of cancer information sources found on, 178*fig*
    See also Internet
"why me" experience, 129
woman patients. *See* female patients

PRETEST KEY

Cancer in Women

1.	d	Chapter 1
2.	b	Chapter 2
3.	c	Chapter 3
4.	c	Chapter 3
5.	b	Chapter 4
6.	c	Chapter 4
7.	a	Chapter 5
8.	b	Chapter 5
9.	c	Chapter 6
10.	c	Chapter 6
11.	b	Chapter 6
12.	b	Chapter 7
13.	c	Chapter 8
14.	c	Chapter 8
15.	b	Chapter 9
16.	c	Chapter 9
17.	d	Chapter 9
18.	c	Chapter 10
19.	a	Chapter 10
20.	a	Chapter 11

NOTES

Western Schools® offers over 1,800 hours to suit all your interests – and requirements!

Cardiovascular
Cardiovascular Nursing: A Comprehensive Overview ....32 hrs
A The 12-Lead ECG in Acute Coronary Syndromes ....42 hrs

Clinical Conditions/Nursing Practice
A Advanced Assessment ....35 hrs
Airway Management with a Tracheal Tube ....1 hr
Asthma: Nursing Care Across the Lifespan ....28 hrs
Auscultation Skills ....38 hrs
— Heart Sounds ....20 hrs
— Breath Sounds ....18 hrs
Care at the End of Life ....3 hrs
Chest Tube Management ....2 hrs
Clinical Care of the Diabetic Foot ....8 hrs
A Complete Nurses Guide to Diabetes Care ....37 hrs
Diabetes Essentials for Nurses ....30 hrs
Death, Dying & Bereavement ....30 hrs
Essentials of Patient Education ....30 hrs
Healing Nutrition ....24 hrs
Hepatitis C: The Silent Killer (2nd ed.) ....3 hrs
HIV/AIDS ....1 or 2 hrs
Holistic & Complementary Therapies ....18 hrs
Home Health Nursing ....30 hrs
Humor in Healthcare: The Laughter Prescription ....20 hrs
Orthopedic Nursing: Caring for Patients with
     Musculoskeletal Disorders ....30 hrs
Osteomyelitis ....2 hrs
Pain & Symptom Management ....1 hr
Pain Management: Principles and Practice ....30 hrs
A Palliative Practices: An Interdisciplinary Approach ....66 hrs
— Issues Specific to Palliative Care ....20 hrs
— Specific Disease States and Symptom
        Management ....24 hrs
— The Dying Process, Grief, and
        Bereavement ....22 hrs
Pharmacologic Management of Asthma ....1 hr
Seizures: A Basic Overview ....1 hr
The Neurological Exam ....1 hr
Wound Management and Healing ....30 hrs

Critical Care/ER/OR
Ambulatory Surgical Care ....20 hrs
Basic Nursing of Head, Chest, Abdominal, Spine
     and Orthopedic Trauma ....20 hrs
A Case Studies in Critical Care Nursing ....46 hrs
Critical Care & Emergency Nursing ....30 hrs
Hemodynamic Monitoring ....18 hrs
A Nurse Anesthesia ....58 hrs
— Common Diseases ....20 hrs
— Common Procedures ....21 hrs
— Drugs ....17 hrs
A Practical Guide to Moderate Sedation/Analgesia ....31 hrs
Principles of Basic Trauma Nursing ....30 hrs

Geriatrics
Alzheimer's Disease: A Complete Guide for Nurses ....25 hrs
Nursing Care of the Older Adult ....30 hrs
Psychosocial Issues Affecting Older Adults ....16 hrs

Infectious Diseases/Bioterrorism
Avian Influenza ....1 hr
Biological Weapons ....5 hrs
Bioterrorism & the Nurse's Response to WMD ....5 hrs
Bioterrorism Readiness: The Nurse's Critical Role .... 2 hrs
Infection Control Training for Healthcare Workers ....4 hrs
Influenza: A Vaccine-Preventable Disease ....1 hr
Smallpox ....2 hrs
West Nile Virus (2nd ed.) ....1 hr

Oncology
Cancer in Women ....30 hrs
Cancer Nursing (2nd ed.) ....36 hrs

Pediatrics/Maternal-Child/Women's Health
A Assessment and Care of the Well Newborn ....34 hrs
Attention Deficit Hyperactivity Disorders
     Throughout the Lifespan ....30 hrs
Diabetes in Children ....30 hrs
End-of-Life Care for Children and Their Families ....2 hrs
Induction of Labor ....8 hrs
Manual of School Health ....30 hrs
Maternal-Newborn Nursing ....30 hrs
Menopause: Nursing Care for Women
     Throughout Mid-Life ....25 hrs
A Obstetric and Gynecologic Emergencies ....44 hrs
— Obstetric Emergencies ....22 hrs
— Gynecologic Emergencies ....22 hrs
Pediatric Nursing: Routine to Emergent Care ....30 hrs
Pediatric Pharmacology ....10 hrs
Pediatric Physical Assessment ....10 hrs
A Practice Guidelines for Pediatric Nurse Practitioners ....46 hrs
Women's Health: Contemporary Advances and Trends ....30 hrs

Professional Issues/Management/Law
Documentation for Nurses ....24 hrs
Medical Error Prevention: Patient Safety ....2 hrs
Nurse Leadership ....25 hrs
Ohio Law: Standards of Safe Nursing Practice (3rd ed.) ....1 hr
Surviving and Thriving in Nursing ....30 hrs
Understanding Managed Care ....30 hrs

Psychiatric/Mental Health
A ADHD in Children and Adults ....8 hrs
Antidepressants ....1 hr
Antipsychotics ....1 hr
Anxiolytics and Mood Stabilizers ....1 hr
Basic Psychopharmacology ....5 hrs
Behavioral Approaches to Treating Obesity ....13 hrs
A Bipolar Disorder ....10 hrs
A Borderline Personality Disorder ....21 hrs
A Child/Adolescent Clinical Psychopharmacology ....12 hrs
A Childhood Maltreatment ....10 hrs
A Clinical Psychopharmacology ....10 hrs
Depression: Prevention, Diagnosis, and Treatment... ....25 hrs
A Evidence-Based Mental Health Practice ....22 hrs
A Geropsychiatric and Mental Health Nursing ....40 hrs
A Integrating Traditional Healing Practices ....35 hrs
IPV (Intimate Partner Violence) (2nd ed.) ....1 or 3 hrs
A Mindfulness and Psychotherapy ....25 hrs
A Multicultural Perspectives in Working with Families ....27 hrs
A Obsessive Compulsive Disorder ....9 hrs
A Problem and Pathological Gambling ....9 hrs
Psychiatric Nursing: Current Trends in Diagnosis ....30 hrs
Psychiatric Principles & Applications ....30 hrs
A Schizophrenia ....5 hrs
A Suicide ....21 hrs
A Trauma Therapy ....11 hrs
A Treating Explosive Kids ....14 hrs
A Treating Victims of Mass Disaster and Terrorism ....6 hrs

REV. 9/24/07